Considerations in Non-Caucasian Facial Plastic Surgery

Guest Editor

SAMUEL M. LAM, MD, FACS

FACIAL PLASTIC SURGERY CLINICS OF NORTH AMERICA

www.facialplastic.theclinics.com

February 2010 • Volume 18 • Number 1

SAUNDERS an imprint of ELSEVIER, Inc.

W.B. SAUNDERS COMPANY
A Division of Elsevier Inc.

1600 John F. Kennedy Blvd., Suite 1800, Philadelphia, PA 19103-2899

http://www.theclinics.com

FACIAL PLASTIC SURGERY CLINICS OF NORTH AMERICA Volume 18, Number 1
February 2010 ISSN 1064-7406, ISBN 978-1-4377-1819-5

Editor: Joanne Husovski
Developmental Editor: Theresa Collier

Facial Plastic Surgery Clinics of North America (ISSN 1064-7406) is published quarterly by Elsevier Inc., 360 Park Avenue South, New York, NY 10010-1710. Months of issue are February, May, August, and November. Business and Editorial Offices: 1600 John F. Kennedy Blvd., Suite 1800, Philadelphia, PA 19103-2899. Periodicals postage paid at New York, NY, and additional mailing offices. Subscription prices are $306.00 per year (US individuals), $437.00 per year (US institutions), $344.00 per year (Canadian individuals), $524.00 per year (Canadian institutions), $412.00 per year (foreign individuals), $524.00 per year (foreign institutions), $149.00 per year (US students), and $207.00 per year (foreign students). Foreign air speed delivery is included in all *Clinics* subscription prices. All prices are subject to change without notice. POSTMASTER: Send address changes to *Facial Plastic Surgery Clinics*, Elsevier Health Sciences Division, Subscription Customer Service, 3251 Riverport Lane, Maryland Heights, MO 63043. **Customer service: 1-800-654-2452 (US and Canada); 1-314-447-8871 (outside US and Canada); Fax: 314-447-8029; E-mail:journalscustomerservice-usa@elsevier.com (for print support); journalsonline support-usa@elsevier.com (for online support).**

Reprints. For copies of 100 or more of articles in this publication, please contact the Commercial Reprints Department, Elsevier Inc., 360 Park Avenue South, New York, NY 10010-1710. Tel.: 212-633-3812; Fax: 212-462-1935; E-mail: reprints@elsevier.com.

Facial Plastic Surgery Clinics of North America is covered in *MEDLINE/PubMed* (*Index Medicus*).

Contributors

CONSULTING EDITOR

J. REGAN THOMAS, MD, FACS
Professor and Chairman, Department of
Otolaryngology, University of Illinois at
Chicago, Chicago, Illinois

GUEST EDITOR

SAMUEL M. LAM, MD, FACS
Director, Willow Bend Wellness Center, Lam
Facial Plastic Surgery Center and Hair
Restoration Institute, Plano, Texas

AUTHORS

BABAK AZIZZADEH, MD, FACS
The Center for Facial & Nasal Plastic Surgery,
Beverly Hills; Attending Surgeon, Facial Plastic
& Reconstructive Surgery, Cedars-Sinai
Medical Center; Assistant Clinical Professor of
Surgery, Division of Head & Neck Surgery,
David Geffen School of Medicine at UCLA,
Los Angeles, California

RAMI K. BATNIJI, MD, FACS
Attending, Department of Plastic Surgery,
Hoag Hospital; Batniji Facial Plastic Surgery,
Newport Beach, California

WILLIAM J. BINDER, MD, FACS
Facial Plastic and Reconstructive Surgery,
Beverly Hills; Assistant Clinical Professor,
Department of Head and Neck Surgery, UCLA
School of Medicine; Attending Surgeon,
Department of Head and Neck Surgery, Cedars
Sinai Medical Center, Los Angeles, California

PAUL J. CARNIOL, MD
Clinical Associate Professor, University of
Medicine and Dentistry of New Jersey,
Newark; Summit, New Jersey

ROXANA COBO, MD
Private Practice, Facial Plastic Surgery,
Centro Médico Imbanaco; Coordinator,
Service of Otolaryngology, Centro Médico
Imbanaco, Cali, Colombia

BRUCE F. CONNELL, MD
Clinical Professor of Surgery, University of
California, Irvine, College of Medicine,
Irvine, California

VALÉRIE CÔTÉ, MD
Department of Otolaryngology–Head and Neck
Surgery, McGill University, Montreal, Canada

NABIL FANOUS, MD, FRCS(C)
Department of Otolaryngology–Head and Neck
Surgery, McGill University, Montreal;
Department of Surgery, Sherbrooke University,
Sherbrooke; The Canadian Institute of
Cosmetic Surgery, Montreal, Quebec, Canada

MONTE O. HARRIS, MD
Founder, Center for Aesthetic Modernism,
Chevy Chase, Maryland; Clinical
Assistant Professor, Department of
Otolaryngology–Head and Neck Surgery,
Georgetown University Medical Center;
Department of Dermatology,
Howard University College
of Medicine, Washington,
District of Columbia

HARRY S. HWANG, MD
Chief Resident, Department of
Otolaryngology–Head and Neck Surgery,
University of California, San Francisco, San
Francisco, California

AMIR M. KARAM, MD
Director, Carmel Valley Facial Plastic Surgery;
Clinical Faculty, Division of Otolaryngology-
Head and Neck Surgery, Department of
Surgery, University of California,
San Diego, School of Medicine,
San Diego, California

EMINA KARAMANOVSKI, MD
Hair Transplant Coordinator, Lam Institute for
Hair Restoration, Plano, Texas

DAVID W. KIM, MD, FACS
Clinical Associate Professor, Facial Plastic
Surgery, Department of Otolaryngology–Head
and Neck Surgery, School of Medicine,
University of California, San Francisco, San
Francisco, California

SAMUEL M. LAM, MD, FACS
Director, Willow Bend Wellness Center,
Lam Facial Plastic Surgery Center and
Hair Restoration Institute, Plano, Texas

KIMBERLY J. LEE, MD
Assistant Clinical Professor, Department of
Otolaryngology–Head and Neck Surgery,
University of California, Los Angeles School of
Medicine, Los Angeles; Attending Surgeon,
Division of Otolaryngology, Cedars-Sinai
Medical Center, Beverly Hills, California

GRIGORIY MASHKEVICH, MD
Assistant Professor, Department of
Otolaryngology–Head and Neck Surgery,
Division of Facial Plastic and Reconstructive
Surgery, New York Eye & Ear Infirmary, New
York, New York

KIM MURRAY, MD
University of Medicine and Dentistry of New
Jersey, Newark, New Jersey

PAUL S. NASSIF, MD, FACS
Assistant Clinical Professor, Department of
Otolaryngology, University of Southern
California School of Medicine; University of
California, Los Angeles School of Medicine,
Los Angeles; Partner, Spalding Drive Cosmetic
Surgery and Dermatology, Beverly Hills,
California

JOE NIAMTU III, DMD
Cosmetic Facial Surgery, Richmond, Virginia

STEPHEN W. PERKINS, MD
Clinical Associate Professor, Indiana University
School of Medicine, Department of
Otolaryngology; Meridian Plastic Surgeons,
Indianapolis, Indiana

PETER RULLAN, MD
Medical Director, Dermatology Institute, Chula
Vista, California

JOSEPH K. WONG, MD, FRCS(C)
Director, Advanced Aesthetic Plastic Surgery
Centre, Toronto, Ontario, Canada

HEATHER WOOLERY-LLOYD, MD
University of Miami School of Medicine,
Miami, Florida

**WOFFLES T.L. WU, MBBS, FRCS,
FAMS (Plast Surg)**
Consultant Plastic Surgeon, Camden Medical
Centre, Singapore; Honorable Head,
Department of Plastic Surgery, Zhejiang
Provincial Peoples Hospital, Hangzhou, China

ALICE S. ZHAO, BA
University of Medicine and Dentistry of New
Jersey, Newark, New Jersey

A. JOSHUA ZIMM, MD, FACS
Attending Surgeon, Department of
Otolaryngology-Head and Neck Surgery,
Manhattan Eye, Ear, and Throat/ Lenox Hill
Hospital, New York, New York

Erratum

David A. Caplin, MD

In the November 2009 issue of *Facial Plastic Surgery Clinics of North America* on facelift, Dr David A. Caplin's affiliations were incorrectly published. Dr Caplin is Clinical Instructor at Washington University, St Louis, and in private practice at Parkcrest Plastic Surgery, 845 North New Ballas Court, Suite 300, St Louis, MO 63141, USA. His e-mail address is: Gfts27@aol.com.

Facial Plast Surg Clin N Am 18 (2010) v
doi:10.1016/j.fsc.2009.12.001

Contents

Supratarsal crease fixation in the Asian patient can provide a more open-eyed, awake look without compromising their ethnic appearance. A conservative supratarsal crease height and conservative to no removal of postseptal fat help to ensure this natural-appearing result. With the full-incision method, consistently excellent results have been achieved with durable crease fixation despite a prolonged recovery time. The supratarsal crease fixation provides an excellent method for the younger patient seeking cosmetic eyelid enhancement. However, for the aging Asian patient, the complexity of the strategy is greater.

The population of the United States is becoming increasingly more diverse as there is an ever expanding influx of various ethnic groups and races that comprise the general population. As a result, the singular concept of Nordic beauty that dominated the United States media throughout the middle of the twentieth century has given way to a more diverse multiracial aesthetic. There is also a growing trend in aesthetic surgery toward ethnic feature preservation and avoidance of a "westernized" look that was more popular in previous years. Today's facial plastic surgeon must be familiar with these trends and aesthetic goals within this rapidly growing patient population. This article describes the anatomy of the Asian and Latino face and describes the techniques of midface alloplastic augmentation.

Methods of alloplastic forehead augmentation using soft expanded polytetrafluoroethylene (ePTFE) and silicone implants are described. Soft ePTFE forehead implantation has the advantage of being technically simpler, with better fixation. The disadvantages are a limited degree of forehead augmentation and higher chance of infection. Properly fabricated soft silicone implants provide potential for larger degree of forehead silhouette augmentation with less risk of infection. The corrugated edge and central perforations of the implant minimize mobility and capsule contraction.

This article discusses and presents options related to the cosmetic reduction of enlarged lips, primarily in ethnic populations. No formal study is performed. The author presents a literature review and discusses his personal 26-year experiences in lip surgery. When basic tenets are followed, cosmetic lip reduction is a predictable procedure with very little morbidity. Although lip augmentation is a popular cosmetic procedure, a certain percentage of the population desires smaller lips. Reduction cheiloplasty is a safe and predictable procedure that has been performed over a half century. This procedure is relatively simple and has a moderate learning curve. Cosmetic lip reduction is safe and effective, and has a high level of patient acceptance when certain diagnostic and treatment criteria are fulfilled.

Racial genetics play a significant role in determining a patient's response to any skin treatment. Contrary to traditional skin classifications, the new genetico-racial classification takes into consideration the racial origins of patients, as manifested in both their skin color and their feature contour characteristics, rather than their skin color alone. According to this new classification, patients may belong to 1 of 6 categories, originating from the 3 ancient continents: Africa, Europe, and Asia. In this article the Asian category, as well as its subcategories, are approached in a radically different way. This new geneticoracial classification ushers in a "paradigm shift" in the way Asian patients are perceived before, during, and after skin treatments. The new geneticoracial classification advances that Asians are excellent candidates to most peels and laser treatments, as long as their genetic disposition and their anticipated responses to those treatments are understood and respected.

> With the growth of new technology and products over the last 10 years, there has been an increased ability to improve a patient's appearance with procedures that can be performed in an office setting, including laser procedures. Demand for these procedures has grown among all ethnic groups. Patients with ethnic skin can have varying response to lasers. This factor should be considered when planning their treatment. Patients with ethnic skin are at greater risk for laser energy absorption by melanin, postinflammatory hyperpigmentation, and loss of pigment due to laser effects on melanin production leading to hypopigmentation. Therefore, any laser therapy should be planned carefully, especially in the treatment of patients with darker skin types.

> This article focuses on chemical peels for darker skin types. All races comprise a range of Fitzpatrick skin color types: light skin types in African Americans, Asians, Middle Easterners, and Latinos and dark skin types in whites. With the focus on Fitzgerald skin types IV to VI, this article discusses chemical peels, providing current information on types of peels, detailed techniques, preoperative and postoperative care, complications, hazards, and nuances of management.

> Botulinum toxin A is a highly efficacious and cost-effective, nonsurgical option for reducing the width and shape of the lower face and jawline. The results can vary from the subtlest thinning of the face to an extremely thin, cachectic appearance. Many nuances can be achieved. The administration is simple, and the process takes barely 5 minutes in an office setting. Botulinum toxin A can also be effectively used to reduce the bulk of an enlarged parotid gland without affecting saliva production.

> Traumatic injury resulting in nasal deformity poses unique challenges to the surgeon. Optimal management requires careful preoperative analysis and thoughtful surgical planning. The goals of rhinoplasty are to correct both cosmetic and functional

problems that may not have otherwise been an issue prior to the injury. Although it is overly simplistic to group all individuals from one ethnicity as having one type of nose, the rhinoplasty surgeon must understand the common variations of nasal anatomy seen in various races of individuals. This article discusses ethnic anatomic differences in the non-Caucasian nose in the context of posttraumatic nasal deformity. The various rhinoplasty techniques and strategies to address these issues are reviewed.

Asian rhinoplasty is one of the most challenging ethnic rhinoplasties that plastic surgeons perform because of the thick skin and soft-tissue envelope. There are three goals: pleasing the patient, achieving an aesthetically appealing result, and preserving a natural look. Of these goals, the most arduous is to satisfy the patient, as many patients have unrealistic goals and may desire an extremely narrow Western nose. Furthermore, patients may bring in celebrity or model photographs and expect that outcome, even though it may not be suitable for their face or appear over-resected and pinched. The surgeon's most important task is to attempt to persuade the patient that this result is nonfunctional, esthetically unfit, and difficult to achieve with their skin. For ethnic surgery, a clear and thorough grasp of nasal anatomy, function, and surgical techniques is paramount. An extensive preoperative discussion, including expectations, outcomes, and a detailed list of potential complications with the patient can prevent physician-patient miscommunication. Before surgery, it is essential to review the office examination, previous operative summary, photographs, nasal analysis sheet, problem list, and plan before proceeding with the surgical treatment.

Rhinoplasty is one of the most common facial plastic procedures performed in the Hispanic/mestizo ethnic group. Today, emphasis is placed on ethnic and cultural backgrounds, definition of facial and nasal characteristics, and a clear understanding of patients' desires. This article highlights the different types of problems encountered in mestizo patients. It describes a graduated approach to the nose whereby support structures of the nose are strengthened by careful placement of sutures and grafts, trying to achieve greater definition and support without necessarily making the nose look bigger.

We are in the midst of truly changing times, as patients of African descent actively embrace facial cosmetic surgery. Gaining surgical consistency in patients of African descent has proven to be elusive and unpredictable for many rhinoplasty surgeons. Surgical success relies on the surgeon's ability precisely to identify anatomic variables and reconcile these anatomic realities with the patient's expectations for aesthetic improvement and ethnic identity. An appreciation for underlying heritage provides a link culturally to connect with prospective patients and serves as a tool for establishing realistic aesthetic goals. This article highlights the significance of exploring ancestry in the rhinoplasty consultation; identifies key anatomic variables in the nasal tip, dorsum, and alar base; and reviews surgical logic that has facilitated the achievement of consistent, balanced aesthetic outcomes.

Middle Eastern Rhinoplasty   201

Babak Azizzadeh and Grigoriy Mashkevich

The ethnic appearance of the Middle Eastern nose is defined by several unique visual features, particularly a high radix, wide overprojecting dorsum, and an amorphous hanging nasal tip. These external characteristics reflect distinct structural properties of the osseo-cartilaginous nasal framework and skin–soft tissue envelope in patients of Middle Eastern extraction. The goal, and the ultimate challenge, of rhinoplasty on Middle Eastern patients is to achieve balanced aesthetic refinement, while avoiding surgical westernization. Detailed understanding of the ethnic visual harmony in a Middle Eastern nose greatly assists in preserving native nasal-facial relationships during rhinoplasty on Middle Eastern patients. Esthetic alteration of a Middle Eastern nose follows a different set of goals and principles compared with rhinoplasties on white or other ethnic patients. This article highlights the inherent nasal features of the Middle Eastern nose and reviews pertinent concepts of rhinoplasty on Middle Eastern patients. Essential considerations in the process spanning the consultation and surgery are reviewed. Reliable operative techniques that achieve a successful aesthetic outcome are discussed in detail.

Facial Plastic Surgery Clinics of North America

RELATED INTEREST

Oral and Maxillofacial Surgery Clinics, February 2009 (Vol. 21, No. 1)
Complications in Cosmetic Facial Surgery
Joseph Niamtu III, MD, *Guest Editor*

THE CLINICS ARE NOW AVAILABLE ONLINE!

Access your subscription at:
www.theclinics.com

Preface

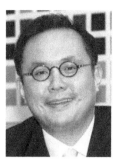

Samuel M. Lam, MD
Guest Editor

The makeup of today's facial plastic surgery patient is as diverse as ever with a larger percentage of patients from various ethnicities seeking cosmetic enhancement. This edition of *Facial Plastic Surgery Clinics* focuses on a broad range of non-White groups, including African, Hispanic, Asian, and Middle Eastern individuals, with coverage of important topics ranging from cultural considerations, rejuvenation of the aging face, ethnic lip reduction, hair restoration, to rhinoplasty techniques. In-depth discussion of the management of difficult-to-treat ethnic skin is covered with an introduction to a new paradigm for ethnic skin and safe and effective treatment strategies using advanced lasers and traditional peels.

This edition draws from an international cadre of experts on the non-White face from a diversity of disciplines including facial plastic surgery, plastic surgery, and dermatology. Given the growing interest from non-White patients today, this edition of *Facial Plastic Surgery Clinics* should serve as an indispensable reference source for the contemporary aesthetic surgeon of the face. I hope you reap benefits from the assiduous work that my colleagues and I have put into this year-long labor of love.

Samuel M. Lam, MD
Dallas, Texas, USA

Facial Plast Surg Clin N Am 18 (2010) xiii
doi:10.1016/j.fsc.2009.11.017

facialplastic.theclinics.com

A New Paradigm for the Aging Face

Samuel M. Lam, MD

KEYWORDS
• Fat transfer • Facial rejuvenation • Ethnicity

Commonalities and differences exist for managing the aging face of the ethnic and nonethnic individual. This article explores the intersection and divergence of strategies for facial rejuvenation through the filter of a new paradigm for the aging face. This new paradigm is, in effect, the opposite of traditional lifting- and excisional-based rejuvenative surgery. Using facial fat transfer, adding to the face rather than subtracting from it, defines the new paradigm. Although facial fat transfer is universally applicable to almost any individual who undergoes aging, it is particularly beneficial for the ethnic face as a standalone procedure on many counts. First, many ethnic individuals of varying origins have greater skin melanin content that serves as a protective barrier against solar aging, which can create cutaneous elastosis and dyschromias. Accordingly, the aging process, particularly in dark-skinned individuals, can be almost entirely a manifestation of volume depletion with little evidence of gravity and skin damage. In addition, fat transfer can be used as a sculpting method to soften ethnic features and facial shape to create a more balanced appearance. This topic is studied in more depth in this article. Facial fat transfer can be a potent and primary method for reversal of aging in ethnic and nonethnic populations.

Before the role of facial fat transfer in different ethnicities can be understood, the logic behind its use in all individuals must be considered. Adding more adipose to an eyebag, fat to an already ptotic brow, or fat to a seemingly heavy jawline seems counterintuitive. Accordingly, how facial fat transfer is perhaps a revolution in thinking and approach to the aging face (in short a new paradigm) must be defined at the outset. The best way to regard facial fat transfer is to begin with the educational process of understanding and perceiving negative space. For example, rather than seeing the steatoblepharon of an eyebag, the eyebag can be considered to represent the fat that remains after a great percentage of fat has dissipated along the orbital rim and midface. Similarly, instead of seeing drapage of upper-eyelid skin and a ptotic brow, it can be envisaged that the bony orbital rim becomes more exposed over time and that the convexity of the brow contour needs to be restored rather than elevated due to perceived gravity (which in reality plays a negligible role in the brow). The best way to understand this phenomenon of deflation rather than gravity is to start with the patient's old photograph, which in almost every case exemplifies a fuller brow contour rather than an elevated one. The brow is one of the most difficult areas to understand that deflation rather than gravity is at play. The reader is encouraged to think of the brow as a balloon that deflates over time creating the perceived effect of sagging; filling would give the best results.

Currently, I rarely perform a browlift, because I find that it is simply unnecessary and, in many cases, counterproductive. The longer, almond-shaped eye of youth gives way to a bonier, rounder look that is exacerbated by browlifting and aggressive traditional blepharoplasty. In almost every circumstance, periorbital fat transfer is the mainstay of rejuvenative intervention that I rely on, and, in conjunction, I occasionally perform traditional blepharoplasty to enhance my fat transfer result rather than as a substitute for it. I perform an upper-eyelid blepharoplasty with a fat transfer for the upper-eyelid/brow complex only when it is warranted, which is in approximately 1 in 5 patients. I prefer a selective skin-only blepharoplasty,

Willow Bend Wellness Center, Lam Facial Plastic Surgery Center & Hair Restoration Institute, 6101 Chapel Hill Boulevard, Suite 101, Plano, TX 75093, USA
E-mail address: drlam@lamfacialplastics.com

Facial Plast Surg Clin N Am 18 (2010) 1–6
doi:10.1016/j.fsc.2009.11.001
1064-7406/10/$ – see front matter © 2010 Elsevier Inc. All rights reserved.

removing 2 to 3 mm of redundant skin, in the following cases:

1) When the eyelid skin hangs at or below the ciliary margin
2) When the skin edge appears "crêpey" and irregular, or preferably an upper eyelid that manifests both of these conditions

The reason to remove the extra skin in the case of skin irregularity is apparent. The reason to remove skin when the skin hangs at or below the ciliary margin is to minimize the drooping eyelid look if some of the fat resorbs and fails to achieve the desired esthetic objective.

With lower-eyelid steatoblepharon, the need to remove fat from the perceived eyebag is rarely indicated and the need to remove redundant skin almost never arises. I prefer to perform fat grafting alone for the lower eyelid in almost every case but, in approximately 1 in 10 cases, I perform a concurrent transconjunctival lower-eyelid blepharoplasty to manage the extra fat that will not, most likely, be sufficiently camouflaged with fat grafting to the inferior orbital rim. The situation in which I prefer a transconjunctival blepharoplasty with fat grafting to the inferior orbital rim involves eyebags that are so protuberant that they extend well beyond the orbital rim in an anterior-posterior position. In fastidious individuals who want the absolute best results for the lower eyelid, I offer to perform a concurrent lower-eyelid blepharoplasty but still try to manage expectations that there might nevertheless be some remaining perceived steatoblepharon. I almost never remove extra skin from the lower eyelid but instead choose to manage rhytids and flaccidity of the lower eyelid with skin resurfacing and botulinum toxin therapy. I find that traditional skin-muscle flap blepharoplasty carries too high a risk of changing the shape of the eye by altering the lateral canthus even slightly in any direction (medially, laterally, inferiorly, or superiorly).

Many patients (and surgeons) are surprised at how much the midface affects the look of the eyes. The gaunt, flattened terrain of the aged midface can contribute more significantly than almost any other facial feature, including the eyelids themselves, to the tired appearance of an eye. To help patients (and surgeons) appreciate the effect that a fuller midface contour has on the look of the eyes, I gently nudge the cheek into a fuller, rounder contour by pushing it up from below with my thumb to simulate volume (not lifting) and have the patient see that, with this maneuver, even though the lower-eyelid contour may be worsened, the eyes look more alert and

the face looks markedly more rested in appearance. To understand why a malar implant fails to rejuvenate the midface, one must understand how an aged midface ages. With volume loss to the midface as people age, the bony malar eminence becomes more exposed (ie, the bony prominence is the hallmark of aging). A solid implant on the malar eminence worsens this bony look and thereby exacerbates aging. Fat transfer covers the bony prominence and blends it in with the surrounding contour depressions. Similarly, midface lifts fail to work because they lift deflated tissue upward and stretch the skin more over exposed bony terrain, which ultimately does not resolve the core issue, that is, volume depletion of the midface.

I mentally divide the central cheek into 3 zones (minus the buccal area, to be discussed later). The central anterior cheek, which corresponds with maximal cheek deflation along the mediosuperior to inferiolateral line of the malar ligament, is perhaps the most important region to fill for aging in most individuals. Pushing this area too forcefully can create an overexuberant appearance to the cheek and also over feminize a masculine face. The lateral cheek is defined as the region that overlies the malar bony eminence. In gaunt narrow faces, I prefer to augment this region more aggressively than in heavier faces or in individuals with prominent cheekbones. Trying to balance a face is an underlying objective with any facial esthetic endeavor (ie, creating harmony between various sizes of neighboring facial structures, without greatly disturbing personal identity). The lateral cheek also serves as an important area to augment for men to create a more structured outer cheek shape that can be masculinizing. The lower, medial, anterior cheek, which rests directly above the nasolabial groove and partially defines the upper border of the nasolabial fold, should almost never be augmented. It tends to become more pronounced in heavier individuals and makes the cheek look ptotic and heavy. Accordingly, in more heavily set individuals, placing fat more superiorly and centrally can offset this heavy appearance and create a relative narrowing of the face. Modest amounts of fat should be used in order not to create too fat a face.

The buccal area can be one of the most important areas to fill or one of the most important areas to avoid. In the heavier patient, the buccal region appears full and heavy. Filling the central upper anterior cheek as mentioned can make the buccal area appear smaller in these individuals. However, in the gaunt face, the buccal area can be a central focus to enhance to make the face appear more youthful. Most often, traditional perspectives for the aging face concentrate on the upper, mid, and lower faces; however, I look at the buccal area as an important transition point between the middle and lower faces. Unifying the face that becomes more markedly disjointed and separate with aging is an important goal in facial rejuvenation, and filling the buccal area facilitates this goal by unifying the stark transition between an augmented cheek and an augmented and lifted lower face. Mentally, I have divided the buccal region into 3 zones: the medial buccal hollow, the central buccal hollow, and the lateral (subzygomatic) buccal hollow (which I also refer to more colloquially as the backfill zone).

The central buccal hollow is self-evident and corresponds to the most obvious central buccal depression, which can be a focal point of interest for filling. In more aged individuals who have lost dentition, I conceptualize a more medial extension of the buccal hollow that corresponds with the upper arch of teeth/maxilla. If this area is filled, the labiomandibular groove (marionette) line can be temporarily exacerbated for several weeks, or with aggressive augmentation can be permanently worsened. The patient should be aware of this possibility. In my opinion, fat grafting is not a reliable option to fill linear fold defects like the nasolabial groove or the labiomandibular groove. Other options must be used to manage the fold with more consistent outcomes. The gaunt patient is particularly helped by filling the lateral buccal hollow, which corresponds with the region that falls immediately inferior to the zygomatic arch/bony malar eminence. Patients who have had a standard SMAS-ectomy rhytidectomy and who have lost volume to the outer face and are already predisposed toward being gaunt are greatly assisted by filling this lateral backfill region. In any circumstance, after augmenting the midface/cheek region, the surgeon may create a relative buccal hollow that should be addressed at that point to soften this accentuated transition. Women do not aspire to looking fat, so buccal augmentation must be undertaken after meticulous and detailed consent and discussion with a patient.

The chin/anterior jawline is another important area to augment in the aged face. A lower face and neck lift can manage the jowl and the neck but the patient may still not appear as refreshed as possible. A chin implant is also not necessarily the answer, as can be understood through the concept of the inverted U. Most surgeons and patients are focused on the jowl and the labiomandibular groove as the problem areas; however, a new concept that I have developed focuses on the inverted U shape of bony exposure that occurs with aging. The upper anterior chin that lies just

medial to the labiomandibular groove should be the focus of attention, as this depression creates the starkest relief of aging but is also the least understood or managed. The lower limb of the inverted U corresponds to a region known as the prejowl depression; that is, the recess of soft tissue immediately in front of the jowl itself.

As mentioned earlier in this article, to understand these concepts the surgeon must begin to see negative space well. Seeing positive space problems such as the jowl and the fold addresses only part of the problem with aging. Seeing negative space (hollowness, bone exposure) is integral to a successful vision and the design of a treatment protocol. An extended chin implant helps to address the lower limb (prejowl) of the inverted U but worsens the upper limb of the U, which can be one of the most important areas to work on. Fat grafting to the jawline can eliminate the need for a lower facelift or significantly improve a facelift result.

An area that I address less commonly is the lateral mandible; however, it can be an important area to fill in select individuals. For instance, the most common indication that I have to address the lateral mandible is found in the older patient who has in the past undergone a lower SMAS-ectomy rhytidectomy that has caused further worsening of volume loss across the lateral mandible, where the bony prominence of the mandible is completely exposed leading to more aging. When the buccal area is filled in these individuals, the picture still seems incomplete, given the extended lower lateral loss in the mandible. Filling the lateral mandible can support the buccal fill by creating a more unified extension of the buccal fill. A second indication is loss of bone in the lateral mandible, which is typically present following previous orthognathic mandibular advancement. The patient can look cheek-heavy, which would only be worsened with anterior cheek filling, without support to the lower lateral face. The concept of facial balance is reiterated here. Finally, a prominent jowl in an individual who refuses to undergo a proper rhytidectomy can be better effaced by filling in front of (prejowl) and behind (postjowl) the jowl itself. The only caution is that many individuals who exhibit a prominent jowl may also be slightly more heavily set in the jowl and mandate a more targeted approach to the immediate postjowl defect without significant lateral extension so as not to widen the face and render it heavier in appearance.

There are some important major limitations of fat transfer. First, fat grafting is principally intended to manage soft-tissue loss of the face and not necessarily bony weaknesses. For more predictable projection of the mandible, an alloplastic chin implant is still mandated with or without fat grafting. The cheek region can almost always be better managed in aging simply with fat grafting, as minor bony weaknesses can be camouflaged with soft-tissue augmentation with fat transfer. Similarly, minor degrees of chin retrusion can also be camouflaged with fat grafting. However, excessive fat transfer to the chin to address what a chin implant would otherwise have done better, will most likely create a fat-appearing chin, which is obviously unesthetic. Second, fat transfer is not indicated to manage lip augmentation, which causes unduly protracted edema/distortion and is associated with a high resorption rate. As mentioned earlier, grafted fat also has too soft a consistency to consistently lift away the labio-mandibular and nasolabial groove depressions.

I have likened fat grafting to hair grafting, because of their similar nature, trajectory, and outcomes, to help individuals better understand fat grafting using the model of hair transplantation. Fat grafting and hair transplantation use a tiny micrograft that is suspended in a network of surrounding native tissue that requires ingrowth of blood supply to mature and grow over time. Accordingly, fat grafting results (if done properly with surviving grafts) look best approximately 2 years following fat transfer when the graft is fully vascularized. Using the model of hair restoration, a transplanted hair graft survives for the first few days via plasmatic imbibition. Over the following few months, the graft continues to survive using a process of primary then secondary inosculation. Only after 6 months is the graft formally supplied via neovascularization. At that point, the hair graft grows and improves and continues to do so for approximately 18 months. Fat grafting looks good for the first month to 6 weeks because of edema that mimics a fat-grafting result. However, at 3 months, when all swelling has dissipated and the fat graft has not fully established its blood supply, it may not look so good. Starting at approximately 6 months, the fat-grafting result begins to improve steadily for approximately another 12 to 18 months just as a hair transplant result does (obviously only if the surgeon can assure graft survival). Because fat is not a bioinert

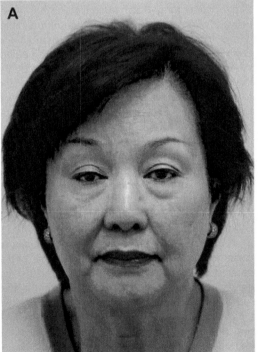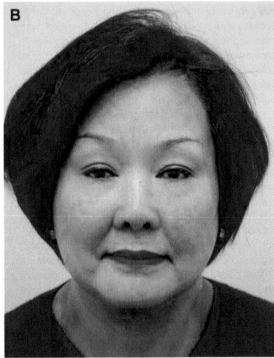

Fig. 1. This Chinese patient (my mother) shows a more prominent steatoblepharon and a high crease height due to fat involution. She would have had a terrible result with any kind of browlift or skin removal from the upper eyelid. Instead, she underwent a concurrent transconjunctival blepharoplasty and full facial fat transfer, including to the inferior orbital rim, brow, and upper-eyelid region. She also has a wider, heavier lower face. By filling fat into the periorbital region, anterior cheek, and anterior chin, the face can ultimately look more dimensional (less flat) and less wide. She also underwent a corset platysmaplasty to improve her neck contour.

substance like injectable hyaluronic acid, it must be respected as a live graft. Weight changes can influence the result, so obese individuals or those with poorly controlled weight, are not necessarily good candidates. Using fat to fill small surface defects, like acne scars, is unadvisable because the live graft may create bumps and lumps as the fat grows asymmetrically in these areas. Similarly, using fat to fill asymmetric facial defects is potentially fraught with problems if the fat graft gains robust blood supply or if the patient's weight fluctuates. It is as important to understand these limitations as it is to understand the esthetic benefits of fat transfer.

With this foundation of understanding, the different way in which fat transfer can be applied to the ethnic face compared with the nonethnic face can be understood. The term *ethnic* encompasses a broad demography including Asian, African, Hispanic, and Middle Eastern. However, some universal concepts may be applicable. In certain ethnicities, such as Asian and related ethnicities, a wider facies may be the norm. In these cases, fat grafting may be considered a less-than-ideal treatment option. On the contrary, fat grafting can be used to accentuate the chin and anterior cheek to effectively narrow the facial shape (**Fig. 1**). In addition, in more melanin-protected races, volume depletion can be the principal, or only, manifestation of significant aging. By addressing this element of aging, most of the aging can be effectively corrected.

The Asian eyelid is a special topic of interest for me, and one that is difficult for the Occidental surgeon trying to manage this condition. I have divided the aging Asian eyelid into 3 categories for better understanding of how blepharoplasty or fat grafting may be used to rejuvenate this element safely and naturally. The 3 categories are:

1) Aging Asian eyelid with a natural supratarsal crease
2) Eyelid without a crease
3) Eyelid with an existing surgically created supratarsal crease.

The Asian eyelid that naturally has a crease may seem easy to correct; simply lift the brows and perform a traditional standard blepharoplasty. The problem with this technique is that the

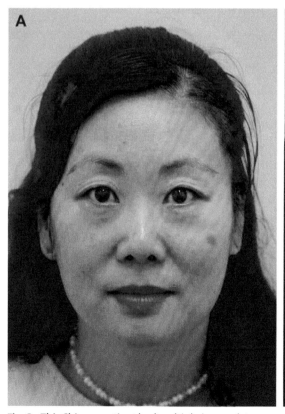
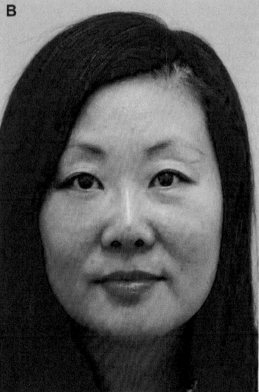

Fig. 2. This Chinese patient had multiple incomplete or partial creases, which, as the text states, should be treated as if she has no crease at all. In addition, she has a negative vector eye shape. She was rejuvenated with only full facial fat transfer and is shown before (*A*) and after (*B*) the procedure.

supratarsal crease will be unnaturally elevated via 1 or both of these techniques. In whites, who may have a naturally high crease, the result may not be unnatural (but could still change the appearance of their youthful countenance). In Asians, the result can be unnatural. The eyelid crease can actually go up with aging as fat loss creates upward retraction of skin. Fat transfer can be used to lower the crease (see **Fig. 1**). In general, fat grafting for the aging Asian eyelid with a crease is still the principal mechanism by which the crease position is maintained or lowered. Only if the skin hangs at or below the ciliary margin do I consider an adjunctive, albeit conservative, blepharoplasty in conjunction with fat transfer. In the aging Asian eyelid without a crease, the options become more difficult. Just cutting skin without a supratarsal crease can lead to scarring because there is no crease to hide the incision within and also limit any improvement, as the palpebral fissure in an Asian eyelid without a crease is already narrow. If fat is removed from the postseptal compartment without formal crease creation, the risk is unpredictable and there is the possibility of unintended partial crease formation by the preseptal tissues adhering to the postseptal tissues.

In the Asian eyelid without a crease, there are only 2 options in my opinion: create a suptarsal crease via a double-eyelid blepharoplasty or perform fat transfer (**Fig. 2**). The real problem with creating a supratarsal crease in the older individual is that the eyelid shape will change and the individual may not desire a crease. The recovery period can be long following incision-based Asian blepharoplasty. In these circumstances fat grafting alone can be the best option.

Finally, the aging Asian eyelid with a previously man-made crease, especially one made during the era of Westernization in the 1980s when a lot of skin and fat were removed, can be a particularly difficult problem. From a distance, the eyelid already looks somewhat fake, even if the crease has fallen lower over time. The reason for this is that the thicker brow skin has draped downward giving the eyelid shape an unnatural thick appearance. Just removing eyelid skin can further unmask the previously over-resected eyelid tissue by making the crease high again and also worsening the thick appearance of the eyelid contour. For these reasons, a previously over-cut Asian eyelid should not be addressed through a browlift or skin removal blepharoplasty because the condition will worsen. In these circumstances, fat transfer is the only safe option.

SUMMARY

Fat transfer has become the primary method for facial rejuvenation in my clinical practice for all ethnicities. This technique can be effectively used to address panfacial volume loss so long as artistry, technical skill, and an in-depth understanding of fat grafting changes over the years are well applied and understood. Fat grafting can replace many traditional facial rejuvenation techniques or serve as an important adjunct to excisional and lifting procedures to temper the degree of excision and lifting that are required.

FURTHER READINGS

Lam SM. Aesthetic facial surgery for the Asian male. Facial Plast Surg 2005;21:317–23.

Lam SM. Aesthetic strategies for the aging Asian face. Facial Plast Clin North Am 2007;15:283–91.

Lam SM, Glasgold MJ, Glasgold RA. Complementary fat grafting. Philadelphia: Lippincott, Williams, Wilkins; 2006.

McCurdy JA Jr, Lam SM. Cosmetic surgery of the Asian face. 2nd edition. New York: Thieme Medical Publishers; 2005.

Shirakabe Y, Suzuki Y, Lam SM. A new paradigm for the aging Asian face. Aesthetic Plast Surg 2003;27: 397–402.

Shu T, Lam SM. Liposuction and lipotransfer for facial rejuvenation in the Asian patient. Int J Cosmet Surg Aesthetic Dermatol 2003;5:165–73.

Lower Facial Rejuvenation in the Non-Caucasian Face

Bruce F. Connell, MD

KEYWORDS

• Facelift • Mid-face • Rejuvenation • Neck lift

It is now possible for refinement of the details concerning the diagnosis of face and neck problems, along with the ability to restore a natural appearance 15 or 20 years younger with minimal detectability of surgical incisions.

INCISION PLACEMENT

Incisions should only be as short or long as needed to produce the desired results (**Fig. 1**). In all non-Caucasian patients (**Fig. 2**), the careful placement of the incision within the first color change from the cheek to the helix of the ear almost always results in a nondetectable scar, whereas if that location is anterior by 3 or 4 mm there will be a visible scar because one would see a color change, the scar, another color change, and still another color change. This common error has been noted by the author in non-Caucasians as well as Caucasians who have much redness to their skin. The chances of a nondetectable scar placed along the edge or margin of the helix is almost always undetectable, whereas a scar placed on the tragus or anterior to the tragus frequently results in a change in pigmentation or a change in color match of the cheek skin to the tragus skin, which makes it obvious that the person has had a facelift from across the dining table and frequently even from across the room.

For a nonoperated appearance the earlobe should have a transition from the earlobe as a pedicle of skin, so that there is not a scar at the junction of the earlobe with the thick cheek skin. In the postauricular area in both Caucasians and non-Caucasians, incisions along the hair have much less possibility of creating a visible problem with alopecia caused by hair shift than making the incision above the occipital hair. An exception to this would be for neck corrections in patients who have no skin to be discarded because the excessive neck skin goes into the concavity formed by the new neck contour (see **Fig. 1**). The abandonment of the traditional erroneous concept that a pressure dressing is necessary for hemostasis or for healing of the postsurgical neck has almost completely eliminated skin vascular problems including sloughs behind the ears. Excision of skin of the face as well as the neck, and also in the occipital area, requires a closure with less than no tension. The author usually describes the edges as "kissing" when finished except for perhaps 3 small points. In many patients the neck cannot be improved without lifting the face because the facial deep tissues have fallen into the neck. These patients can have support of the superficial musculoaponeurotic system (SMAS) holding up the weight of the skin, which eliminates skin tension in the temporal area as well as the preauricular areas. The positioning of the patient so that the chin-neck angle is at 90° when the occipital skin is excised means that the scar will have less tension. If the patient's chin is elevated when the skin is excised, the resulting tension when the patient looks downward will create a large scar in the occipital area. Another error frequently seen for both non-Caucasians and Caucasians is the excision of skin in a direction perpendicular to the long axis of the sternocleidomastoid. Even in a 90-year-old patient there is no excessive skin in

University of California Irvine, College of Medicine, 2200 East Fruit Street, 101, Santa Ana, CA 92701, USA
E-mail address: drbconnell@aol.com

Facial Plast Surg Clin N Am 18 (2010) 7–17
doi:10.1016/j.fsc.2009.11.002
1064-7406/10/$ – see front matter © 2010 Elsevier Inc. All rights reserved.

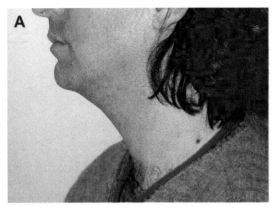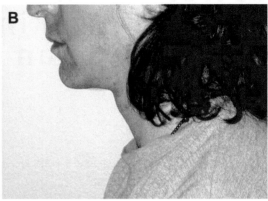

Fig. 1. (A) Neck contour correction with open liposuction of subcutaneous fat, removal of submental subplatysmal fat and tangential excision of 95% of the huge digastric muscle anterior bellies. Only a 2.3-cm transverse skin incision posterior to the submental crease was needed. No transection of platysma muscle. (B) One year postoperative view.

this direction when the head is moved from side to side.

It is essential to make elevation and separation of the skin from the SMAS and platysma muscle with gentle handling of the tissues. This action permits deep layer support with good skin flap subdermal vascularity. Protection of arterial and venous drainage for the elevated skin flaps permits minimal swelling and discoloration. Postoperative tissue swelling would interfere with the skin blood supply and lymphatic drainage, and should be prevented by precise and near atraumatic surgical technique. Precise elevation of skin flaps with little trauma is made easier by using transillumination. Skin flap trauma with resultant histamine release can be caused by prolonged excessive retraction or forceful scissor shoving, which releases much histamine. Avoiding histamine release and postoperative swelling permits the possibility of safer facelifts for smokers, diabetics, and older individuals.

Separation of the skin from the SMAS carries the advantage that the skin and SMAS can be moved along separate vectors and under different tension. This skin-SMAS separation produces a better rejuvenation and a natural appearance. Different vectors of tissue shifting for skin and deep layer support require a high degree of surgical skill to elevate the flaps without thinning the SMAS flap. Unfortunately, use of the SMAS for rejuvenation is not an easy surgical technique. Skill in precise separation of the overlying tissues from the SMAS is essential. This dissection must neither thin the SMAS nor injure the subdermal plexus of arteries and veins. The SMAS is always

thick enough to hold sutures unless the dissection technique thins or removes some of the SMAS while elevating the skin flap (Fig. 3). If during the surgical dissection the ability to recognize the SMAS layer and precisely to uncover the intact SMAS is lacking, other less efficient techniques for deep layer support must be used. For most patients, a satisfactory facelift result requires modification of the deep layer support of the SMAS, fascia, and platysma (Fig. 4). When used appropriately, the SMAS will move cheek fat into the eyelid-cheek depression, changing the direction of the nasojugal groove from the diagonal position of old age to the horizontal position of youth, while the malar rotation point provides more malar prominence (Fig. 5).

For non-Caucasian facelift procedures relying on tightening of aging skin flaps in an attempt to elevate and support sagging, deep tissues often have early recurrence of the original deformities. Skin tension results in wide and visible scars. Skin is elastic, and when pressure or weight is applied the skin will stretch. Skin will not support fat and muscles except for a short period of time. The inelastic SMAS can provide sustained support of the deep tissues. To minimize visible scars, redundant skin is excised and the skin closure is made under less than normal skin tension. The difference in tension is noted when the patient is looking downward, looking upward, or turning the head. The restoration of youthful contours is created by restoring the SMAS and attached muscles as well as the facial fat to the same youthful position, and permits a rejuvenated appearance without a tight or postsurgical appearance.

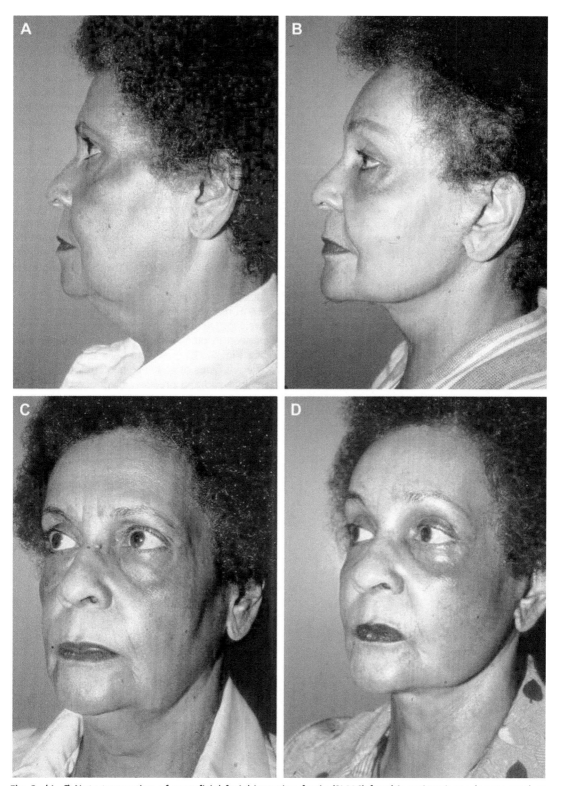

Fig. 2. (*A, C*) Note transection of superficial facial investing fascia (SMAS) for this patient is too low to produce periorbital rejuvenation SMAS facelift. No platysma muscle transection or digastric muscle excision. (*B, D*) Five months postoperative view.

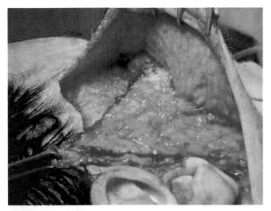

Fig. 3. Hammock support to submental area by SMAS liberation from malar, masseter, parotid fascia, and mandibular ligament.

SUPERFICIAL MUSCULOAPONEUROTIC SYSTEM

A primary facelift patient always has been found to have a SMAS strong enough to give excellent support to the submental area, depressed angles of the mouth, nasolabial folds, nasolabial grooves, and midface if a high SMAS transection is made. In addition, the high SMAS transection and freeing the smile creases (crow's feet) reduces excessive skin of the lower eyelid, and can change the diagonal direction of the nasojugal groove from the countenance of old age to the transverse direction of youth. Shortening the lower eyelid can be accomplished only if the smile crease attachments from the skin to the orbicularis oculi muscle are released. The lateral component of the orbicularis oculi, which pulls the lateral eyebrow downward forcefully when smiling, is released by careful transection of only the portion of the muscle acting as a depressor of the orbicularis oculi muscle (depressor orbicularis lateralis). When this transection is made, a muscle flap of orbicularis can add additional support to the lower eyelid by advancing the lower cut edge in a superolateral direction and suturing it to the periosteum. The midface elevation and the sling effect on the submental area by a shift of the SMAS produces excellent submental contour improvement and support (see **Fig. 4**). The midface support by the SMAS results in little or almost no postoperative swelling. There is no risk of lower eyelid ectropion as seen in other mid-facelift surgical techniques (see **Fig. 3**). To make the neck appear youthful, different types of aesthetic neck deformities must be analyzed and precisely diagnosed. An attractive and pleasing appearance requires a well-contoured neck. The neck can indicate age, health,

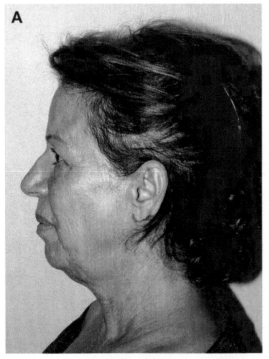
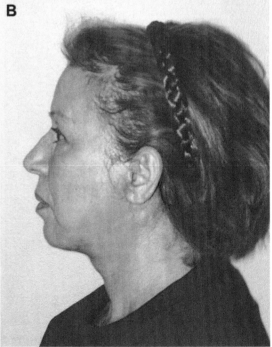

Fig. 4. (*A*) Latina patient for facelift with surgery including high SMAS facelift for midface support and submental support along with transection of the platysma muscle at the hyoid. Ninety-percent tangential excision of the digastric anterior bellies. (*B*) Three months postoperative view.

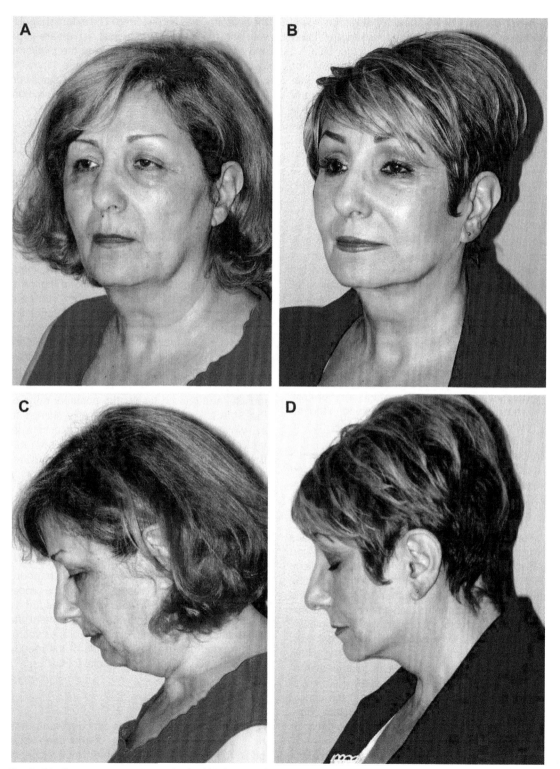

Fig. 5. (*A*, *C*) Far Eastern patient who had high SMAS for support to the lower eyelids, nasojugal crease, elevation of the angle of the mouth, and midface submental support. There was 90% tangential excision of digastric muscle anterior bellies. (*B*, *D*) Thirteen months postoperative view.

disease, fitness, obesity, beauty, elegance, masculinity, femininity, vitality, strength, and sensuality.

Liposuction and tightening of neck skin is not enough to achieve maximum restoration. Skin tightening will not overcome problems in the deep layer. Rejuvenation by using deep layer facelift techniques includes support with transection of the SMAS at the top or above the zygomatic arch. Often, platysma muscle contour correction and support is needed. The neck lift component of a facelift includes correction of excessive skin, platysma muscle laxity, short platysma muscle, subcutaneous or subplatysmal fat, the anterior belly of the digastric muscle hypertrophy, and large submandibular glands. Tightening of skin over these problems does not correct them. A contour problem frequently not diagnosed is the double chin caused by large anterior bellies of the digastric muscles (Fig. 6). For younger patients who have no sagging subcutaneous tissues and skin of the face, a submental incision alone for digastric muscle reduction is adequate. Submental double chin correction for many patients includes the following components:

1. Tangential removal of 95% of the anterior belly is accomplished by passing a curved hemostat beneath the portion of the muscle to be excised.
2. The muscle is then transected with needle cautery at the insertion at the chin and reflected.
3. The muscle is separated near the sling with a needle coagulating current.

Patients with vertically short platysmal muscles or bands are treated by muscle interruption and release at the level of the cricoid cartilage (Fig. 7). The vertical SMAS incision overlying the parotid is 1 to 2 cm anterior to the ear and continues to become the platysmal incision within the avascular 1 cm anterior to the sternocleidomastoid muscle. When complete platysmal transection is planned, the incision is passed within the approximately 1-cm wide avascular area anterior to the anterior border of the sternocleidomastoid muscle, and crosses the neck at the cricoid level. Anterior submental platysmal muscle edge-to-edge approximation along with invagination is planned.

When elevating the platysma from the tail of the parotid to the anterior border of the sternocleidomastoid, a safety space from the marginal mandibular nerve is maintained by using blunt surgical sponge dissection. This dissection is more tedious in secondary procedures in which the anatomy may be distorted. The external jugular vein and the transverse cervical nerves are large and easy to identify. By transecting the platysma low in the neck, accentuation of the larynx is avoided, and there will be a smooth transition with a concave curve from the neck to submental area.

Approximation of the submental platysma muscle completes the 3-vector sling formed by the upward cheek-SMAS shift and rotated SMAS flap to mastoid fascia.

Allis clamp traction to elevate and provide tension to the SMAS layer make dissection safe and easy because scissors will follow the tense SMAS plane, leaving the nerve down more than 1 cm. The vertical limb of the SMAS incision is then made, with the assistant stabilizing the SMAS flap with 2 Allis clamps. The SMAS is carefully elevated until the desired result and motion at the upper nasolabial fold, philtrum, outward turning of the lateral vermillion of the upper lip, elevation of the angle of the mouth, elimination of the jowls, and support to the submental area are achieved. This procedure usually does not require an extended dissection across the cheek.

Once freed from the malar bone, masseter muscle, and parotid fascia, the posterior edge of the SMAS flap is grasped by 3 Allis clamps to see which directional shift produces the best facial result. This direction is often with a superior rotation about its malar pivot point. The superior SMAS flap margin is sutured to the temporalis fascia. The SMAS overlapping augments the zygomatic arch and adds fullness to the temporal concavity, which becomes deeper with aging. This SMAS cheek flap moves good quality SMAS over and below the zygomatic arch where, in the future or often 12 to 15 years later, a secondary SMAS incision could be made through good-quality SMAS fibrous tissue. Folding the upper edge of the flap downward is not needed to provide thicker fixation tissue or to augment the zygomatic arch, and may limit the proper vector for elevation of a depressed angle of the mouth, upper cheek, and upper nasolabial fold.

NECK LIFT

A neck lift allows the precious subcutaneous fat to be preserved and problems of the deep layer origin to be appropriately treated. Neck rejuvenation sometimes requires a facelift if there is downward descent of the subcutaneous fat forming jowl lines and if the tissues of the face have descended into the neck. When a neck lift is performed with a needed facelift, a more balanced and natural

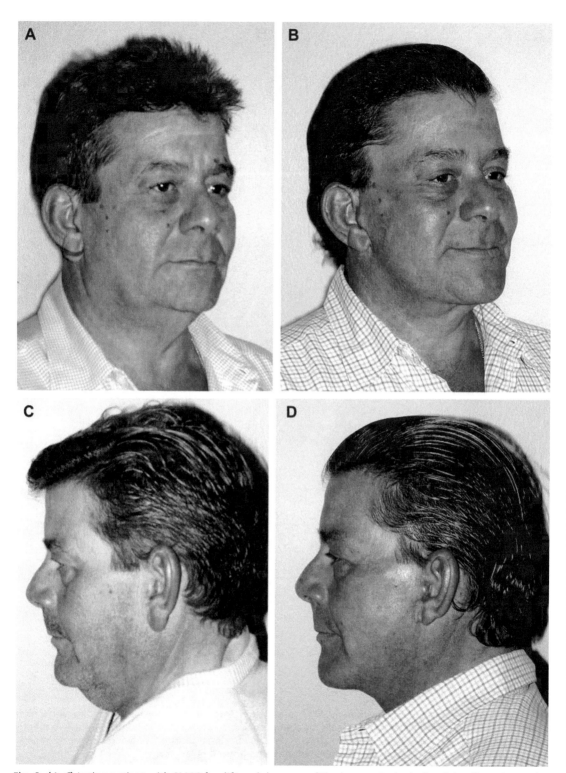

Fig. 6. (*A, C*) Latino patient with SMAS facelift and decrease of the large anterior belly of the digastric muscles. Decrease in length of old appearing earlobes. (*B, D*) Five months postoperative view.

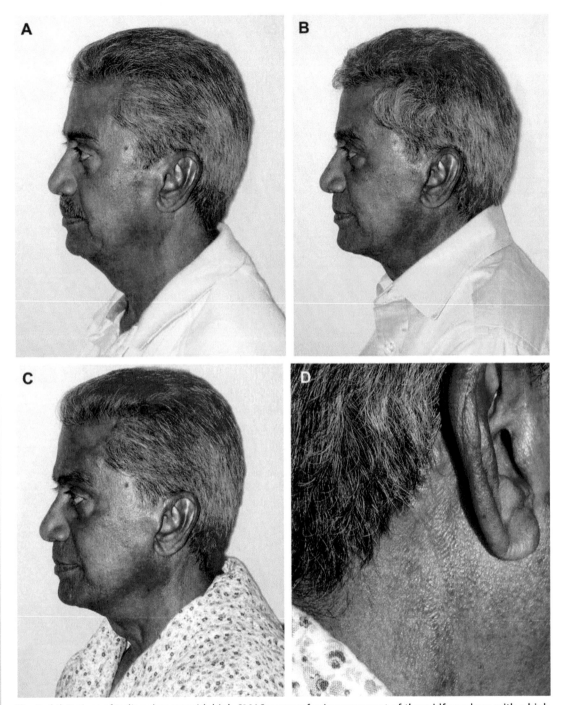

Fig. 7. (*A*) Patient of Indian descent with high-SMAS surgery for improvement of the midface along with a high-SMAS transection to give support to the cheeks including transection at the level of the hyoid. (*B*) Two months postoperative view. (*C*) Twelve months postoperative view. (*D*) Occipital incision following hairline 12 months post operation. The patient is healing well, the scar not being noticed by anyone.

rejuvenation is obtained. Often, a significant amount of redundant skin must be excised using periauricular incisions, with removal of excessive face and neck skin along with a face and neck lift. A precisely performed neck lift allows skin to be excised without skin tightness, and provides a more sustained and natural appearing improvement when deep layer support is used. On occasion, chin implants can improve the results but cannot by themselves produce the best neck contour.

Although the author avoids it, many surgeons perform the submental Z-plasty neck lift. This procedure may create a visible scar location that may be detected when the patient looks from side to side or upward. There are usually better ways to improve the neck without making anterior neck Z-plasties.

The submental incision is often made 1 to 1.5 cm posterior to the submental crease. This location is better than using the submental crease, which accentuates a "witch's chin" and is immobile. When the osseocutaneous connection from the bone to the skin is released, this submental crease disappears forever. The posterior position for the incision heals better than when placed closer to the chin. Male patients are asked not to shave for 1 or 2 days so that the inclination of the beard hairs can be followed with the knife for the hairs to grow through the incision. If perpendicular incisions are made, there may be a loss of 2 rows of hair bulbs, which may cause loss of beard stippling in the submental area, which in turn appears to be a scar even though it is only skin without hair.

Platysmal muscle transverse transection should be performed at the level of the cricoid cartilage or lower, and never at the level of the hyoid. Transection higher than the cricoid level may result in visible cut muscle edges, a depression in this area, and muscle dysfunction. The extent of platysmal transection depends on the type of bands or the type of short platysma muscle present. Precise SMAS liberation from the attachments at the malar, masseter, parotid gland fascia, and the anterior mandibular ligament attachments results in improved submental support, which is long lasting and visible at the time of surgery.

A frequently used technique for deep layer support using the SMAS includes a high transection at the superior edge of the zygomatic arch or higher and a transposition of a flap to the mastoid fascia. A superior, third flap[1] could be used to obtain the precise vector needed for elevation of the angle of the mouth, flattening of the nasolabial fold, and changing the nasojugal groove from the diagonal configuration of old age to the horizontal of youth. If preoperatively it is noted that the prominent gland is large, producing an objectionable contour, and is not ptotic, resection of the protruding portion of the gland can be performed through the submental incision after the platysmal muscle is opened in the midline.

Why and when is submandibular gland reduction indicated? Large submandibular glands may disrupt the attractive neck contour in thin necks or in patients who have had prior neck surgery. If the glands are hidden by submental fat, lax platysmal muscle, and redundant skin, surgical correction of these problems may permit the glands to be revealed and pleasing neck contours disrupted. Preoperative palpation is an important part of the preoperative evaluation of the neck. For surgical correction, the large submandibular glands are exposed through a submental incision between the chin crease and hyoid. The platysmal muscle is opened in the midline and reflected. The capsule of the submental gland is incised in the inferior one-third portion, and resection of the gland is made within the capsule. The submental incision in the midline of the platysmal muscle is closed by invagination with 1 or 2 layers of interrupted 4-0 nylon sutures. Seldom is excessive muscle excised in the midline. The most important part of the surgical procedure for minimizing scar detection is excision of skin in such a manner that no tension exists. The deep layer maintains the support. Basic concepts include the realization that skin is a covering layer and not a supporting one. Only skin that is truly excessive should be excised.

SUTURE CLOSURE

Use of the SMAS/platysmaplasty deep layer support has made possible tension-free precise closure of facelift incisions with no tension at the helix, tragus, and earlobe, thus producing a great reduction in detectable scars. Sutures used are usually 4-0 nylon. Attention to detail is the key to a result of the best quality.

Dressings were once thought to prevent edema, seromas, and hematomas. Fortunately for patients, most surgeons now acknowledge that this is not true. Although some surgeons claim their dressings provide increased patient comfort and improvements in neck contours, experience and common sense argue against these convictions. There are many rational arguments against the use of a facelift dressing. The most obvious of these is the danger of placing pressure on delicate skin flaps. Facial and neck pressure dressings will not reduce edema, and most bandages create a tourniquet effect, which decreases venous and lymphatic return and contributes to edema. In addition, a tight neck or facelift dressing is not comfortable.

POSTOPERATIVE INSTRUCTIONS

After surgery, a good position that ensures an open cervicomental angle is one in which the patient sits with "elbows on knees" and a book or computer on another chair. This posture allows activities such as reading, writing, eating, and watching television. Any time that compromise of the postauricular flap is noted, one should check to ensure that a tight closure has not created lateral tension across its base, strangling it. If in doubt, offending sutures should be removed without hesitation, because secondary healing is always superior to slough. When seated, the patient's head must rest against the wall or head-rest to relax the posterior neck muscles, or the posterior neck will ache later.

Sutures are removed as indicated, usually in stages over a period of 6 to 9 days. Fine sutures are removed from areas of low tension first, usually on postoperative days 3 and 5. Half-buried vertical mattress sutures are removed later over postoper-ative days 5 to 10. Sutures in relatively higher tension areas at the sideburn and behind the ear are removed last.

COMPLICATIONS

The author's experience has shown that longer and more extensive facelift procedures have not resulted in an increased rate of complications. Hematomas, the most common complication re-ported in the literature, are thought to be more common in men. Because the author's procedures are long and tend to outlast the effect of epineph-rine, bleeding is usually discovered and corrected before wound closure. During the past 30 years, only one male patient and no female patient under-going a facelift has been returned to surgery from the recovery room for evacuation of a hematoma.

There have been no zygomatic buccal nerve injuries, one marginal mandibular nerve palsy, and one permanent injury to the frontotemporal branch of the facial nerve during this period. Three patients experienced temporary unilateral weak-ness of the frontalis muscle, but all recovered without residual effects within 12 weeks. Four patients had temporary unilateral weakness of the lower lip depressor muscle even though it is not required that patients stop smoking.

Skin necrosis is extremely rare. In only 5 cases has it exceeded 1 cm, and in all cases was less than 2 cm. This rarity is attributed to precise plan-ning, atraumatic and gentle skin handling, lack of skin tension due to support of the SMAS, and a thoughtful postoperative plan of care, including no pressure dressings, for all patients.

SUMMARY

SMAS use for non-Caucasians is the same for Caucasians and is of 2 types—adequate use to obtain the best results possible, and limited use. This concept directs attention to the artistic goal rather than focusing on technique by using terms such as a high, low, or extended SMAS. If the SMAS is used with precision, substantial periorbi-tal rejuvenation can be achieved along with decreased excessive lower eyelid skin, support of periorbital fat of the lower eyelids, improvement in smile creases, and restoration of the nasojugal grove to the horizontal direction of youth from the diagonal direction of the aged appearance, along with change from the long, oval, older appearance of the lower eyelid to a shorter youth-ful appearance. A youthful appearing neck as well as rejuvenation of the upper third of the face is important for patient satisfaction following a facelift procedure. Each patient deserves safe surgery and the best possible result.

REFERENCE

1. Connell BF, Semlacher RA. Contemporary deep layer facial rejuvenation. Plast Reconstr Surg 1997;100(6): 1513–23.

FURTHER READING

Connell BF. Facial rejuvenation. In: Brent B, editor. The artistry of reconstructive surgery. St. Louis (MO): CV Mosby; 1987. p. 365–81.

Connell BF, Hosn W. Importance of the digastric muscle in cervical contouring: an update. Aesthet Surg J 2000;20:12–6.

Connell BF, Marten TJ. Surgical correction of crow's feet. Clin Plast Surg 1993;20:295.

Connell BF, Marten TJ. Facelift. In: Cohen M, editor. Mastery in plastic surgery. Boston: Little, Brown & Co; 1994. p. 1873–902.

Connell BF, Marten TJ. Deep layer technique in cervico-facial rejuvenation. In: Psillakis J, editor. Deep face-lifting techniques. New York: Thieme Medical Publishers, Inc; 1994. p. 161–90.

Connell B, Miller SR, Gonzalez-Miramontes H. Skin and SMAS flaps for facial rejuvenation. In: Guyuron B, editor. Plastic surgery: indications, operations, and outcomes. St. Louis (MO): CV Mosby, Inc; 2000. p. 2583–607.

Connell BF, Shamoun JM. The significance of digastric muscle contouring for rejuvenation of the submental area of the face. Plast Reconstr Surg 1997;99(6): 1886–950.

Furnas D. The retaining ligaments of the cheek. Plast Re-constr Surg 1987;11:163.

Guerrerosantos J. The role of the platysma muscle in rhy-tidoplasty. Clin Plast Surg 1983;10:449.

Guyuron B. Problem neck, hyoid bone and submental myotomy. Plast Reconstr Surg 1992;90:830.

Hamra ST. The deep plane rhytidectomy. Plast Reconstr Surg 1990;86:53.

Ristow B. Milestones in the evolution of facelift techniques. In: Grotting JC, editor. Reoperative aesthetic and reconstructive plastic surgery. St. Louis (MO): Quality Medical Publishing, Inc; 1995. p. 191.

Stuzin JM, Baker TJ, Gordon HL. The relationship of superficial and deep fascia fascias relevance to rhytidectomy and aging. Plast Reconstr Surg 1992;89:3.

Pennisi VR, Klabunde EH, Pierce GW. The preauricular flap. Plast Reconstr Surg 1965;35:552–6.

Brent B. Total auricular construction with sculpted costal cartilage. In: Brent B, editor. The artistry of reconstructive surgery. St. Louis (MO): CV Mosby Company; 1987. p. 113–28.

Upper and Midfacial Rejuvenation in the Non-Caucasian Face

Rami K. Batniji, MD[a,b],*, Stephen W. Perkins, MD[c,d]

KEYWORDS

- Endoscopic brow lift • Botulinum toxin
- Filler augmentation • Midface lift
- Lower lid blepharoplasty • Upper blepharoplasty

In the nineteenth century, Johann Friedrich Blumenbach popularized the term "Caucasian" to describe a distinct group of people from the Caucasus region with specific craniofacial features. Although the Caucasus region lies between Europe and Asia and includes Russia, Georgia, Armenia, Azerbaijan, and Iran, the term Caucasian has since been used to describe those individuals of European origin. Although age-related changes have some similarities between Caucasians and non-Caucasians, there are also some distinct differences. In this paper, the authors discuss treatment options, surgical and nonsurgical, for rejuvenation of the upper face and midface, including the periorbital region. For the purposes of this paper, the term non-Caucasian includes African American, Middle Eastern, and Asian ethnicities.

FACIAL ANALYSIS
The Upper Third of the Face

The ideal eyebrow shape was defined as an arch where the brow apex terminates above the lateral limbus of the iris, with the medial and lateral ends of the brow at the same horizontal level.[1] This definition has been further refined to provide a framework for the analysis of the upper third of the face and subsequent treatment options for forehead rejuvenation.[2] Biller and Kim[3] studied the ideal location of the eyebrow apex in Asian and white women. Their findings suggested that neither the ethnicity of the models nor the ethnicity of the volunteers who analyzed the eyebrow position had a significant role in determining the ideal eyebrow position. A survey of plastic surgeons and cosmetologists regarding eyebrow shape in women by Freund and Nolan[4] found that a medial eyebrow at the level of the supraorbital rim was ideal and that brow lifting techniques tend to elevate the medial eyebrow above this level. Increasing eyebrow height with age has been previously reported, and this phenomenon has been attributed to habitually contracting the frontalis muscle. Therefore, an overly elevated brow may not only result in a surprised appearance but also impart an aged countenance.[5]

During the evaluation of the upper eyelid, the forehead should be assessed for ptosis, as this may confound the diagnosis of upper eyelid dermatochalasis. The surgeon should evaluate the upper eyelid to rule out the contribution of blepharoptosis. The position of the upper eyelid should ideally rest at the level of the superior limbus. If unilateral blepharoptosis is identified, the surgeon must rule out blepharoptosis in the contralateral eye, as Herring's Law may apply in this situation. The Asian upper eyelid has several distinct anatomic characteristics including low, poorly defined or absent eyelid crease, narrow palpebral fissure, and/or epicanthal fold.[6]

a Batniji Facial Plastic Surgery, 361 Hospital Road, Suite #329, Newport Beach, CA 92663, USA
b Department of Plastic Surgery, Hoag Hospital, Newport Beach, CA, USA
c Meridian Plastic Surgeons, 170 West 106th Street, Indianapolis, IN 46290, USA
d Indiana University School of Medicine, Department of Otolaryngology, Indianapolis, IN, USA
* Corresponding author.
E-mail address: info@drbatniji.com (R.K. Batniji).

Facial Plast Surg Clin N Am 18 (2010) 19–33
doi:10.1016/j.fsc.2009.11.015
1064-7406/10/$ – see front matter © 2010 Elsevier Inc. All rights reserved.

facialplastic.theclinics.com

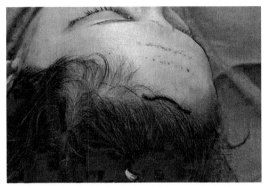

Fig. 1. The trichophytic incision is approximately 4 cm in length and is made at the midline following the natural irregular contour of the hairline. Laterally on each side a 3- to 4-cm incision is made 2 cm posterior to the temporal hairline recession at a location demarcated by the lateral canthus and temporal line.

The Lower Lid/Midface Complex

Evaluation of lower eyelid position and laxity is an essential part of the examination. The ideal position of the lower eyelid margin is at the inferior limbus.[7] A snap test and lid distraction test are key components to the evaluation of lower eyelid laxity. A snap test is performed by grasping the lower eyelid and pulling it away from the globe. When the eyelid is released, the eyelid returns to its normal position quickly; however, in a patient with decreased lower eyelid tone, the eyelid returns to its normal position more slowly. The lid distraction test is performed by grasping the lower eyelid with the thumb and index finger; movement of the lid margin greater than 10 mm demonstrates poor eyelid tone and an eyelid tightening procedure is indicated. A Schirmer test is indicated if there is concern about dry eye syndrome. Progressive loss of elastic fibers and collagen organization lead to dermatochalasis (loss of skin elasticity and subsequent excess laxity

of lower eyelid skin).[8] In addition, the orbital septum weakens with age leading to steatoblepharon (pseudoherniation of orbital fat).[9] Orbicularis oculi muscle hypertrophy is also associated with age-related changes of the upper and lower eyelid complex.[10]

The tear trough is also known as the nasojugal groove and is defined as the natural depression extending inferolaterally from the medial canthus to approximately the midpupillary line.[11] A hollowness may be present lateral to the midpupillary line and parallel to the infraorbital rim; this has been referred to by various names, including the lid/cheek junction. Various anatomic explanations for the tear trough deformity have been provided in the literature, including an attachment of orbital septum to arcus marginalis at the level of the orbital rim, a gap between the levator labii superioris alaeque nasi muscle and the orbicularis oculi muscle, and loss of facial fat in the tear trough or pseudoherniation of fat superior to the tear trough. The tear trough and lid/cheek junction occur inferior to the orbital rim and arcus marginalis.

TREATMENT OPTIONS
Brow/Forehead

Nonsurgical options for brow/forehead
There are several nonsurgical options available for the rejuvenation of the brow/forehead, including neuromodulators, dermal fillers, and autologous fat grafting. For example, Lambros reported volumizing the brow with hyaluronic acid fillers to give more youthful appearance to the brow/periorbital region.[12]

Surgical options and technique for brow/forehead
Many techniques for surgical rejuvenation of the upper third of the face have been described in the literature. Although the open technique via a coronal or trichophytic approach has been the

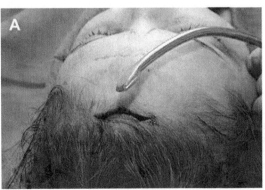
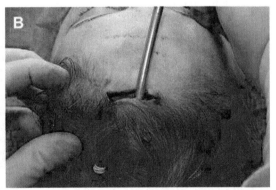

Fig. 2. (*A*) The Ramirez EndoForehead parietal elevator (Snowden Pencer, Tucker, GA) is used to elevate the forehead and temporal skin in a subgaleal plane. (*B*) The elevation is continued approximately 5 cm posterior to the incision sites.

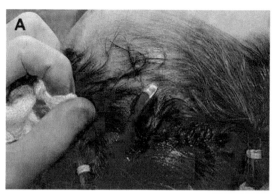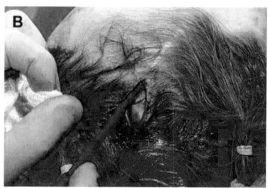

Fig. 3. (*A*) A custom-made curved elevator is positioned into the temporal region through the lateral incision to divide the conjoint tendon. (*B*) Dissection of this temporal region is performed down to an area slightly superior to the zygomatic arch and lateral canthus.

standard with which all other techniques have been compared, our preferred method for surgical rejuvenation of the brow is the endoscopic brow lift. Botulinum toxin injected into the corrugator supercilii and procerus muscles at least 2 weeks before endoscopic brow lift. The combination of chemical ablation of the depressor muscles with botulinum toxin A and myotomy of the depressor muscles during the endoscopic forehead lift acts synergistically not only to maintain the elevated forehead position but also to treat the nasoglabellar furrows. The addition of botulinum toxin may also lessen the chance of return of depressor muscle function compared with myotomy or myectomy alone.

One noticeable effect of the endoscopic brow lift is an elevation of the hairline. Although this is an acceptable result for most patients, persons who have high hairlines (greater than 5 to 6 cm) may not wish to move the hairline more posterior. We perform a technique combining a short 3- to 4-cm trichophytic incision with endoscopic equipment to lift the forehead in patients who present with brow ptosis and high hairlines.[13] This technique includes a trichophytic incision that is approximately 4 cm in length and is made at the midline following the natural irregular frontal hairline contour in a scalloped fashion. Laterally, on each side, a 3- to 4-cm vertical incision is made 2 cm posterior to the temporal hairline recession at a location demarcated by the lateral canthus and temporal line (**Fig. 1**). Initially, flap elevation is made in a subgaleal plane (**Fig. 2**). The elevation is performed approximately 5 cm posterior to the incision sites; the posterior elevation not only minimizes the development of scalp rolls but also mobilizes the posterior flap, allowing for closure of the trichophytic incision without elevating the hairline. The temporal region is elevated in a plane between the temporoparietal fascia and the superficial layer

of the deep temporal fascia, and the conjoint tendon is then divided (**Fig. 3**). Dissection of this temporal region is performed down to an area slightly superior to the zygomatic arch and lateral canthus. The frontal branch of the facial nerve is protected because the plane of dissection is between the temporoparietal fascia and the superficial layer of the deep temporal fascia. Following this, elevation is made in a subperiosteal plane down to a level of 2 cm above the supraorbital rim (**Fig. 4**) and the arcus marginalis is then elevated. Arcus marginalis elevation is performed with the nondominant hand functioning as a guide to the level of the supraorbital rim and the location of the supraorbital foramina (**Fig. 5**). This elevation is performed in the region of the glabella down to the nasion. Once the arcus marginalis is elevated, an endoscope is used to provide visualization; and the conjoint tendon is further divided with curved endoscopic scissors (Accurate Surgical & Scientific Instruments Corp, Westbury, NY) down to the level of the sentinel vein (**Fig. 6**). Care is then taken to identify and preserve the supraorbital

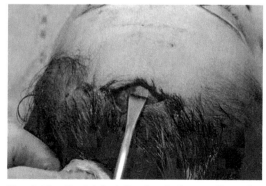

Fig. 4. The Daniel EndoForehead elevator (Snowden Pencer) is used to elevate the brow in a subperiosteal plane down to a level 2 cm above the supraorbital rim.

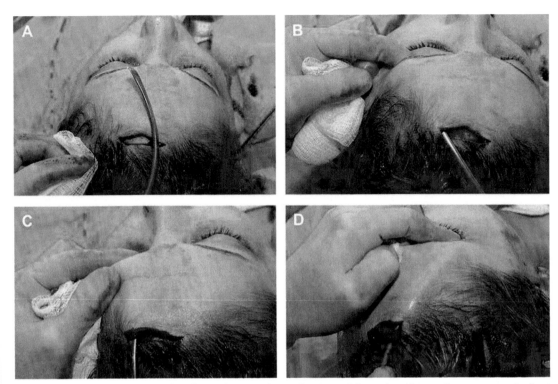

Fig. 5. (*A*) The Ramirez EndoForehead A/M dissector (Snowden Pencer) is used to elevate the arcus marginalis at the level of the supraorbital rim. (*B–D*) The elevation is performed with the nondominant hand functioning as a guide to the level of the supraorbital rim and the location of the supraorbital foramina.

neurovascular bundle (**Fig. 7**). With a custom-made reusable electrode knife tip, the periosteum is incised in a horizontal direction at the level of the supraorbital rim (**Fig. 8**). Myotomy of the corrugator supercilii and procerus muscles is performed with the electrode knife tip. Because the motor nerve to the corrugator supercilii muscle runs within the substance of the lateral orbicularis oculi muscle,

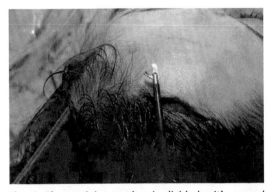

Fig. 6. The conjoint tendon is divided with curved endoscopic scissors (Accurate Surgical and Scientific Instruments Corp). This aspect of the procedure is performed under visualization using a 30-degree endoscope, which is placed through the lateral incision.

we perform a lateral myotomy of the orbicularis oculi muscle not only to weaken the orbicularis oculi muscle but also to interrupt the innervation to the corrugator supercilii muscle. In an effort to camouflage the trichophytic incision, we not only bevel the incision but also de-epithelialize the posterior flap. A 2- to 3-mm strip of epidermis from the posterior flap is excised (**Fig. 9**). The anterior flap of the trichophytic incision is lifted up, and vertical incisions are made through the anterior flap. Staples are placed at these positions to approximate the anterior and posterior flaps. The excess skin and soft tissue from the anterior flap are then excised in a beveled manner; the bevel is directed from posterior to anterior (**Fig. 10**). The staples are then removed and hemostasis is achieved with bipolar electrocautery. Fixation with sutures via bone tunnels of the outer cortex of the skull is performed. The bone tunnels are made with the Browlift Bone Bridge system and drill bit with a 2-mm diameter and 25-mm guard (Medtronic Xomed Surgical Products, Jacksonville, FL). Two bone tunnels are created at the trichophytic incision site in a horizontal direction, whereas bone tunnels are created in the vertical direction at the lateral incisions (**Fig. 11**). Using the drill bit with a 25-mm guard, there have been

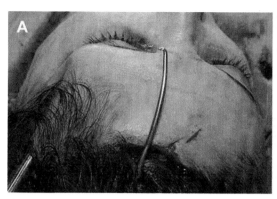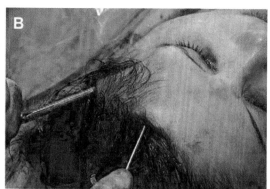

Fig. 7. (A) The subperiosteal elevation is completed at the level of the supraorbital rim using the Isse elevator. (B) The trichophytic incision provides easy access to the level of the supraorbital rim despite the high anterior hairline and double convexity of the forehead.

no instances of cerebrospinal fluid leaks or other intracranial complications. If significant bleeding is encountered from the bone tunnel site, hemostasis is achieved with Bone Wax (Ethicon, Somerville, NJ), and new bone tunnels are created. A 2-0 polyglactin suture (Vicryl) is used for fixation from the bone tunnel to the galea and subcutaneous tissue of the anterior flap to achieve lifting of the medial forehead at the trichophytic incision site. Very minimal lifting is performed medially so that the medial brow may remain at the level of the supraorbtial rim. The lateral forehead is lifted with the suture from the bone tunnel to the galea and the subcutaneous tissue at the most anterior aspect of the lateral incision on both sides (**Fig. 12**). This suture not only lifts the lateral forehead but also reapproximates the edges of the lateral incision. The lateral incision is closed with staples. The trichophytic incision is closed in a layered fashion (**Fig. 13**). With meticulous closure,

the trichophytic incision is well camouflaged (**Fig. 14**).

Upper Eyelid

Treatment of the non-Caucasian upper eyelid depends on several factors, of which ethnicity is paramount. Is the non-Caucasian individual Asian, Middle Eastern, or African American? Within the Asian population, there are distinct differences in perceived beauty and motivation for rejuvenation of the upper eyelid based on culture and whether that patient is Korean, Chinese, or Japanese.[14] If a natural crease is present in the aging Asian upper eyelid, volume enhancement and conservative excision of excess skin would benefit the patient, whereas a patient who has undergone a previous procedure and who has a surgically created crease may benefit from volume enhancement alone, and a patient without a crease may benefit from double eyelid surgery. Does the patient have a history of keloid formation? If so, a nonincision suture technique for double eyelid surgery may be an option; however, this treatment has a higher relapse rate compared with incision techniques and fixation. Incision techniques have the benefit of addressing the epicanthal fold in the Asian upper eyelid with an epicanthoplasty.[15]

In the non-Asian, non-Caucasian patient, a traditional upper eyelid blepharoplasty is an excellent option to treat upper eyelid dermatochalasis and steatoblepharon. The preoperative assessment of the patient seeking rejuvenation of the upper and/or lower eyelid complex includes a history to evaluate for systemic disease processes, such as collagen vascular diseases and Grave disease, dry eye symptoms, and visual acuity changes. It is important to delineate whether the changes to the upper and/or lower lids are related to age-related changes to the eyelids (dermatochalasis and

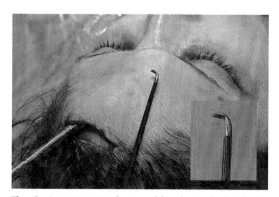

Fig. 8. A custom-made reusable electrode knife tip (inset shows tip of instrument) is used to incise the periosteum at the level of the supraorbital rim and perform myotomy of the procerus, corrugator supercilii, and orbicularis oculi muscles.

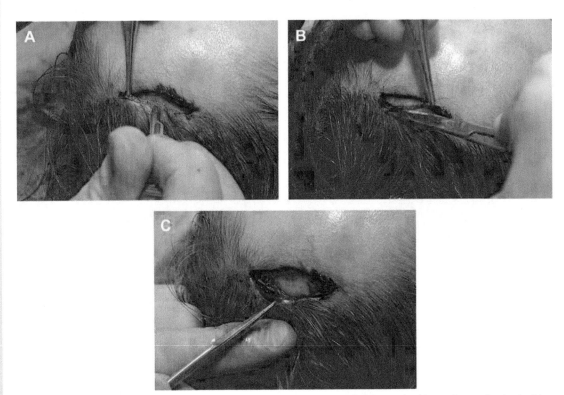

Fig. 9. A 2- to 3-mm strip of epidermis from the posterior flap is excised. (*A*) A scalpel is used to make the incision through the epidermis. (*B*) Sharp curved scissors are then used to complete the excision of the strip of epidermis. (*C*) The intact dermis, subcutaneous tissue, and hair follicles after removal of the epidermal layer.

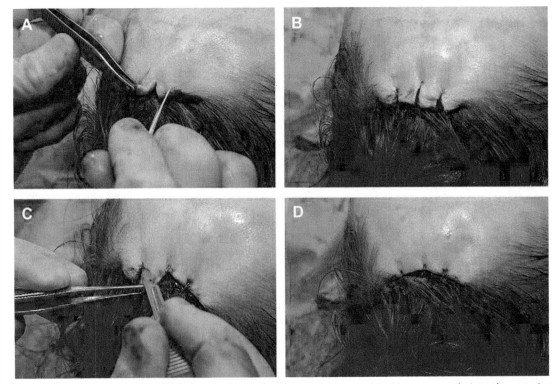

Fig. 10. Sequential resection of the anterior flap is performed. (*A*) Vertical incisions are made into the anterior flap, and (*B*) staples are placed to approximate the anterior and posterior flaps. (*C*) The excess skin and soft tissue from the anterior flap is then excised in a beveled (posterior to anterior) manner. (*D*) The result after this skin excision.

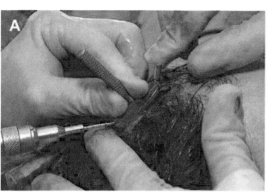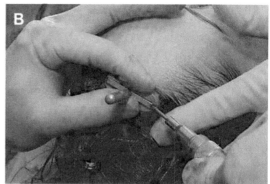

Fig. 11. The Browlift Bone Bridge system (Medtronic Xomed Surgical Products) and drill bit with a 2-mm diameter and a 25-mm guard is used to make a vertically oriented tunnel at the lateral incision (A) and 2 horizontally oriented bone tunnels at the trichophytic incision (B).

steatoblepharon) or a manifestation of a systemic process, such as allergy or an endocrine disorder. For example, a patient with Grave disease may have upper eyelid retraction and exophthalmos, but the myxedematous state of hypothyroidism may mimic dermatochalasis. Therefore, thyroid-stimulating hormone (TSH) level should be obtained if a thyroid disorder is suspected. If any unusual history is gleaned from the preoperative assessment, it may be prudent to obtain an ophthalmologic evaluation before undertaking blepharoplasty. The limitations of blepharoplasty and the role of adjuvant procedures must be discussed with the patient. For example, the patient

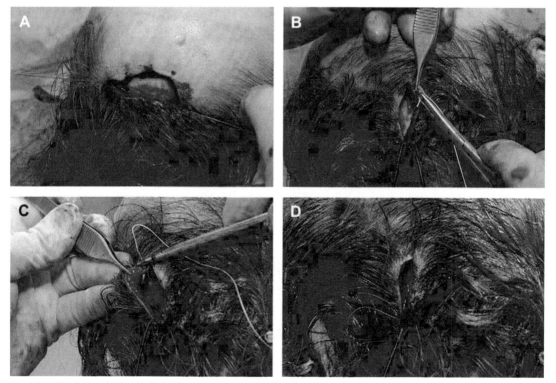

Fig. 12. (A) A 2-0 polyglactin (Vicryl) suture is used for fixation from the bone tunnel to the anterior flap of the trichophytic incision. (B, C) At the lateral incision, fixation is achieved with suture from the bone tunnel to the most anterior aspect of the lateral incision on both sides. (D) This suture not only lifts the lateral forehead but also reapproximates the edges of the lateral incision. The suture is passed through galea to achieve proper tissue strength for elevation and fixation.

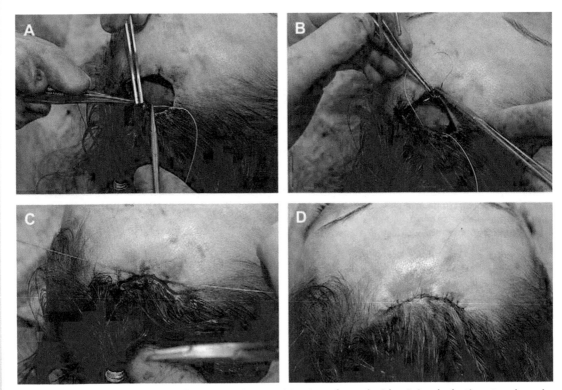

Fig. 13. (*A, B*) Meticulous closure of the trichophytic incision is performed with a 3-0 polyglactin suture in an interrupted buried fashion to obtain deep-tissue reapproximation. (*C*) The assistant further mobilizes the posterior flap to allow closure of the wound without moving the hairline more posteriorly. Further subcutaneous reapproximation is achieved with 4-0 polydioxanone. (*D*) Following this maneuver, skin closure with proper eversion of the skin edges is achieved with a 5-0 blue polypropylene (Prolene) suture in a running interlocked manner.

seeking periorbital rejuvenation with significant crow's feet may benefit from botulinum toxin treatment, whereas the patient with fine wrinkling, crepe paper skin may achieve significant improvement with skin resurfacing.

Surgical technique for the upper eyelid

The surgeon must be meticulous in the surgical markings for upper eyelid blepharoplasty prior to surgery as a difference of 1 to 3 mm (mm) from one eyelid to the next may create noticeable asymmetries. Therefore, the surgical markings for both upper eyelids are made using a fine tip marker and small calipers. With the patient looking up, the supratarsal crease is identified and measured from the eyelid margin using small calipers; this denotes the location of the inferior limb of the surgical marking. This measurement ranges

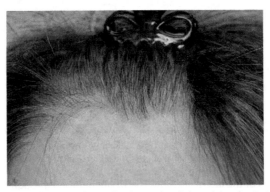

Fig. 14. Postoperative photograph showing the esthetic result of the trichophytic incision at 12 months.

from 8 to 12 mm from the lid margin (10–11 mm in women; 8–9 mm in men) (**Fig. 15**). The inferior limb of the marking is curved gently and parallels the lid margin; the inferior limb of the marking is carried medially to within 1 to 2 mm of the punctum and laterally to the lateral canthus. If the marking is carried along the curve of the eyelid crease lateral to the lateral canthus, the final closure scar line will bring the upper eyelid tissue downward, thus resulting in a hooded appearance. In an effort to avoid this unsightly result, the marking sweeps diagonally upward from the lateral canthus to the lateral eyebrow margin (**Fig. 16**). This modification of the lateral incision makes it easy for women to camouflage the incision with makeup. Medially, the nasal-orbital depression should not be violated as an incision in this area may result in a webbed scar; ending the incision medially within 1 to 2 mm of the punctum avoids this result. Next, the superior limb of the surgical marking is made. This is facilitated by using smooth forceps to pinch the excess amount of upper eyelid skin so that the lashes roll upward (**Fig. 17**). The surgeon's contralateral hand is used to reposition the eyebrow superiorly to isolate the perceived contribution of brow ptosis from upper eyelid dermatochalasis. Alternatively, if the patient is undergoing a forehead lift at the same time as the upper eyelid blepharoplasty, the surgeon may elect to perform the forehead lift first and then to measure the appropriate amount of upper eyelid skin excision necessary to provide rejuvenation of the upper eyelid complex while minimizing the risk of lagophthalmos.

Typically, isolated upper eyelid blepharoplasty can be performed under local anesthesia with

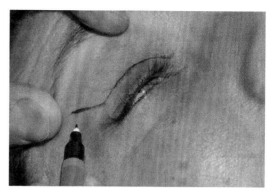

Fig. 16. The marking sweeps diagonally upward from the lateral canthus to the lateral eyebrow margin.

intravenous sedation. Lidocaine 2% with epinephrine (1:50,000) is infiltrated deep to the skin but superficial to the orbicularis oculi muscle, thus minimizing the risk of ecchymosis caused by the injection of local anesthesia. Stabilization of the skin in the eyelid is paramount to making the skin-only incision of the upper eyelid; therefore, an assistant is required to place tension on the skin. A round-handled scalpel with a #15 Bard-Parker blade is ideal for following the curves of the surgical markings in the upper eyelid. Once the skin incision is made, the skin is then sharply dissected from the underlying orbicularis oculi muscle with the blade or dissecting beveled scissors. The preseptal orbicularis oculi muscle is then evaluated. If it is atrophic or very thin, then the muscle need not be excised; however, most often, a thin strip of preseptal orbicularis oculi muscle is excised medially, thus exposing the fat compartments. If the muscle is robust, then the excision is performed along the entire length of the eyelid.

Attention is then directed to the pseudoherniation of orbital fat. If there is fullness of the upper eyelid, a conservative approach to removal of fat is followed to avoid a hollowed or sunken appearance to the upper eyelid. A small opening is made in the orbital septum overlying the middle and medial fat compartments. Gentle pressure on the globe reveals redundant fat from each compartment. Using Griffiths-Brown forceps, the herniated fat is grasped from its respective compartment; and, unless the patient is under general anesthesia, the fat is infiltrated with local anesthesia to minimize discomfort associated with subsequent electrocautery and excision of the redundant fat (**Fig. 18**). Meticulous hemostasis is of utmost importance not only to maintain a clear operative field but also to minimize the risk of postoperative bleeding. Once fat removal from both

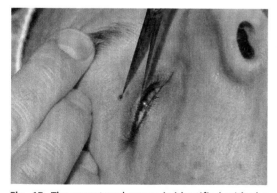

Fig. 15. The supratarsal crease is identified with the patient looking upward; the supratarsal crease is then measured from the lid margin using small calipers. This measurement denotes the location of the inferior limb of the surgical marking and ranges between 8 and 12 mm.

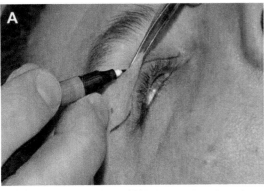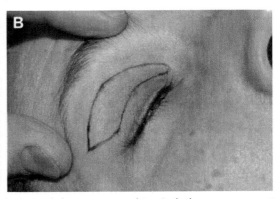

Fig. 17. The superior limb of the surgical marking is made. Smooth forceps are used to pinch the excess amount of upper eyelid skin to roll the eyelashes upward (*A*). The superior limb is connected with the inferior limb medially and laterally (*B*).

compartments is completed, bipolar electrocautery is used to ensure hemostasis before wound closure.

The preferred technique for skin closure is as follows (**Fig. 19**): 7-0 blue polypropylene suture is used in an interrupted fashion to reapproximate the skin edges. Whereas a 6-0 mild chromic or fast-absorbing gut suture may create an inflammatory response and subsequent milia, a 7-0 sized suture rarely produces milia. The upper eyelid

blepharoplasty incision closure is then completed with a running 6-0 blue polypropylene suture in a subcuticular fashion with knots tied at the medial and lateral aspects of the incision (**Fig. 20**).

Lower Eyelid

Nonsurgical rejuvenation options

Many methods have been used to efface the tear trough deformity including fat grafts, injections

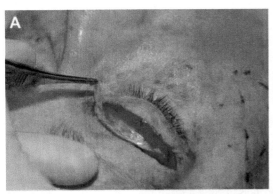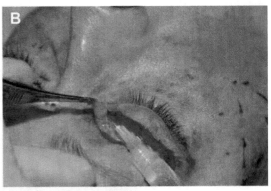

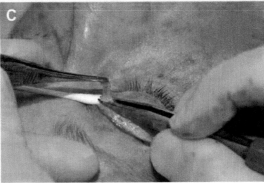

Fig. 18. A small opening is made in the orbital septum to access the middle and medial fat compartments. Gentle pressure on the globe demonstrates redundant fat from each compartment; forceps are used to grasp the herniated fat (*A*). Local anesthesia is infiltrated at the base of the herniated fat (*B*) and then the base is cauterized (*C*). Excision of the fat is then performed at the cauterized base.

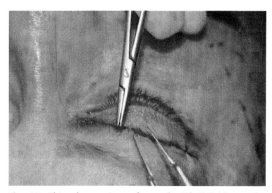

Fig. 19. Skin closure is performed with 7-0 blue polypropylene sutures used in an interrupted fashion to reapproximate the skin edges; the remainder of the skin closure is performed with 6-0 blue polypropylene suture in a subcuticular fashion with knots tied at the medial and lateral ends.

with fat or injectable fillers,[16] and alloplastic implants.[17] Treatment of lower eyelid fine lines and wrinkles may be treated with skin resurfacing; however, the non-Caucasian patient may have a tendency for pigmentation issues after resurfacing. Therefore, pre- and posttreatment of the skin with a bleaching agent and/or retinoid must be considered. A nonablative resurfacing procedure decreases the risk of pigmentation issues in the non-Caucasian patient compared with ablative procedures. Fractionated technologies (both CO_2 and erbium) may have a prominent role in skin resurfacing of non-Caucasian skin.

Surgical technique for lower eyelid

Lower eyelid blepharoplasty may be performed via a transconjunctival or transcutaneous approach. Among the transcutaneous approaches, the skin-muscle flap is our preferred technique. The indications for this technique include true vertical excess of lower eyelid skin, orbicularis oculi muscle

hypertrophy, and the presence of pseudoherniation of orbital fat. The incision is 2 mm inferior to the lower eyelid margin and extends from the lower punctum medially to a position 6 mm lateral to the lateral canthus; lateral extension of the incision to this position minimizes rounding of the canthal angle. Following the skin incision, fine curved scissors are used to dissect through the orbicularis muscle at the lateral aspect of the incision (**Fig. 21A**). Then, blunt scissors are positioned posterior to the muscle at the lateral aspect of the incision and, with spreading motions of the blunt scissors, the skin-muscle flap is elevated off the orbital septum along an avascular plane (**Fig. 21B**). The subciliary incision is then completed using the scissors in a beveled manner to ensure the preservation of the pretarsal portion of the orbicularis oculi muscle, thus minimizing the risk of postoperative lower eyelid malposition. Small openings are made in the orbital septum to obtain access to the orbital fat compartments. Gentle palpation of the globe results in herniation of orbital fat through these openings of the orbital septum. Bipolar electrocautery is used to cauterize the fat pad before excision; before cauterization, local anesthesia is infiltrated into the fat pocket to minimize pain. This procedure is performed for the lateral, middle, and medial fat pockets. Gentle palpation of the globe following resection of orbital fat allows for reassessment of orbital fat. A conservative approach to fat resection is maintained to avoid the creation of a sunken appearance. Then, the skin-muscle flap is repositioned. If mildly sedated, the patient is asked to open his or her mouth and look upward; this maneuver allows for maximal separation of the wound edges and subsequent conservative resection of skin and muscle. On the other hand, if the patient is completely sedated, single-finger pressure at the inferomedial portion of the melolabial

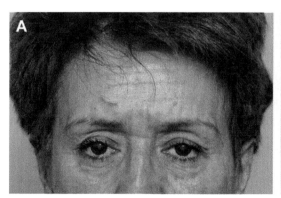

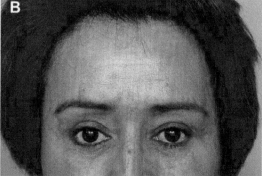

Fig. 20. An example of a patient before (*A*) and after (*B*) upper eyelid blepharoplasty. This patient underwent concomitant endoscopic browlift and lower eyelid blepharoplasty.

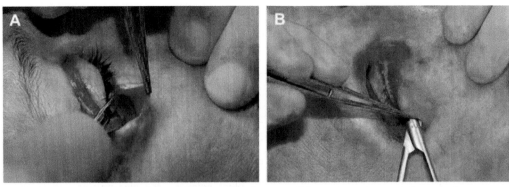

Fig. 21. (A) The incision is situated 2 mm inferior to the lower eyelid margin and extends from the lower punctum medially to a position 6 mm lateral to the lateral canthus. Following the skin incision, fine curved scissors are used to dissect through the orbicularis muscle at the lateral aspect of the incision, thus exposing the orbital septum. (B) Outwardly beveled blunt scissors are introduced posterior to the muscle at the lateral aspect of the incision and, with spreading motions of the blunt scissors, the skin-muscle flap is effectively elevated off the orbital septum along an avascular plane to the level of the inferior orbital rim inferiorly and the incision superiorly.

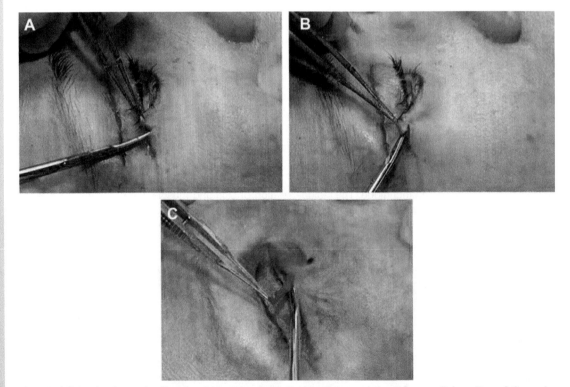

Fig. 22. (A) Maximal stretch effect is achieved by single-finger pressure at the inferomedial portion of the melolabial mound. Then, an inferiorly directed segmental cut is made at the lateral canthus to determine the amount of excess skin and muscle to excise. A tacking suture is placed to maintain the position of the skin-muscle flap. (B) The overlapping skin and muscle are excised. Conservative resection decreases the incidence of postoperative lower eyelid malposition. (C) If orbicularis oculi muscle hypertrophy is evident, an additional 1-2 mm strip of muscle is resected to prevent overlapping of muscle and subsequent ridge formation during closure of the subciliary incision.

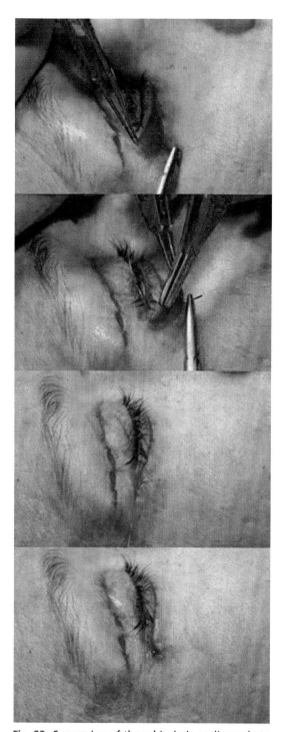

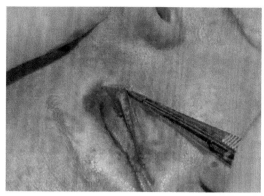

Fig. 24. The subciliary incision is closed with 7-0 blue polypropylene suture at the lateral canthus in a simple interrupted fashion; the remainder of the incision is closed with 6-0 mild chromic suture in a running fashion.

mound creates the same maximal stretch effect. Following this maneuver, an inferiorly directed segmental cut is made at the lateral canthus to determine the amount of excess skin to excise (**Fig. 22**A). A tacking suture is placed to maintain the position of the skin-muscle flap; eyelid scissors are then used to excise the overlapping skin (**Fig. 22**B). If orbicularis oculi muscle hypertrophy is evident, a 1- to 2-mm strip of muscle is resected to prevent overlapping of the muscle and ridge formation during closure of the subciliary incision (**Fig. 22**C). Conservative resection of skin and muscle decreases the incidence of postoperative lower eyelid malposition. In addition, suspension of the orbicularis oculi muscle to the periosteum

Fig. 23. Suspension of the orbicularis oculi muscle to the periosteum of the lateral orbital rim at the tubercle with 5-0 polyplyconate (Maxon) maintains proper eyelid position.

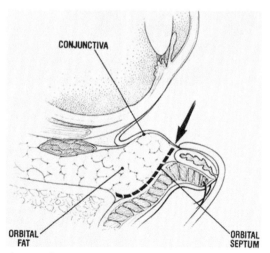

Fig. 25. The preseptal approach to the transconjunctival blepharoplasty relies on an incision located inferior to the tarsus and not deep to the inferior fornix, thus allowing for a more anterior to posterior approach to the fat pockets.

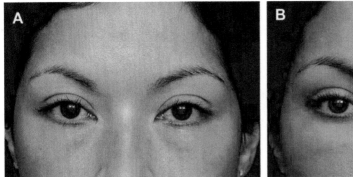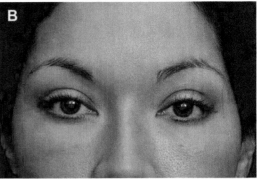

Fig. 26. Lower blepharoplasty via transconjunctival approach: (*A*) preoperatively and (*B*) postoperatively.

of the lateral orbital rim assists in maintaining proper eyelid position (**Fig. 23**). If there is evidence of festoons or malar mounds, an extended lower eyelid blepharoplasty is performed inferior to the infraorbital rim; the redundant orbicularis oculi muscle and/or malar mounds are addressed by advancing the entire skin-muscle flap and suborbicularis oculi fat (SOOF) unit superiolaterally.[18] Following muscle suspension, the subciliary incision is closed (**Fig. 24**) with 7-0 blue polypropylene

suture at the lateral canthus in a simple interrupted fashion; the remainder of the incision is closed with 6-0 mild chromic suture in a running fashion.

Compared with the transconjunctival approach, the transcutaneous method can correct true vertical excess of lower eyelid skin and orbicularis oculi hypertrophy. However, there are specific indications for the transconjunctival approach.[19] For example, young patients with excellent elasticity, presence of hereditary pseudoherniation of

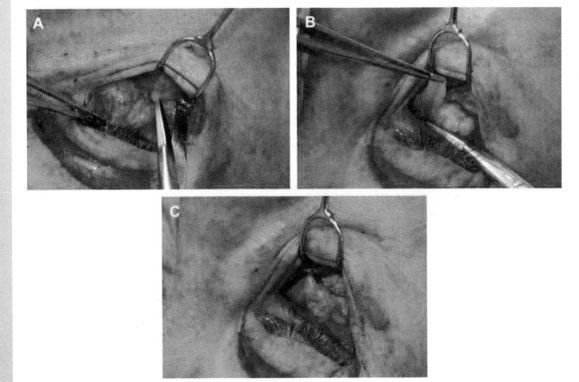

Fig. 27. Fat transposition. A pocket is created posterior to the orbicularis oculi muscle but anterior to the periosteum (*A*). The medial fat pocket is released from the surrounding orbital septum (*B*) and subsequently sutured over the infraorbital rim into the previously made pocket with 6-0 polyglycolic acid (Dexon) (*C*).

orbital fat, and no evidence of skin excess are ideally suited for the transconjunctival approach. In addition, patients with Fitzpatrick skin types V–VI may benefit from the transconjunctival approach, as the transcutaneous lower eyelid blepharoplasty scar may depigment in these patients. The transconjunctival approach results in transection and release of the inferior retractor muscles, thus allowing for a temporary rise in the lower eyelid position. This fact makes the transconjunctival approach an ideal procedure for secondary lower eyelid blepharoplasty.[20] During transconjunctival blepharoplasty, a preseptal approach is maintained via an incision located inferior to the tarsus and not deep in the inferior fornix, which allows for a more anterior to posterior access to the fat pockets (**Figs. 25** and **26**).[21]

Transposition of pedicled orbital fat over the orbital rim is an excellent adjunct to lower eyelid blepharoplasty for patients with a tear trough deformity.[22] Fat transposition is performed with lower eyelid blepharoplasty extending below the infraorbital rim. Once the orbital fat from the medial pocket is isolated from the orbital septum, it is transposed over the orbital rim and positioned into a pocket posterior to the orbicularis oculi muscle and anterior to the periosteum to efface the tear trough deformity. The transposed orbital fat is then secured to the periosteum using interrupted 6-0 polyglycolic acid (Dexon) sutures (**Fig. 27**). The contour of the orbital fat is then softened using bipolar electrocautery. The lower eyelid blepharoplasty is then completed as previously described.

SUMMARY

The non-Caucasian face has many unique attributes, including skin tone, texture, elasticity, skin thickness, and subcutaneous fat content. These differences may place the patient at increased risk for scarring and pigmentation issues. There are various nonsurgical and surgical procedures for rejuvenation of the non-Caucasian face. The selection of the proper treatment must be coupled with a thorough understanding of the age-related changes that occur in the non-Caucasian face to meet and hopefully exceed the patient's expectations.

REFERENCES

1. Westmore M. Facial cosmetics in conjunction with surgery. Paper presented at the Aesthetic Plastic Surgical Society Meeting. Vancouver, British Columbia (Canada) May 7, 1974.

2. Schreiber JE, Singh NK, Klatsky SA. Beauty lies in the "eyebrow" of the beholder: a public survey of eyebrow aesthetics. Aesthet Surg J 2005;25:348–52.

3. Biller JA, Kim DW. A contemporary assessment of facial aesthetic preferences. Arch Facial Plast Surg 2009;11(2):91–7.

4. Freund RM, Nolan WB III. Correlation between brow lift outcomes and aesthetic ideals for eyebrow height and shape in females. Plast Reconstr Surg 1996;97:1343–8.

5. Gunter JP, Antrobus SD. Aesthetic analysis of the eyebrows. Plast Reconstr Surg 1997;99:1808–16.

6. Seiff SR, Seiff BD. Anathomy of the Asian eyelid. Facial Plast Surg Clin North Am 2007;15:309–14.

7. Moses JL. Blepharoplasty: cosmetic and functional. In: McCord CD, Tantenbaum M, Nunery W, editors. Oculoplastic surgery. 3rd edition. New York: Raven Press; 1995. p. 285–318.

8. Friedman O. Changes associated with the aging face. Facial Plast Surg Clin North Am 2005;13:371–80.

9. Rankin BS, Arden RC, Crumley AL. Lower eyelid blepharoplasty. In: Papel ID, editor. Facial plastic and reconstructive surgery. 2nd edition. New York: Thieme; 2002. p. 196–207.

10. Bernardi C, Dura S, Amata PL. Treatment of orbicularis oculi muscle hypertrophy in lower lid blepharoplasty. Aesthetic Plast Surg 1998;5:349–51.

11. Loeb R. Fat pad sliding and fat grafting for leveling lid depressions. Clin Plast Surg 1981;8:757–76.

12. Lambros V. Volumizing the brow with hyaluronic acid fillers. Aesthet Surg J 2009;29(3):174–9.

13. Perkins SW, Batniji RK. Trichophytic endoscopic forehead-lifting in high hairline patients. Facial Plast Surg Clin North Am 2006;14:185–93.

14. Lam SM. Aesthetic strategies for the aging Asian face. Facial Plast Surg Clin North Am 2007;15(3):283–91.

15. Park JI, Park MS. Park Z-epicanthoplasty. Facial Plast Surg Clin North Am 2007;15(3):343–52.

16. Kane MA. Treatment of tear trough deformity and lower lid bowing with injectable hayaluronic acid. Aesthetic Plast Surg 2005;29(5):363–7.

17. Flowers RS. Tear trough implants for correction of tear trough deformity. Clin Plast Surg 1993;20:403–15.

18. Becker FF, Deutsch BD. Extended lower lid blepharoplasty. Facial Plast Surg Clin North Am 1995;3: 189–94.

19. Perkins SW. Transconjunctival lower lid blepharoplasty. Facial Plast Surg Clin North Am 1995;3:175–87.

20. Fedok FG, Perkins SW. Transconjunctival blepharoplasty. Facial Plast Surg 1996;12:185–95.

21. Perkins SW, Dyer WK, Simo F. Transconjunctival approach to lower eyelid blepharoplasty: experience, indications, and techniques in 300 patients. Arch Otolaryngol 1994;120:172–7.

22. Goldberg RA. Transconjunctival orbital fat repositioning: transposition of orbital fat pedicles into a subperiosteal pocket. Plast Reconstr Surg 2000; 105:743–8.

Hair Restoration in the Ethnic Patient and Review of Hair Transplant Fundamentals

Samuel M. Lam, MD[a],*, Emina Karamanovski, MD[b]

KEYWORDS

• Hair transplant • Hair restoration
• Ethnic hair restoration • Hair loss

Superior hair restoration requires the application of universal principles along with variations that apply to specific ethnic populations. This article serves as a primer on basic tenets of hair restoration, with additional attention given to the uniqueness and differences in technique and design that are warranted for a wide range of races and ethnicities. Because hair restoration is a complex subject that mandates sophisticated understanding pertaining to the process of hair loss and how to restore lost hair, this article is not intended to provide a broadly encompassing knowledge to enable full engagement in a safe, clinical practice dedicated to hair transplant surgery. However, this article gives prospective surgeons an insight on how to undertake further study and shore up their deficiencies so as to refine knowledge gaps and ensure patient safety and excellent surgical outcomes.

Although this article is geared toward surgeons, like with any surgery, one must first understand when not to operate before one can claim the right to operate on an individual. In short, this brief introduction rapidly outlines cogent limitations that any surgeon must appreciate and understand before starting a practice in hair restoration surgery.

First, hair loss is a progressive disease that involves an expanding region of baldness with dwindling usable hair to transplant into this bald region. (The principle of modern hair restoration is predicated on Norman Orentreich's seminal work in the 1950s that showed that hair grafts transplanted from a region genetically programmed not to be lost, that is, the back and sides of the head, will not be lost even when transplanted into a region that is genetically programmed for hair loss.) One of the greatest fears for transplant surgeons is that they will run out of usable hair to complete the process of hair restoration. This is particularly pertinent in the case of a younger patient with rapidly progressive hair loss, mainly a male patient in his 20s who reveals a pattern that is most likely to become an advanced Norwood class VI or VII. It is the ethical responsibility of every surgeon to understand that hair transplantation in a young male patient is fraught with risks that should be emphasized to the patient, for example, the depletion of donor hair, leaving the surgery unfinished or unnatural results, need for multiple sessions during the patient's lifetime, and the inability to completely shave the head because the donor scar will be revealed. Considering the complexity of the requirements for safe hair restoration in a young patient, the authors advise that the novice surgeon primarily considers medical management as a treatment of choice for young patients.

[a] Willow Bend Wellness Center, Lam Facial Plastic Surgery Center and Hair Restoration Institute, 6101 Chapel Hill Boulevard, Suite 101, Plano, TX 75093, USA
[b] Lam Institute for Hair Restoration, 6101 Chapel Hill Boulevard, Suite 101, Plano, TX 75093, USA
* Corresponding author.
E-mail address: drlam@lamfacialplastics.com (S.M. Lam).

Facial Plast Surg Clin N Am 18 (2010) 35–42
doi:10.1016/j.fsc.2009.11.016

MEDICAL MANAGEMENT OF HAIR LOSS

With pitfalls in mind, one must understand the indication for medical treatment for any male patient who is suffering from hair loss. Because hair loss is a progressive disease, medical treatment is required even for the individual who is contemplating hair restoration surgery; it consists of Food and Drug Administration–approved medications, such as minoxidil (Rogaine) and finasteride (Propecia). These medications slow the progression of hair loss. Their major limitation, other than ongoing cost, is that once they are stopped, the patient's hair loss will revert to the starting pattern, that is, everything he gained during the period he was on the medications is lost.

Although the authors have no options currently besides surgery to restore hair, the results obtained from the use of medications are still significant. Further, medical treatment is most effective in the younger patient with early signs of miniaturization (to be discussed), less effective in patients with more advanced settings of hair loss, and almost completely ineffective in patients who demonstrate "slick baldness" (ie, not even a wispy hair remains). However, medical management offers the ability to restore miniaturized (or vellus) hairs back into thicker, terminal hairs and to slow down the progression of hair loss. Accordingly, even in patients who are contemplating hair restoration, medical management can serve as a potent adjunct to limit further loss and thereby maintain the transplant result to maximal effect, that is, add to the transplanted hairs by maintaining the surrounding original hair.

The nature of male pattern baldness has been discussed in this section. Most men do not advance from thick, terminal hairs to complete baldness. Instead, thick, terminal hairs are slowly converted over time to wispy, vellus hairs (baby hairs) that in turn are shed and lost. Medical management works to reconvert a portion of this type of hair back toward thicker, terminal hairs. Once the hairs are completely gone, they do not grow back. That is why early implementation of medical management is important for anyone who is beginning to lose hair.

Finasteride is an inhibitor of dihydrotestosterone (DHT), which locally causes follicles to miniaturize and shed. Finasteride is an oral medication taken at a dosage of 1 mg/d to retard further hair loss. It is processed through the liver and reduces one's prostate specific antigen by roughly 50%; anyone taking finasteride should alert his or her primary care physician to this fact. It has a very low incidence of sexual side effects, which are reversible on cessation. Finasteride is contraindicated in premenopausal women for risk of birth defects in the male fetus; a woman of childbearing age should not ingest it or handle any crushed pills. Finasteride has shown equivocal benefit in postmenopausal women. It generally takes about 6 to 12 months to start seeing appreciable changes after the start of finasteride.

Minoxidil is a topical medication to be applied to the scalp (not hair) twice a day. Its mechanism of action is unclear, but it is known to convert hairs from the telogen phase into active anagen phase. Accordingly, at times, some hair shedding occurs early in the first few weeks after starting the application as hairs move from telogen to anagen, which should be explained to the patient. Results can be seen earlier in the first few months after the start of minoxidil than with finasteride. The major limitation of minoxidil is contact dermatitis, which can be virtually eliminated in patients who use the brand named Rogaine Foam, which removes the propylene glycol irritant.

FEMALE HAIR LOSS CONSIDERATIONS

More than 30% of women older than 30 years also lose hair even before the onset of menopause.[1] Women can lose hair in a male pattern, diffusely across the hair or in a Christmas tree pattern in which the apex of the "tree" falls along the vertex and the base along the frontal hairline, as described by Olsen.[2] The major problem with hair restoration in women is the need to first understand the underlying process that could account for the hair loss, because although hair loss is predominantly genetic in men, it is not so for women. Besides a small number of females in whom hair loss is genetic, the other reasons for hair loss are usually divided into 2 types: dermatologic and hormonal. Dermatologic evaluation by a dermatologist would be indicated in a woman who exhibits any unusual skin disease that could account for the problem at hand. Basic hormonal workup is indicated in almost every woman to rule out treatable, reversible hormonal diseases, such as hypothyroidism, iron deficiency anemia, autoimmune disorders, and other hormonal imbalances. If no other underlying process is causing hair loss, the first choice of treatment for female hair restoration is 2% minoxidil. The application is topical, the indication is twice a day, and the patient should be alerted to possible initial hair shedding. If the patient is considering hair transplantation, it is highly suggested that she use minoxidil for at least 4 to 6 months before undergoing surgery.

DERMATOLOGIC CONTRAINDICATIONS TO SURGERY FOR HAIR LOSS

This section discusses the broad classification of hair loss diseases that are contraindications for surgery, such as scarring alopecias (eg, discoid lupus, central centrifugal alopecia, traction alopecia), nonscarring alopecias (alopecia areata), and psychological conditions (eg, trichotillomania), and how to recognize these conditions.[3] The surgeon who wants to enter the field of hair restoration surgery and who does not have an in-depth dermatologic background must undergo careful study of these diseases so as to avoid surgery in those patients who are not safe candidates. In addition, surgeons can use their dermatologic colleague and internist more effectively when they encounter a situation that would suggest a contraindication to surgery.

TECHNIQUES IN HAIR TRANSPLANT SURGERY

After understanding the medical side of hair loss, the surgeon should now exercise artistic and technically precise hair restoration techniques. Unlike other types of esthetic surgeries, excellent hair restoration is completely dependent on an excellent surgical team. Likened to building a car, the entire team is important for the success of the outcome. The surgeon's role typically involves deciding on the proper surgical candidate, preparing the donor area for harvesting, designing the hairline, harvesting and closing the donor area, and creating the recipient sites for the eventual hair grafts. The surgical team must perform excellent hair-graft dissection and hair-graft placement. Without these 2 very important components, the hair transplant result can look unnatural or show poor growth. This short section principally focuses on the surgeon's role during hair restoration and briefly touches on the technique of graft dissection and placement. In addition, a focus on the differences in technique as directed toward ethnic populations would be an important consideration, given the emphasis of this presentation.

Hairline Design

The hairline height and shape exhibits the surgeon's artistry and technical knowledge of hair restoration at its zenith. Hairline design is also one of the most important differentiators among various ethnicities, which will be explored in depth after a basic understanding of good hairline design that is more universal in scope is outlined.

The hairline resides at the junction between the horizontal and the vertical plane of the scalp, more specifically at the 45° intersection between these 2 planes. This intersection is the lowest acceptable starting point (central point) for any hairline (but can be scaled upward based on age and degree of existing or projected hair loss) because any hair transplanted below this point corresponds with forehead scalp, which should remain bare. The lateral extent of the anterior hairline falls along an imaginary line drawn through the lateral canthus (lateral points). Hair that resides lateral to this point signifies temporal hair, which also finishes the facial frame and can be as important as the anterior, horizontal hairline in establishing a youthful and balanced result. Once the central point and the 2 lateral points have been fashioned, the points are joined by creating a suppressed saucer-shape design where the central region extending from the central point to the midpupil is flat, from the midpupil toward the lateral canthus is forward convex in design, and the lateral extent beyond lateral canthus point slightly concave to meet the temporal hairline. The degree of suppression and the roundness of the design are based on multiple factors. The younger patient who does not have significant hair loss may tolerate a slightly less-suppressed frontotemporal recession, whereas an individual with more advanced loss would benefit from a more recessed frontotemporal design.

The hairline variations described here pertain to the male hairline; as mentioned earlier, female hair restoration has authentic characteristics and thus lies beyond the scope of this discussion.

Caucasian males tend to exhibit frontotemporal recession. Even in younger patients, the shape of hairline should have some degree of frontotemporal recession designed to accommodate further aging and associated hair loss so that the hair design remains natural over time. It is recommended to design a conservatively high midpoint and receded frontotemporal angles to ensure adequate supply of donor hair needed to cover the increasing demand versus supply ratio occurring in further hair loss progression. With that in mind, the conservatively positioned hairline can be safely lowered in subsequent procedures, but it is very difficult to raise it after establishing a lowered, surgically created one. The reverse temptation is also true for many starting surgeons, that is, to start a hairline so far back that there is no beneficial frame to the face, and thereby the esthetic contribution of hair to the face is lost. Therefore, designing a hairline that is not too high or not too low is a work of art and requires good esthetic judgment.

At the opposite extreme of the hairline for the Caucasian male, an African male exhibits a hairline that is almost straight or straight across forehead with no visible frontotemporal recession (ie, almost a right angle at the frontotemporal junction). A greater degree of recession at this angle is indicated in the advanced balding African male who has limited donor hair but not as limited as his Caucasian counterpart. Because a pronounced frontotemporal recession does not look natural and because shaved hairstyles offer a socially acceptable alternative for the African male (and for other races also), surgical hair restoration may not be a suitable option for a young patient with rapid hair loss. Donor-strip harvesting that creates a visible scar in the closely cropped head must be discussed in advance with a prospective patient, especially with one who may have limited donor hair, ongoing hair loss, and the need to replace an ever-widening field of alopecia, because the strip harvesting may prevent the option of a shaved hairstyle.

Asians tend to have rounder and wider heads, and their hairlines similarly should match this design with a wider arcing central convexity and less-pronounced frontotemporal recessions (with the judgment based on the degree of hair loss and head shape) (**Fig. 1**). The shape of Asian hairline is "flat-convex" in comparison with the Caucasian "round-convex" hairline.

Hispanics can exhibit a full range of hairline shapes depending from where their ultimate racial mix is derived. The term "mestizo" broadly defines how Hispanics in the Western hemisphere can represent an amalgam of white colonial ancestors, indigenous Indian (Native American) populations, and African slave trade heritages. These crossed lineages guide a surgeon to adjust the appropriately modified hairline based on these ancestral constraints.

Although Caucasian and Asian hairlines are positioned to provide a higher frame to the face, a Hispanic hairline can be medium high, and the African hairline takes the lowest-positioned frame. Finally, hairline should be based on Norwood hair loss patterns because hairline and hair loss patterns that fall outside of the Norwood patterns can be unnatural in appearance. Learning these Norwood patterns will help the reader to understand how hair is progressively lost so that it can be proportionately restored.

Donor Harvesting

After hairline design, the next order of business is to harvest the needed donor hair for transplantation. Preparing the area of "safe" donor hair for harvesting requires knowledge of where hair would not be lost over time despite the most advanced stages of male pattern hair loss. This U-shaped fringe can start about 2 cm above the superior helix at its lateral extent and arc backward toward the central occiput in the region of the bony occipital protuberance. Care should be taken to evaluate "retrograde" hair loss from the nape of the neck upward and vertex hair loss that dips downward into usable hair reserves.

Once the region to be harvested has been determined, the hair is shaved flush to the scalp and the hair above taped to restrict interference during harvesting. After the patient is adequately sedated with light intravenous sedation or an oral medication concoction, a ring block consisting of 1% lidocaine with 1:100,000 epinephrine is infiltrated below the planned donor harvest site and around to the forehead below the planned hairline using on average a total of 20 mL for the entire circumference. The next most important task is to infiltrate significant tumescence consisting of 0.01%

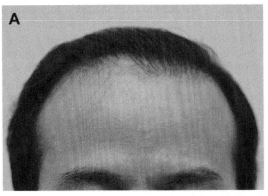 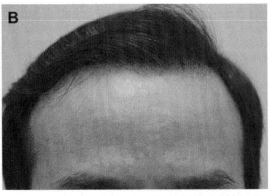

Fig. 1. (*A, B*) An Asian patient who underwent hair restoration to his frontotemporal region in a rounder configuration that matches the shape of most Asian hairline patterns. The angulation of the recipient sites must be exceptionally low to camouflage the appearance of "graftiness" in Asian hair shafts that tend to be thick, round, and straight in nature.

lidocaine with 1:500,000 epinephrine into the subcutaneous plane of the donor area so that the deeper nerve and blood supply are properly protected and the hairs are rigidly in parallel alignment so as to minimize hair transection, that is, damaging hair structure by cutting it inadvertently with blade. On average, the authors use approximately 100 to 200 cm^3 of donor-site tumescence before embarking on the harvest. A multiblade handle outfitted with three No. 10 blades is used to create 2 parallel strips for removal approximately 4.5 to 5.0 mm in width for a total donor-strip width that does not exceed 1 cm. Care is taken to perform the harvest slowly and deliberately, constantly adjusting the insertion angle of the blades so that transection is minimized and the depth of the blades just pass the follicular base staying well above the galea. The lateral extents of the donor strip are tapered to a point so as to facilitate strip removal and subsequent wound closure. The strips are removed and placed into a chilled, saline bath in preparation for graft dissection. Before wound suturing, a trichophytic closure technique is performed by trimming off 1 mm of the bottom skin edge with serrated microscissors (in the patient without excessive wound tension) so as to permit hairs to grow through the scar and thereby minimize scar visibility over time.[4] The unspoken rule in hair restoration is to remove previous scar in any subsequent procedure. Therefore, the authors tend to avoid a trichophytic closure in a patient who is expected to come back in a year or two for additional hair restoration for 2 reasons: first, because the wound closure tension is slightly increased with a trichophytic closure; second, hair that grows in the vicinity of the scar may have a distorted direction and thereby diminish yield. The wound is then closed with a 3-0 nylon suture in a running, nonlocking fashion so that the suture passes only through the midfollicular depth. Deeper bites tend to ensnare the follicles and cause follicular entrapment. Sutures are removed 10 days after transplant surgery. The authors prefer to perform the donor harvest with the patient sitting upright in a chair that can swivel down the headrest for optimal occipital accessibility. After suturing and before recipient site creation, 20 mL of 0.25% bupivacaine with 1:100,000 epinephrine is infiltrated as a ring block circumferentially around the head where lidocaine was injected at the outset so as to prolong the anesthesia for the operative case and thereafter.

Although donor harvesting progresses almost identically for all ethnicities, an important consideration in the African population is the risk of hair transection, given the curlier nature of the hair shaft. Accordingly, the authors often perform either 2-blade harvesting (rather than 3-blade) or a free-hand single-blade harvesting so as to limit the potential risk of hair transection (**Fig. 2**).

Recipient Site Creation

The patient is placed in the supine position for recipient site creation. The surgeon at this point collaborates with the team to determine how many grafts are to be obtained during graft dissection, for example, how many single follicular unit grafts (FUGs) containing 1, 2, 3, and 4 hairs and how many double follicular unit grafts (DFUGs) containing 4 to 8 hairs. Grafts that contain multiple follicular units are an advanced topic of consideration, because improperly angled and spaced grafts and those that are poorly camouflaged by inadequate rows of FUGs, along with a poorly chosen patient, can lead to an artificial looking

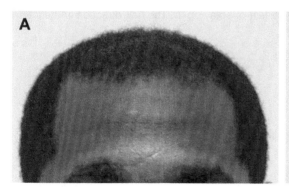 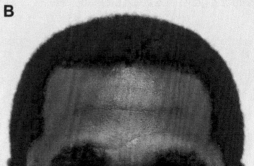

Fig. 2. (*A, B*) African American hair restoration requires more care with donor harvesting and graft dissection to minimize transection of the curlier hair shaft. The curlier nature of the hair shaft provides superior hair density in the transplanted region, requiring fewer grafts to attain the same esthetic result in an individual with finer, straighter hair. Of note, the patient underwent a previous hair transplant elsewhere and did not gain the desired degree of density.

result. However, DFUGs can greatly decrease graft dissection time and achieve, in the right patient, increased visual hair density much more readily than that a total FUG transplant can accomplish (a bias that the authors carry) (**Fig. 3**).

In general, the author (SML) starts by creating recipient sites in the posterior limit of the hairline zone, that is, approximately 3 to 4 cm behind the anterior hairline, for several reasons. If multiunit grafts (MUGs) are used, it is far easier to interdigitate smaller FUG sites among existing MUG sites than the other way around (**Fig. 4**). Starting with the anterior-most extent of the hairline and moving backward can create a result that is too linear, which is unnatural. The author prefers to first build up the central density/posterior hairline limit by creating few rows of stronger 3 to 4 hair grafts and then going posteriorly toward the vertex until the central midscalp is properly filled. Smaller 2-hair FUGs are then interdigitated forward to cover the anterior portion of the hairline. Between 5 and 10 rows of 2-hair grafts are created (depending on the numbers obtained by graft dissection and the planned hairline design), making certain that the hairline seems to be a finely tuned irregular line but not so jagged in a macro fashion that it looks like a sawtooth pattern. The small irregular undulations of the hairline should not exceed 1 to 3 mm in depth and should not follow any visible pattern. The finishing touch involves placing 1 to 2 rows of 1-hair grafts with a few, free-floating "sentinel" hairs that reside anterior to the hairline to complete the blurring effect on the hairline, because a hairline should appear like a line from a distance but not as a line under close inspection.

Recipient site creation also greatly expresses the artistry and care of the surgeon, as the surgeon literally creates the pattern, density, distribution, angle, and direction of these sites that will guide the transplant team of assistants to place the matching grafts into these premade sites.

Hair angle

To understand how to create recipient sites, the surgeon should laboriously study natural hair angles, which may be easier to observe in a non-balding gentleman who has closely cropped hair. By such observation, hair angles can be matched so that results are of optimal density, distribution, and naturalness.

With the patient in a supine position, the surgeon's hand is in a more natural position during the site creation, which, in return, matches very low and anterior hair angles. The exit angle of the transplanted hair vis-à-vis the scalp determines the natural appearance of the result. The low angle creates a shadow effect on the transplanted hair on the scalp, which thereby creates visual appearance of hair density and limits the appearance of baldness. When the visibility of the exit angle is greatly reduced, the transplanted result can look much more natural. The most important area to keep a very low angle (in almost any race) is the anterior hairline and the first few centimeters that fall immediately behind that hairline as well as the central forelock. It is preferable that the starting surgeon maintains low hair angles all the way to the midscalp to minimize a "grafty" appearance that can develop with angles that are too high.

Hair direction

Besides hair angles, the hair direction is also very important to consider when creating recipient sites. The hair direction involves the radial orientation of the recipient site vis-à-vis the midline. In general, 95% of the hairline and central midscalp density should be oriented straight forward rather than like radial spokes of a wheel (see **Fig. 4**). Creating perfectly forward-angled recipient sites helps to facilitate easy combing, mimics natural hair direction, and more importantly, optimizes visual hair density because the hairs do not book-leaf or splay open. The hair direction in the lateral

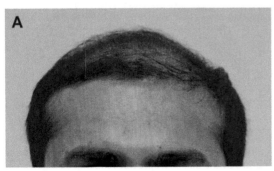
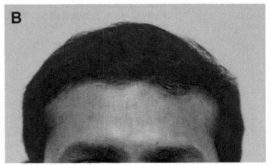

Fig. 3. (*A, B*) An Indian patient who underwent principally multiple follicular unit grafting to achieve remarkable visual density in a single session of hair restoration. FUGs were placed along the perimeter to soften the hairline and transition to the crown region.

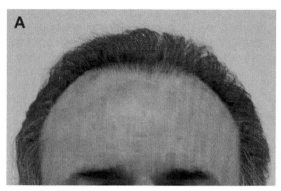
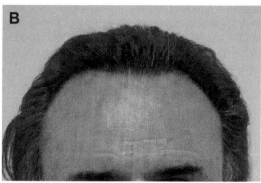

Fig. 4. (*A, B*) Sagittally created recipient sites in a Middle Eastern patient with the first 6 to 7 rows of FUGs tightly interlocked with the larger DFUG sites behind them that in turn compose the central midscalp region. Of note, the patient underwent a previous hair transplant elsewhere and did not gain the desired degree of density. The patient also originally had an unnatural hairline design in which the angles were placed too perpendicularly with respect to the scalp.

hump (upper central temple), anterior temporal angle, lateral crease, vertex transition point, and vertex/crown all follow predictable patterns defined by nature. The hair angles and directions change in these areas, and the explanation of their subtleties lies beyond the scope of this article; the surgeon is encouraged to understand how hair grows differently in each of these regions before deciding to embark on a career in hair restoration surgery.

Hair pattern

The hair pattern is defined by the arrangement of recipient sites vis-à-vis one another. All recipient sites should be created in a tightly interlocking fashion so that each row is staggered from the row in the front and behind it; doing so permits several benefits. Firstly, the grafts can be more tightly arranged. Secondly, the grafts will not compete for surrounding space as much, that is, when the graft is inserted into the site, the surrounding native tissue expands and hence has less of a chance of pushing out the neighboring graft. Thirdly, and most importantly, the staggered orientation permits irregular naturalness and maximal visual density because the viewer will have difficulty identifying rows of hair and have a much harder time seeing bald scalp through multiple staggered rows of hair. The opposite creates perfect aligned hairs with parallel, see-through spaces between them, producing not only a visible but also an unnatural result.

Graft Dissection and Graft Placement

Graft dissection and placement are usually performed by a surgical team. The correct graft dissection and placement are critical because if donor tissue or hair grafts are damaged during the dissection or placement, the result will be affected. During graft dissection, the donor tissue is slivered, trimmed, and hair groupings divided into individual grafts. The tissue and dissected grafts are kept moist at all times and handled with care because if desiccated hair follicles are destroyed, the growth of transplanted hair is diminished. In case of poor tissue and graft handling, the hair shaft may be transected, resulting in poor growth, or hair shaft may be traumatized, resulting in growth of unnatural kinky hair.

Graft placement is a process during which hair grafts are inserted into premade recipient sites. The proper graft placement requires not only correct graft handling but also critical judgment for graft distribution and the knowledge of hair curl orientation. During the process of insertion, the individual grafts are handled with care, maintaining their moisture and avoiding squeezing hair follicles with forceps or forcibly pushing grafts into sites. All improper actions would result in unnatural to poor hair growth. For example, it is important to know natural hair distribution so that a 2- or 3-hair graft is not placed into a site dedicated for 1-hair graft and vice versa for 2 reasons: first, larger grafts placed in the very front would look unnatural; and second, a large graft placed into a small site would grow compressed and contribute to an unnatural result. In addition, hair curls slightly downward, and the person placing grafts has to keep in mind the importance of matching the hair curl with the natural hair growth pattern; otherwise hair would grow in multiple directions, forming undesirable cowlicks, thus resulting in unnatural looks and dissatisfied patients.

In regard to the ethnic differences relevant to the process of graft dissection and placement, there is no significant difference in the principles of tissue and graft handling or the surgical technique used. Only the dissection of the African donor tissue may require use of a curved blade instead of a straight blade (to match the hair curl), which is made by bending a single-edge prep blade.

SUMMARY

Hair transplant in the ethnic patient follows similar universal guidelines for safe hair transplant surgery, which beginner hair transplant surgeons must fully appreciate and master as a prerequisite in their career. However, differences do exist that are important to understand when approaching the diverse ethnicities that abound. Principally, the surgeon should grasp the nuances in hairline shape that differentiate one race from another and create a hair transplant result that appears natural for that race. Other subtleties regarding donor harvesting, recipient site creation, graft dissection, and graft placement that applied to different ethnicities should also be kept in mind.

REFERENCES

1. Unger W, Shapiro R, editors. Hair transplantation. 4th edition. London (England): Informa Healthcare; 2004.
2. Olsen EA. Disorders of hair growth. 2nd edition. Columbus (OH): McGraw-Hill Professional; 2003.
3. Shapiro J. Hair loss: principles of diagnosis and management of alopecia. London (England): Informa HealthCare; 2001.
4. Frechet P. Minimal scars for scalp surgery. Dermatol Surg 2007;33:45–55.

Supratarsal Crease Creation in the Asian Upper Eyelid

Samuel M. Lam, MD[a],*, Amir M. Karam, MD[b,c]

KEYWORDS

- Supratarsal crease • Eyelid • Blepharoplasty • Asian

What makes blepharoplasty on Asian patients unique is the management of the supratarsal crease. Although the presence of a supratarsal crease is a naturally occurring anatomic finding in the Asian population, many of those who lack this anatomic trait will often seek surgical creation de novo . The desire to have a double eyelid is largely cultural, as this feature is considered attractive.

The primary goal of this procedure is not only to create a supratarsal crease but also to create a crease that is consistent with the natural configuration present in the population. From a surgical point of view, this requires a thorough understanding of the natural crease shape and characteristic and mastery of the unique skills required to create it. Asian upper-eyelid blepharoplasty has a rich and complex history. The first reported case was performed and reported in the late nineteenth century.[1,2] Since then, several innovative surgeons began to describe their techniques and concepts. The era of westernization upper blepharoplasty, which focused on creating a high supratarsal crease consistent with the White norm, has given way to methods that preserve ethnic characteristics. The current strategies can be broadly categorized into suture-based, full-incision, and partial-incision techniques.

The method that is advocated in this article is the full-incision technique. The rationale for this preference can be summarized as follows:

(1) Relative permanence compared with other methods

(2) No need to rely on any buried permanent sutures to hold the fixation
(3) Ease in identifying postseptal tissues through a wider aperture
(4) Ability to modulate excessive skin (dermatochalasis) in the aging eyelid.

The major drawback of the full-incision method is the protracted recovery time, in which the patient can look grossly abnormal for 1 to 2 weeks, and still not entirely natural for months, if not a full year. Scarring has proven to be a nonissue if the delicate tissues near the epicanthus are carefully avoided. In the authors' opinion, the incision line is more difficult to observe with the full-incision than with the partial-incision method because there is no abrupt ending as is apparent with the more limited-incision technique.

OPERATIVE TECHNIQUE
Determination of the Eyelid Crease Position

The first step is designing the proposed eyelid crease. There are several variations ranging from inside fold (the medial incision terminates lateral to the epicanthus) and outside fold (the medial incision extends medial to the epicanthus by 1–2 mm). There are 2 variations to the shape of the incision. The first is an oval shape (slight flare of the crease height laterally above the ciliary margin) versus rounded, in which the line runs parallel to the ciliary margin. Our preference is for the inside fold paired with an oval configuration (**Fig. 1**).

[a] Willow Bend Wellness Center, Lam Facial Plastic Surgery Center & Hair Restoration Institute, 6101 Chapel Hill Boulevard, Suite 101, Plano, TX 75093, USA
[b] Carmel Valley Facial Plastic Surgery, San Diego, CA, USA
[c] University of California, San Diego School of Medicine, 4765 Carmel Mountain Road, Suite 201, San Diego, CA 92130, USA
* Corresponding author.
E-mail address: drlam@lamfacialplastics.com (S.M. Lam).

Facial Plast Surg Clin N Am 18 (2010) 43–47
doi:10.1016/j.fsc.2009.11.004
1064-7406/10/$ – see front matter © 2010 Elsevier Inc. All rights reserved.

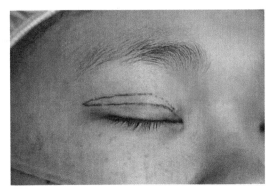

Fig. 1. The surgical marking of the inside fold paired with an oval configuration.

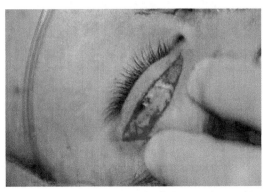

Fig. 2. Incision and removal of the overlying skin. Note that the obicularis muscle is left down at this stage. A no. 15 blade is used to incise the skin down through the orbicularis oculi muscle.

Surgical Marking

The patient should be placed in the supine position and the upper-eyelid skin is held taut to the point that the eyelashes are just beginning to evert. The supratarsal crease should be marked at a distance of 7 mm from the ciliary crease to create a natural, low crease design (which constitutes the naturally occurring shape). The degree of skin excision to be performed should err on the side of conservatism with about 3 mm between the upper and lower limbs.

Anesthesia

Deep sedation should be avoided, as patient cooperation is vital to ensure symmetry toward the end of the procedure. A mixture of 0.5 mL of 1% lidocaine with 1:100,000 epinephrine and 0.5 mL of 0.25% bupivicaine with 1:100,000 epinephrine attached to a 30-gauge needle is used to infiltrate the upper-eyelid skin by raising 2 to 3 subcutaneous wheals, which are then manually distributed by pinching the skin along the entire length of the incision. This method avoids threading the needle and limits the chance of a hematoma that can lead to difficulty in gauging symmetry during the procedure. A total of only 1 mL of the local anesthesia mixture described earlier is infiltrated along each proposed incision to maintain symmetry.

Surgical Exposure

A no.15 blade is used to incise the skin down through the orbicularis oculi muscle, taking care not to pass the blade much further than that initial depth (Fig. 2). Bipolar cautery is used to coagulate the vascular arcades that run perpendicularly across the incision line to limit unnecessary bleeding and thereby mitigate swelling and distortion during this delicate procedure. The depth of

the incision can be further deepened with the no.15 blade down toward the orbital septum before removing the skin island with curved iris scissors. Additional cautery is used as needed. At this point, the same procedure is performed on the contralateral side and is continued in this alternating fashion to ensure symmetry.

The same iris scissors are then used to excise an additional 1 to 2 mm strip of tissue along the inferior edge of the wound to remove any remaining orbicularis oculi fibers and some initial fibers of the underlying orbital septum (Fig. 3).

With the assistant gently balloting the eyeball above and below the incision line to help herniate the postseptal adipose, the surgeon makes a small fenestration along the lateral extent of the wound edge just at the point where the strip of orbicularis was previously removed. With the countertraction and balloting of the eyeball mentioned earlier, the surgeon continues to excise thin films of tissue until the yellow postseptal adipose tissue is encountered (Fig. 4). The reason for the small fenestration and the constant attention by the assistant to ballot around the incision to push the

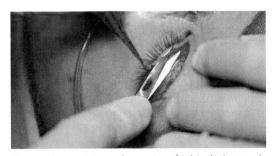

Fig. 3. The excision of a strip of obicularis muscle along the inferior edge of the incision. This excision will expose the underlying septum.

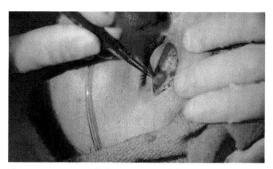

Fig. 4. Exposure of the postseptal fat.

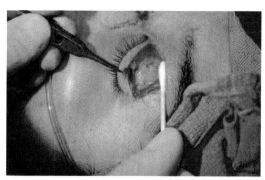

Fig. 6. The postseptal fat is swept away and the levator aponeurosis is fully exposed.

fat through the defect is that identifying the postseptal fat is the safety landmark for avoiding injury to the deeper levator aponeurosis.

Once the fat is identified, a fine-toothed curved mosquito clamp is inserted into the fenestration and gently spread medially to lift the remaining orbital septum away from the deeper fat pad and levator aponeurosis. Repeated entry and exit of the tines through the defect can help ensure that the correct tissue plane of dissection is maintained. With the tines open and the orbital septum tented upward, a bipolar cautery with iris scissors can be used to open the remaining orbital septum to expose fully the deeper postseptal adipose and underlying levator aponeurosis (**Fig. 5**).

A cotton-tipped applicator is used to sweep the preaponeurotic (postseptal) fat pad away from the glistening white levator (**Fig. 6**). At times, a thin posterior leaf of the orbital septum can be seen between the levator and the fat pad. Gentle dissection (using a fine-toothed mosquito clamp followed by scissors) of this thin orbital septum away from the fat pad can be undertaken to reveal the levator more fully. The same technique is undertaken on the contralateral side to this point.

Levator-to-Skin Fixation Sutures

Many surgeons believe that excessive adipose tissue must be removed to attain a more open

eyelid configuration. It is our position that in more than 80% of cases a simple levator-to-skin fixation is all that is necessary to attain the desired eyelid shape configuration and perceived opening of the palpebral aperture. Accordingly, preaponeurotic fat is rarely removed. At this point, the first levator-to-skin fixation suture can be placed.

With the 5-0 nylon loaded backhanded on the needle driver, the patient is asked to open his/her eyes to determine the position of the midpupil on forward gaze so as to place the suture through the upper skin edge at the midpupil. The suture bite is through the entire epidermis and dermis, as this suture will be removed 7 days postoperatively.

With the 5-0 nylon now loaded normally in a forehand fashion, a horizontal bite is placed through the levator at the approximate lower edge of the exposed levator, again aligned at the midpupil (**Fig. 7**). Next, with the 5-0 nylon loaded in a backhand fashion, the final throw of the needle is placed through the lower skin edge, again aligned with the midpupil. The patient is then asked to open his/her eyes after 1 suture knot to determine proper eyelash position (**Fig. 8**). The eyelashes should be slightly everted, and that should be the desired end point. The crease height will seem

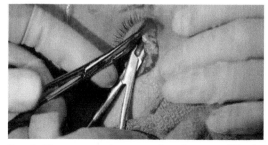

Fig. 5. The use of the mosquito clamp to lift the septum up to protect the underlying levator aponeurosis. An iris scissor is used to divide the septum along the entire length of the incision.

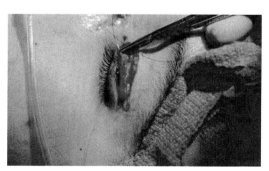

Fig. 7. The positioning of the 5-0 nylon suture used to create the new crease.

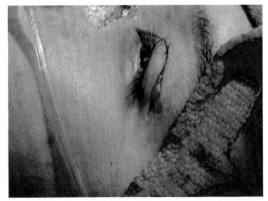

Fig. 8. Once each of the sutures is placed, patients are asked to open their eyes to assess positioning and symmetry.

grossly too high and should not be used as the desired end point. If the eyelash position is deemed appropriate, the remaining 4 square knots are thrown to anchor the suture knot. The same technique is undertaken on the contralateral side, and symmetry of the creases is noted and can be adjusted if necessary. A higher crease is created by placing the horizontal bite through the levator more superiorly, and lowered by placing the suture more inferiorly, along the levator.

With the initial fixation suture placed bilaterally and symmetry observed, the 4 remaining fixation sutures per side can be placed in the same fashion. The second fixation suture is aligned with the medial limbus and the third fixation suture positioned halfway between the lateral limbus and the lateral canthus. Two additional fixation sutures are used between these points to fine-tune any perceived asymmetry. A total of 5 fixation sutures are placed per side. The skin is then approximated with a running, nonlocking 7-0 nylon suture. **Fig. 9** illustrates a patient following the this procedure before and 18 months after the procedure.

POSTOPERATIVE CARE

Postoperative care is straightforward, consisting of icing the eyelid areas for the first 48 to 72 hours and cleansing the incision line twice daily with hydrogen peroxide and dressing it with bacitracin ointment for the first postoperative week. The patient returns on the seventh postoperative day for the removal of all 5 fixation sutures per side (5-0 nylon) and the running skin closure (7-0 nylon). At times the patient may complain of difficulty opening his/her eyes due to excessive edema or temporary levator dysfunction, which disappears over the first several days but can linger even up

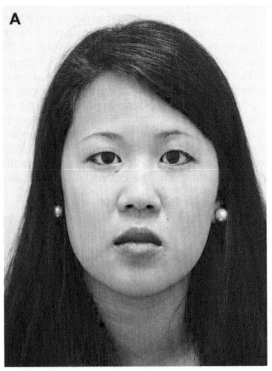
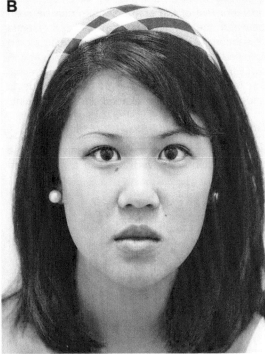

Fig. 9. Before (*A*) and after (*B*) comparison of a 24-year-old Chinese woman 1.5 years after a full-incision double-eyelid procedure.

to 3 to 6 weeks following the procedure. The patient is reassured that it often takes 1 full year to achieve a natural crease configuration owing to persistent pretarsal edema that can linger for many months. Narrow rectangular-shaped eyeglasses can camouflage some of the exorbitant edema in the immediate postoperative period; and, for female patients, mascara can be used to help hide the abnormal height of the crease during the initial few months following the surgery.

SUMMARY

Supratarsal crease fixation in the Asian patient can provide a more open-eyed, awake look without compromising their ethnic appearance. A conservative supratarsal crease height and conservative to no removal of postseptal fat help to ensure this natural-appearing result. With the full-incision method, the senior author (SML) has been able to achieve consistently excellent results with durable crease fixation despite a prolonged recovery time. The supratarsal crease fixation provides an excellent method for the younger patient seeking cosmetic eyelid enhancement. However, for the aging Asian patient, the complexity of the strategy is greater; for details regarding this approach the reader is referred to the senior author's accompanying article in this publication entitled *A New Paradigm for the Aging Face*.

REFERENCES

1. Lam SM. Mikamo's double-eyelid blepharoplasty & the westernization of Japan. Arch Facial Plast Surg 2002;4:201–2.
2. McCurdy JA Jr, Lam SM. Cosmetic surgery of the Asian face. 2nd edition. New York: Thieme Medical Publishers; 2005.

Midface Alloplastic Augmentation in the Asian and Latino Patient

A. Joshua Zimm, MD[a,b],
William J. Binder, MD[c,d,e],*

KEYWORDS

- Midface augmentation • Alloplastic augmentation
- Asian facial cosmetic surgery
- Latino facial cosmetic surgery

In recent years, the population of the United States has become more diverse as there is an ever expanding influx of various ethnic groups and races that comprise the general population. According to the US Census Bureau, the nation will be more racially and ethnically diverse, as well as older, by 2050. The non-Caucasian population is projected to be 235.7 million out of a total United States population of 439 million by mid century. Today, Asians make up 5% (15.3 million) of the United States population. This figure is expected to nearly double to 9% (39.5 million) by 2050. The Latino, or Mestizo population now comprises 15% of the population of the United States (45.9 million). By 2050, it is expected to increase to 30% of the population (131.7 million).[1] As a result, the singular concept of Nordic beauty that dominated the United States media throughout the middle of the twentieth century has given way to a more diverse multiracial aesthetic, as championed in the entertainment industry, with the choice of multicultural fashion models that grace the runways and print media.[2] In addition, there is a growing trend in aesthetic surgery toward ethnic feature preservation and avoidance of a "westernized" look that was more popular in previous years. Today's facial plastic surgeon must be familiar with these trends and aesthetic goals within this rapidly growing patient population. This article describes the anatomy of the Asian and Latino face and describes the techniques of midface alloplastic augmentation.

There are various facial characteristics that present unique challenges in the Asian patient. A review of these characteristics will prove helpful to frame this discussion. Asian skin is thicker and contains greater collagen and pigmentation. The Asian face is also subjected to different gravitational and directional forces due to an overall wider midfacial skeletal structure, increased malar fat, and a weaker chin.[3] The midface in Asian patients is typified by dense fat both superficial and deep to the superficial musculoaponeurotic system (SMAS). The combination of increased superficial fat and a thicker dermis lessens the incidence of superficial rhytids in Asian patients. The fat and fibrous connections between the SMAS and parotidomasseteric fascia decrease the amount of soft tissue ptosis in

[a] 1421 Third Avenue, 4th Floor, New York, NY 10028, USA
[b] Department of Otolaryngology-Head and Neck Surgery, Manhattan Eye, Ear, and Throat/Lenox Hill Hospital, 210 East 64th Street, 3rd floor, New York, NY 10065, USA
[c] Facial Plastic and Reconstructive Surgery, 120 South Spalding Drive, Suite 340, Beverly Hills, CA 90212, USA
[d] Department of Head and Neck Surgery, UCLA School of Medicine, Los Angeles, CA, USA
[e] Department of Head and Neck Surgery, Cedars Sinai Medical Center, Los Angeles, CA, USA
* Corresponding author. Facial Plastic and Reconstructive Surgery, 120 South Spalding Drive, Suite 340, Beverly Hills, CA 90212.
E-mail address: wjbmd8@aol.com (W.J. Binder).

Facial Plast Surg Clin N Am 18 (2010) 49–69
doi:10.1016/j.fsc.2009.11.005
1064-7406/10/$ – see front matter © 2010 Elsevier Inc. All rights reserved.

many Asians. For these reasons, the midface in Asians usually has minimal rhytids and a mild to moderate amount of ptosis as the patient ages. However, because of the dense attachments between the fascial layers, soft tissue surgical rejuvenation procedures usually do not provide as much soft tissue elevation in Asian patients.[4]

The typical facial skeleton in Asians has a strong and wide zygomaticomalar region. The bizygomatic width of these patients measures above average. The lower facial skeleton is often characterized by a weak chin in the anterior-posterior dimension, but the bimandibular width is usually wider in Asians than in Caucasians. In addition, the anterior-posterior distance between the mentum and hyoid bone is typically shorter than in Caucasians. Chin augmentation accordingly is often a useful adjunct to facial rejuvenation surgery in this population (**Fig. 1**). The dental occlusion in Asians can have mild to moderate bimaxillary protrusion that causes the lower lip to be slightly protuberant, which often accentuates and exaggerates their microgenia. The position of the lower lip should therefore not be used as the only factor in judging ideal chin position. Chin augmentation should be performed conservatively, leaving the lower lip slightly protruding to maintain the ethnicity of the Asian face.[4]

Skin incisions in Asians have a greater propensity toward hypertrophic and keloid scars, tend to remain erythematous for a longer period of time, turn hyperpigmented for an unacceptable length of time, or remain hypopigmented.[5] Also, the Asian face tends to be wider and less angular than the Caucasian, similar to a toddler. Except for a portion of the Korean population, the midface tends to be shallower due in part to hypoplasia of the malar bone, with a lower nasal dorsum, fuller eyelids, and a more superficial orientation of the orbital rim. Cultural factors are important in this analysis as well. Prominent malar eminences, or "high cheek bones," which are a celebrated feature of Caucasian women, are often construed as an unfavorable trait in this population. The excessively high malar eminences, found particularly in Koreans, are often considered masculine features and deemed unattractive within their culture.[3]

Latinos, or Mestizos, who represent a mixture of European immigrants and the native populations of the Americas, have a strong mongoloid component in their facial features, and therefore have similar characteristics to Asians. Facial features of this ethnic group include thick sebaceous skin, abundant malar fat, prominent malar eminences, upper eyelid hooding, a broad face, a wide nasal dorsum, a platyrrhine or mesorrhine nose, a wide bigonial angle, and a protrusion of the dental arches that project the upper lip anteriorly resulting in an acute nasolabial angle.[6,7] It should be noted that these are rough generalizations regarding the various races and ethnic groups. Given the extensive interracial mingling in our society, there are various subpopulations within these broad categories.

The use of facial implants began in the 1950s with various primitive cheek and chin implants. Since then, there have been advances in materials, shapes of implants, surgical techniques and, perhaps most importantly, the understanding of the role of volume and skeletal structure in the aging process. The facial skeleton and its corresponding soft tissue form the architecture of the face and neck. Facial implants augment the soft tissue and skeletal framework by replacing volume lost during the aging process, supporting soft tissue and elevating it to a more youthful position.[8] Binder's innovations in the 1980s established midface augmentation with malar/submalar implants as an independent and powerful method for midface rejuvenation by helping restore lost midfacial volume.[9]

During the aging process, there are several characteristic changes in the midface. There is a loss of skin elasticity, soft tissue volume depletion, descent of soft tissue, and a diminution of the dental and skeletal support of the soft tissue envelope.[4] As the malar, buccal, temporal, and infraorbital fat pads atrophy and lose their facial support, these areas become progressively ptotic secondary to gravity. The nasolabial folds become exaggerated, and the infraorbital rim becomes exposed. In conjunction with deepening of the nasolabial and nasojugal folds, submalar hollowness and cavitary depressions occur. These changes initially flatten the midface, which leads to exposure of the underlying bony anatomy creating an aged, fatigued appearance. By elevating, supporting, and replacing lost midface volume, midface implant techniques underscore the notion that the face can be rejuvenated successfully not only via "lifting" procedures but also through the augmentation of the soft tissue and skeletal foundation.[9,10] Alloplastic midface augmentation is especially helpful in the Asian and Latino populations, who as a result of the aging process acquire more significant flattening of the midface, and thus become an ideal group for anterior projection and support of the premaxillary and submalar area.

From a technical point of view, midface augmentation using alloplastic implants is straightforward and bears relatively few risks. The implantation is reversible and may be combined with standard rhytidectomy techniques. The aesthetic benefit is consistent, predictable, and lasting. Midface implants can replace lost volume, reduce midface laxity, and decrease the depth of the nasolabial folds (**Fig. 2**). Submalar

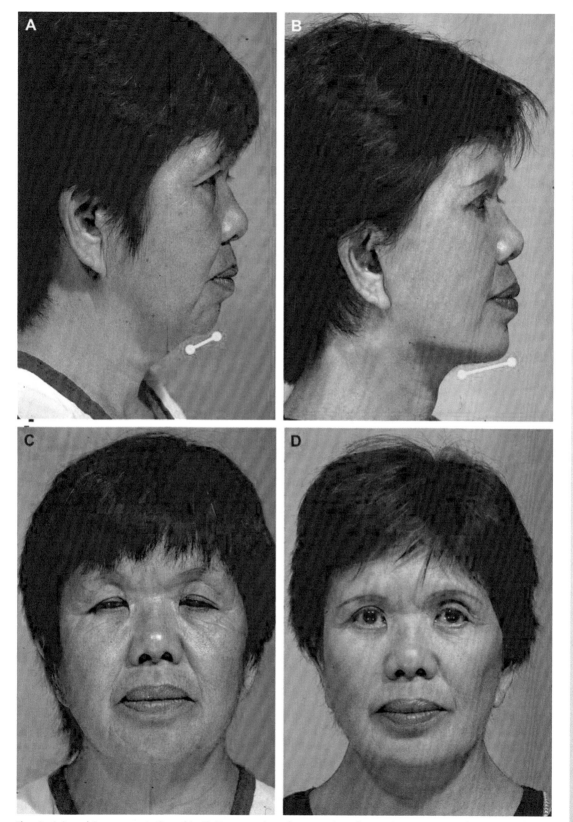

Fig. 1. Asian chin augmentation. (*A, C*) Preoperative photographs of an Asian patient with microgenia and a shortened distance between the mentum and hyoid bone, who underwent a rhytidectomy, chin implant, upper and lower lid blepharoplasty, and perioral dermabrasion. (*B, D*) Postoperative photographs showing improved mandibular projection and lower facial harmony.

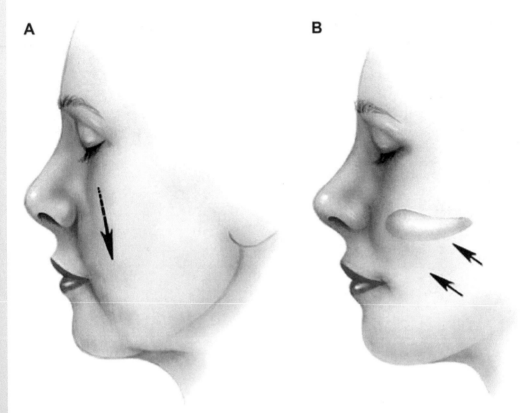

Fig. 2. (*A*, *B*) Suspension effect of midface implants. Midface implants augment the facial skeleton and restore soft tissue volume. The combined effect is to relocate the malar prominence to a more anterosuperior location and restore the hollow regions. (*From* Binder WJ, Azizzadeh B. Aesthetic midface implants. In: Azizzadeh B, Murphy MR, Johnson CM, editors. Master techniques in facial rejuvenation. Philadelphia: Saunders; 2007. p. 197–215; with permission.)

augmentation, performed in isolation, can provide a moderate amount of midfacial rejuvenation in middle-aged patients (age 35 to 45 years) who show early signs of facial aging and atrophy but lack the soft tissue laxity of extensive jowling or deep neck rhytids.[9]

When combined with rhytidectomy, midface alloplastic augmentation can either sharpen or soften angles and depressions of the aging face, which can lead to a more natural look. The implants allow the skin and soft tissue to be draped over a broader, well-defined area after midface augmentation of the bony scaffold (**Fig. 3**). In addition, if placed before facelifting, midface implants reduce lateral traction forces on the oral commissure, which also prevents an unnatural "overoperated" appearance. Finally, undermining of the midface periosteum during implant placement releases the deep attachments of the SMAS to the facial skeleton, thereby allowing greater mobilization and suspension of the ptotic soft tissues. The implant therefore acts as a spacer and prevents rapid reattachment of the periosteum, which keeps the midfacial soft tissues in an elevated and augmented position. As

a result, midface alloplastic augmentation can significantly enhance and prolong the cosmetic outcomes of subperiosteal, sub-SMAS, and deep plane rhytidectomy (**Fig. 4**).[9,11]

Midface augmentation can thus achieve dramatic aesthetic results not achievable through soft tissue suspension techniques alone. Furthermore, many patients with prominent malar skeletons (as in the Asian population) but inadequate submalar soft tissue will benefit from volumetric enhancement of the midface inferior to the prominent zygomatic process. Also, patients having midface augmentation with concomitant revision rhytidectomy will benefit from having decreased downward vertical forces on the lower eyelid. Other procedures such as deep plane facelifting and subperiosteal facelifting can provide viable alternatives to midface alloplasts; however, if problems with volume loss and loss of facial shape are not addressed, the face may appear skeletonized, especially in those with very prominent bone structure and thin skin.[9]

Injectable soft tissue fillers and fat transfer offer another option for improving midfacial aesthetics.

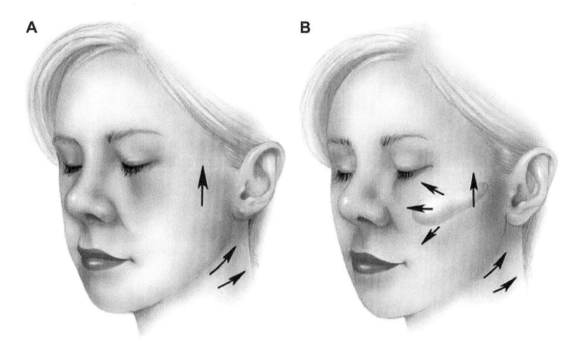

Fig. 3. Convexity effect of midface implants. (*A*) Facelifts generally stretch skin over a flat midface structure in a 2-dimensional pattern. (*B*) Malar and submalar implants augment the bony and soft tissues of a more convex midface region that allows a more natural draping, resulting in a third dimension for facial rejuvenation. (*From* Binder WJ, Kim BP, Azizzadeh B. Aesthetic midface implants. In: Azizzadeh B, Murphy MR, Johnson CM, editors. Master techniques in facial rejuvenation. Philadelphia: Saunders; 2007. p. 197–215; with permission.)

However, the most important difference between fillers and midfacial implants is that implants not only provide support and volume to ptotic soft tissue, they also allow for a fixed 3-dimensional quality to the face and support of the soft tissues that volumetric filling alone cannot achieve. Fillers in the midface in large amounts can migrate laterally and result in an amorphous, overfilled, and unnatural look.[9]

A key anatomic region in the midface is the submalar triangle, which is bordered superiorly by the zygomatic prominence, medially by the nasolabial fold, and laterally by the masseter muscle. This anatomic area represents the most common site of volume loss in the aging midface, especially in Asians and Latinos, but can be corrected readily with alloplastic implants (**Fig. 5**).

PREOPERATIVE ANALYSIS

Preparing for midfacial alloplastic augmentation begins with a thorough history and physical examination followed by digital photographs and optional digital computer imaging. The computer imaging can help the patient identify the exact nature of their concerns and potential benefits of surgery. It is also important to analyze the entire upper and lower face and neck. Basal photos

and apical bird's eye views are especially helpful in identifying midface pathology and can help in selecting midface implants. Preoperative analysis and discussion of soft tissue and skeletal asymmetries is imperative both to prevent exaggeration of these effects postoperatively and to avoid unrealistic patient expectations.[9]

Selecting the appropriate midfacial implant requires an ability to recognize the characteristics of midface deformity (**Table 1**).[10,12] Ideal evaluation requires separate analyses of the bony malar area and the soft tissue component of the submalar region. Patients exhibiting type I deformity with primary malar hypoplasia and adequate midface soft tissue are best suited for malar shell implants that cover the zygoma and contiguous areas. These implants yield an arched appearance and project the cheek laterally. Fine edges gradually blend into the adjacent tissues to avoid abrupt changes in the facial architecture.

The most common deformity of the aging face, especially in Asians and Latinos, is a type II submalar deficiency. This deformity is characterized by normal malar skeletal structure and soft tissue atrophy of the midface. Volume loss and inferior descent of the midface soft tissues leaves an excavated, flattened appearance. Submalar implants are the implants of choice for patients with this deformity.

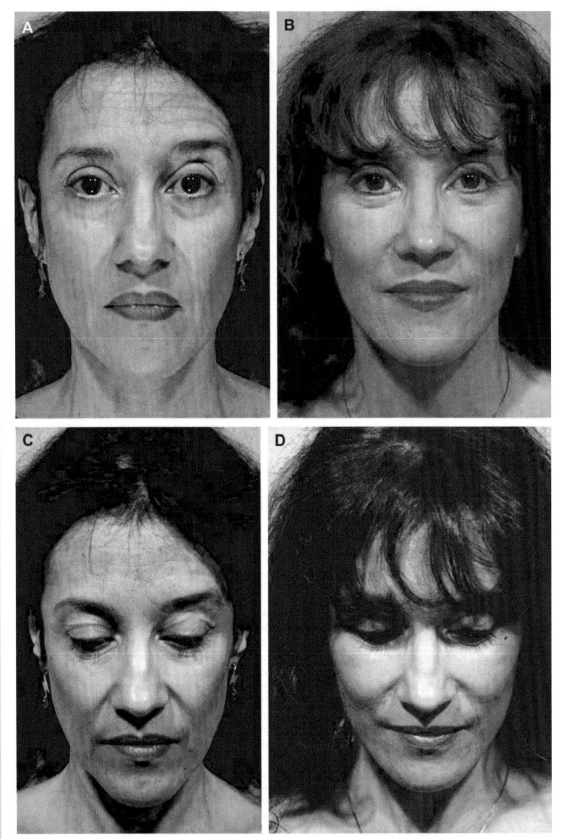

Fig. 4. Rhytidectomy and submalar implants. Preoperative photos (*A, C, E*) in a Latino woman with good midfacial bone structure. The malar eminence is relatively high and sharp adding to the contrast within the submalar region. This patient achieved a significant and long-term benefit from the submalar implant, which can be seen to elevate and support the midface in the postoperative photos (*B, D, F*).

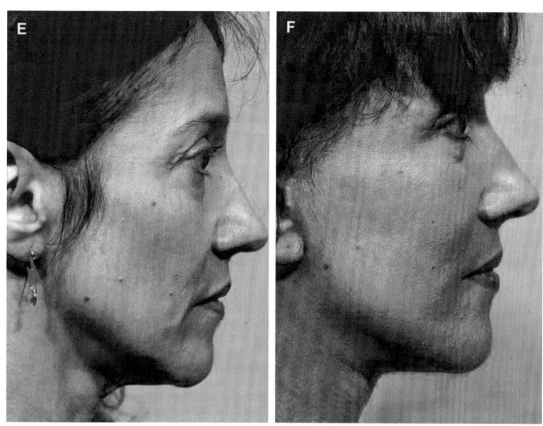

Fig. 4. (*continued*) (*E*) Preoperative side view. (*F*) Postoperative side view.

Type III deficiency is characterized by both a malar and submalar deficiency. The effects of aging are exaggerated in these patients, because they have poor skeletal support that facilitates soft tissue descent toward the nasolabial folds and oral commissure. Combined malar-submalar implants are the treatment of choice for patients with a type III deficiency. Most of these patients will do poorly with a rhytidectomy alone because of this lack of bony support for the suspended soft tissues. Hence, the result of rhytidectomy in these patients without alloplastic augmentation is usually suboptimal and transient at best.[9] In addition, some patients with premaxillary retrusion may require custom implants using computer-aided design (CAD) and manufacturing (CAM) techniques that use a high-resolution computed tomography (CT) scan of the face (**Fig. 6**).[13]

SURGICAL TECHNIQUE
General Guidelines

Available biomaterials for midface augmentation include silicone, polytetrafluoroethylene (Medpor,

Porex Surgical Products, Newnan, GA, USA), and expanded polytetrafluoroethylene (ePTFE). The authors prefer silicone implants because of their flexibility, low infection rates, and ease of insertion and removal.[9,14–19] Despite the occasional use of the subciliary and lateral facelift approach for implant placement, the transoral approach placing the implant in a subperiosteal pocket offers the most advantages. This approach facilitates an easy insertion and direct visualization of all midface anatomic structures, in particular the infraorbital nerve and inferomedially, the submalar space. There is also the advantage of avoiding external scars, and prevention of the potential downward traction on the lower eyelid postoperatively if a subciliary approach is used. The process of capsular fibrosis facilitates tight adherence of the silicone implants to the facial skeleton in the subperiosteal plane, which protects against postoperative implant migration.[9,10] However, a potential disadvantage of the transoral approach is the risk of contamination and wound infection due to the implant's exposure to oral flora. Hence, meticulous surgical technique is of paramount importance.

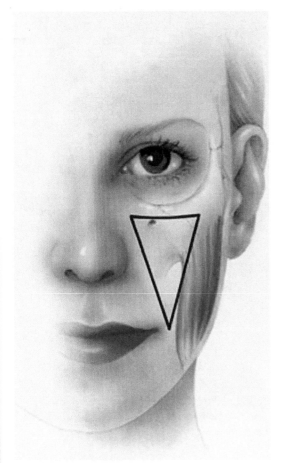

Fig. 5. Submalar triangle. The submalar triangle is bordered superiorly by the zygomatic prominence, laterally by the masseter muscle, and medially by the nasolabial fold; it is the most common area of deficiency with aging. (*From* Binder WJ, Kim BP, Azizzadeh B. Aesthetic midface implants. In: Azizzadeh B, Murphy MR, Johnson CM, editors. Master techniques in facial rejuvenation. Philadelphia: Saunders; 2007. p. 197–215; with permission.)

The type of facial deformity may determine the sequence of procedures when performing alloplastic augmentation and rhytidectomy concurrently. Type I and III patients who require a major malar component to their midface augmentation procedure or have significant facial asymmetry should have their implants performed before the rhytidectomy. This action allows the surgeon to visualize and thus compensate for the structural changes that may not be apparent after facial edema occurs. In this case, the wound is either left open until the end of the rhytidectomy, or a Penrose drain is placed into the oral incisions to prevent the formation of fluid collections. For most Asian or Latino patients, who require only submalar soft tissue augmentation

because of a type II deformity, the operator can perform the rhytidectomy before placement of the implant. In this case, the advantages include the ability to maintain a dry implant pocket, reduction of subperiosteal bleeding, and the capability of closing the intraoral incision immediately following augmentation to reduce the risk of infection. In either situation, local anesthetic is infiltrated into the tissues in a similar manner as if the implant procedure were performed alone.[9]

Preparation for Surgery

Antibiotic prophylaxis with a broad-spectrum oral antibiotic is started 1 day preoperatively. In the holding area, the patient sits upright, and the crucial areas designated for augmentation are clearly marked (**Fig. 7**). The marked areas should illustrate the midfacial volume deficit, areas of depression, infraorbital nerve axis, and the malar eminence. As a general guide, the most medial border of the typical midface implant may be readily identified by marking the position of the infraorbital nerve, which is parallel to the midpupillary line with the patient staring straight ahead. Then the patient should smile widely to assist in determining the most inferomedial position of the implant and thus ensure that there is no interference with the facial mimetic function. The markings should outline the areas of maximal depression that will receive the maximal augmentation. Once the skin is marked, the patient should be shown a mirror to allow he or she to concur that the proposed changes are satisfactory.[9] Of importance is that the markings may vary to some degree from the ultimate placement of the implant, and should not be the sole determining factor for implant placement.

Intravenous antibiotics and steroids are used routinely intraoperatively. After the patient has received adequate anesthesia, whether via general anesthesia or intravenous sedation, the surgeon injects 1% or 0.5% lidocaine with epinephrine into the gingival-buccal sulcus and the midface in the subperiosteal plane. To aid in the even dispersion of the local anesthesia and minimize contour irregularities due to injectate overaccumulation, hyaluronidase (Wydase, Wyeth-Ayerst, Philadelphia, PA, USA) is added to the anesthetic solution and the face is then massaged. The operative site is prepared with povidone-iodine (Betadine, Purdue Frederick, Norwalk, CT, USA) from soaked gauze sponges inserted into the gingival-buccal sulcus at the level of the canine fossa for 10 minutes.[9]

Table 1
Patterns of midface deformity

Type	Description of Deformity	Augmentation Required	Implant Type to Use
Type 1	Primary malar hypoplasia: malar boney deficiency with adequate soft tissue. Face lacks desirable features of angular, well-defined cheeks	Requires primarily lateral projection of the malar eminence; results in high-arched, laterally projected cheeks	Malar implant: shell-type extends into the submalar space for more natural result
Type 2	Submalar deficiency; soft tissue deficiency with adequate malar bone. Face appears dull and flat; most common deficiency of the aging face	Requires anterior projection of the midface and submalar hollow; restores lost midface volume characteristic of a more youthful face	Submalar implant: placed over the anterior maxilla and the masseter tendon, extending into the submalar space
Type 3	Combined malar and submalar deficiency: volume-deficient face with inadequate bony and soft tissues. Marked by premature signs of aging	Requires both anterior and lateral projection of the entire midface and submalar regions	Combined malar-submalar implant: lateral (malar) and anterior (submalar) projection to fill a large midfacial void

From Binder WJ, Azizzadeh B. Malar and submalar augmentation. Facial Plastic Surg Clin North Am 2008;16(1):17; with permission.

Incision and Dissection of the Malar Eminence

Due to the plasticity of the mucosa, insertion of the implant requires only a 3-mm stab incision in the gingival-buccal sulcus over the lateral canine fossa and maxillary buttress (**Fig. 8**). The incision is made in an upward oblique direction, and is carried immediately and directly to the maxillary bone. Bleeding is minimized by compressing the mucosa against the bone. An inferior cuff of mucosa of a minimum of 1 cm facilitates closure at the end of the procedure. Removing dentures during the operation is unnecessary, because they do not interfere with insertion of the implant, and actually direct placement of the incision above the denture to the correct location.[9]

After the initial incision, the periosteum of the anterior maxilla is elevated superiorly and laterally (**Figs. 9** and **10**). Following the preoperative markings, the surgeon uses his or her external free hand to provide crucial guidance to the direction and extent of dissection. The subperiosteal elevation is initiated with the Joseph elevator, which is changed quickly to a broader 10-mm Tessier elevator (**Fig. 11**). This technique enables a greater degree of safety and ease of periosteal dissection. The infraorbital nerve should be identified carefully if the proposed implant is large or bears a significant medial

component. This identification prevents placing the implant over the foramen.[9]

Dissection then is extended laterally to the malar-zygomatic junction and zygomatic arch. The subperiosteal plane is used for dissection, particularly over the lateral zygoma, where branches of the facial nerve traverse just superficial to this plane (**Fig. 12**). Injuring the temporal branch of the facial nerve can be avoided by using gentle blunt dissection over the mid-zygomatic arch, ensuring the dissection is on bone and within the subperiosteal plane. Emphasis is placed on using a broad elevator, which is far safer than a delicate, thin instrument that could more readily puncture the periosteum laterally because of limited visibility during the procedure.[9]

Exposure of the Submalar Triangle and Creation of an Implant Pocket

Patients with type II or III midface deficiencies require exposure of the submalar space. This anatomic depression extends about 3 cm beneath the zygoma. To expose this region, the subperiosteal dissection is continued inferiorly below the zygoma and over the superior tendinous insertion of the masseter muscle. Gentle elevation of the overlying soft tissue from the

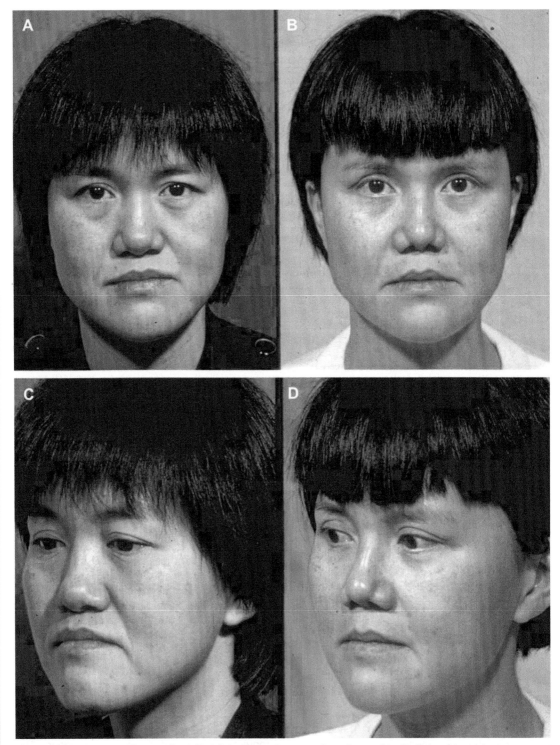

Fig. 6. Custom premaxillary and midfacial implant. Preoperative photos (*A, C, E*) in this patient represent a premaxillary retrusive midface commonly found in the Asian population. Postoperative photos (*B, D, F*) reveal significant improvement in premaxillary projection and midfacial contouring.

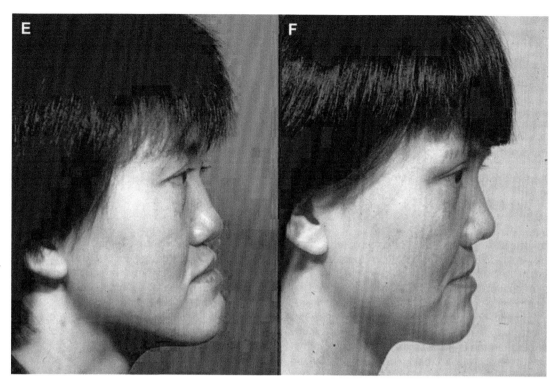

Fig. 6. (*continued*)

deeper plane of the tendon facilitates visualization of the glistening white tendinous attachment of the masseter (**Fig. 13**). The muscle attachments are not divided because they serve as a critical platform for the inferior portion of the submalar implant. The submalar space narrows significantly posteriorly, and is not accessed easily. Careful dissection of the posterior limit can be accomplished by advancing a blunt elevator along the inferior border of the zygomatic arch. Masseter

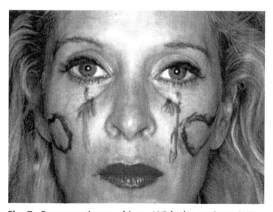

Fig. 7. Preoperative markings. With the patient sitting upright, the areas of midface deficiency requiring augmentation are marked. The infraorbital nerve axis along the midpupillary line designates the medial border of dissection. (*From* Binder WJ, Kim BP, Azizzadeh B. Aesthetic midface implants. In: Azizzadeh B, Murphy MR, Johnson CM, editors. Master techniques in facial rejuvenation. Philadelphia: Saunders; 2007. p. 197–215; with permission.)

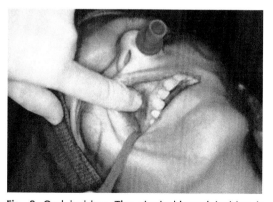

Fig. 8. Oral incision. The gingival-buccal incision is made over the lateral canine fossa. Only 3 mm is required for adequate dissection and exposure of the midface skeleton. A 1- to 1.5-cm cuff of gingiva is maintained inferiorly. (*From* Binder WJ, Kim BP, Azizzadeh B. Aesthetic midface implants. In: Azizzadeh B, Murphy MR, Johnson CM, editors. Master techniques in facial rejuvenation. Philadelphia: Saunders; 2007. p. 197–215; with permission.)

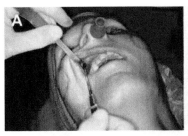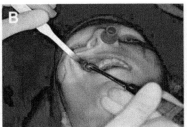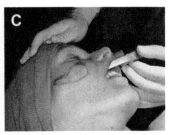

Fig. 9. Periosteal elevation. The periosteum is elevated over the maxilla superiorly and laterally. The borders of the dissection are the masseteric tendon and infraorbital rim (*A–C*). (*From* Binder WJ, Kim BP, Azizzadeh B. Aesthetic midface implants. In: Azizzadeh B, Murphy MR, Johnson CM, editors. Master techniques in facial rejuvenation. Philadelphia: Saunders; 2007. p. 197–215; with permission.)

muscle contraction at its superior border tends to be limited, thereby preventing postoperative implant displacement.[9]

A pocket large enough to accommodate the appropriate implant is created over the malar-zygomatic complex and submalar triangle. The dissected space always should be sufficiently larger than the implant so that the implant can fit into it easily without being compressed by the surrounding tissues, particularly posteriorly. Displacement of the implant can occur if an implant is forced into an inadequately sized pocket, or if the posterolateral portion of the pocket is poorly exposed. In the latter case, constriction of the area will push the implant anteriorly, causing it to migrate or extrude. When the implant is situated in the dissected space, it should sit passively and one generally should be able to move it at least 3 to 5 mm in all directions. After closure of the wound, even after a large pocket is made, the periosteum and soft tissues contract; the pocket immediately closes down around the implant, and the dead space usually is obliterated within 24 to 48 hours.[9,12]

Insertion of the Implant

Preoperative facial analysis along with the type of midface deficiency and the patient's desires typically determines the location and the size of the implant. Selecting the appropriate midface implant should take into account the bulk of the overlying

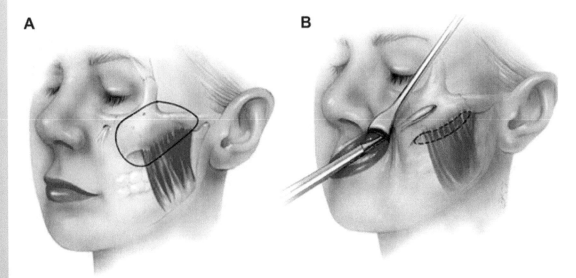

Fig. 10. Periosteal elevation. (*A*) Initial dissection over the anterior maxillary wall. (*B*) The stippled area represents the submalar dissection over the masseteric tendon. The dashed line represents the area that generally is elevated. (*From* Binder WJ, Kim BP, Azizzadeh B. Aesthetic midface implants. In: Azizzadeh B, Murphy MR, Johnson CM, editors. Master techniques in facial rejuvenation. Philadelphia: Saunders; 2007. p. 197–215; with permission.)

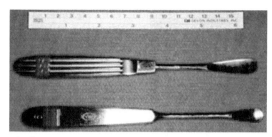

Fig. 11. Instruments: periosteal elevators. Periosteal elevation begins with the Joseph elevator to gain initial access, but most of the dissection should be performed with the 10-mm Tessier elevator. (*From* Binder WJ, Kim BP, Azizzadeh B. Aesthetic midface implants. In: Azizzadeh B, Murphy MR, Johnson CM, editors. Master techniques in facial rejuvenation. Philadelphia: Saunders; 2007. p. 197–215; with permission.)

tissue and formation of the fibrous capsule. Therefore, it is best to choose an implant that is marginally smaller than the desired volume changes. In type II deficiencies, submalar implants generally rest over the anterior face of the maxilla. Type III deformities use combined malar-submalar implants that cover both the malar bony eminence and the submalar triangle. To achieve the desired facial contour changes, positioning an implant in the submalar triangle typically requires greater experience and judgment than is necessary for implants placed over the malar eminence. Regardless of the type of augmentation, however, the end aesthetic result should achieve the desired changes in facial contour and generally correspond to the preoperative facial markings rather than to the underlying skeletal anatomy.[9]

Implants should be soaked in antibiotic solution (bacitracin 50,000 U/L) at the start of the procedure and allowed to remain there until the time

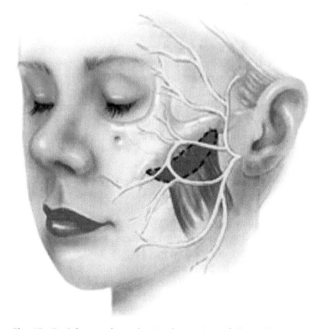
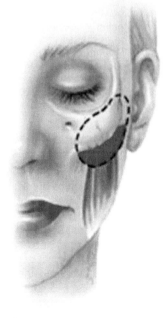

Fig. 12. Facial nerve branches in the region of dissection. It is crucial to dissect in the subperiosteal plane over the zygomatic arch, to avoid injury to the temporal branch of the facial nerve. The use of a broad elevator will help prevent perforation of the periosteum in this region. The buccal branches are also at risk if the region over the masseter is dissected aggressively. (*From* Binder WJ, Kim BP, Azizzadeh B. Aesthetic midface implants. In: Azizzadeh B, Murphy MR, Johnson CM, editors. Master techniques in facial rejuvenation. Philadelphia: Saunders; 2007. p. 197–215; with permission.)

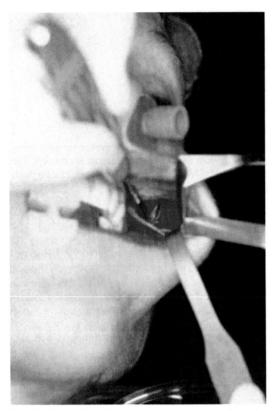

Fig. 13. Submalar triangle and masseteric tendon. The lateral aspect of the dissection will be over the masseteric tendon, inferior to the lateral zygomatic arch. In this region, the soft tissues are elevated gently over the glistening white fibers of the tendon, allowing placement of the tail of the submalar implant. (*From* Binder WJ, Kim BP, Azizzadeh B. Aesthetic midface implants. In: Azizzadeh B, Murphy MR, Johnson CM, editors. Master techniques in facial rejuvenation. Philadelphia: Saunders; 2007. p. 197–215; with permission.)

of insertion. A "no-touch" technique should be used, if possible, to ensure minimal implant handling and reduce the risk of contamination. The surgeon and assistant should also ensure that any powder residue is washed off the surgical gloves. An assortment of different implant sizes and shapes should be available in the operating room, and the surgeon must be capable of customizing the implants via carving (**Fig. 14**). Sizers should be used to determine and confirm the appropriate implant size and shape. Modifications to the implant shape then can compensate for overall size, shape, and facial asymmetry. Shaving an implant as little as 1 mm can impact the final aesthetic results significantly, especially in patients who have thin facial skin,[9] although this is less of a concern in the

Asian and Latino population given their thicker skin and soft tissue.

Assessing for facial asymmetry is critical following insertion of the implants. The operator can use a ruler to measure the distances from the medial border of the implants to the midline. Preexisting facial asymmetry can pose significant challenges and require exquisite attention to the bony and soft tissue topography. In these cases, each implant may need to be contoured or positioned asymmetrically. In addition, patients who have thin skin or prominent facial skeletons may require modifications in the implants, so as to reduce any edges or contours of larger, thicker implants that would otherwise be palpable or cause visible irregularities. Again, this may be less of a concern in the Asian and Latino population. After placing both implants, the surgeon may stand at the head of the table to acquire a more precise assessment of contour asymmetry.[9]

Securing the Implant

To prevent postoperative implant migration, several methods can be used to secure the implant following proper placement. Larger malar or combined malar-submalar implants are not prone to migration and may not require fixation due to their positioning over the zygoma. Nonetheless, it is the authors' recommendation to apply external suture fixation using 1 of 2 techniques. In the indirect lateral suture fixation method, long (10 in [25.4 cm]) double-armed Keith needles on 0-0 silk sutures are passed through the lateral end of the implant (**Fig. 15**). The needles are inserted into the wound and directed posterolaterally; then they exit the temporal region behind the hairline. The implant is then placed into the final position, and the sutures are tied over a cotton roll bolster. This technique works best with malar shell implants in type I deformities by applying a superolateral tension over the implants and maintaining their position over the bony malar-zygomatic eminence.[9]

The second suture method, the direct external fixation method (**Fig. 16**), is better suited for submalar and combined malar-submalar facial implants in type II and III deformities. This method is also the preferred technique when the implants are excessively mobile within the wound pocket or when asymmetrical placement of implants becomes necessary. Midface implants usually have 2 preformed fenestrations, of which the position of the medial fenestration should be marked on the external skin while the implant resides in the subperiosteal pocket. Using

A

B

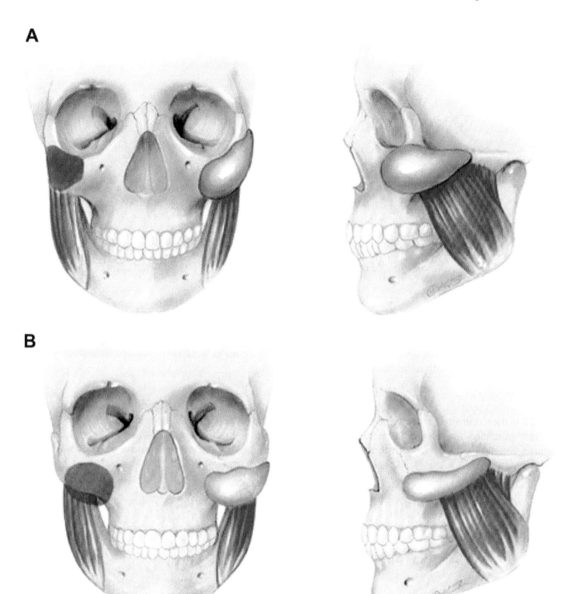

Fig. 14. Implant placement. Malar shell implants for type I deformity rest on top of the malar and zygomatic bone in a more superior and lateral position (*A*). Submalar implants for type II deformity generally lie over the anterior face of the maxilla (*B*).

a right-angle clamp to push the implant upward, underneath the fenestration, the holes can be located, and the resulting external protuberance can be marked on the skin. Symmetry can be confirmed by measuring and comparing the distance of each marking to the midline. After marking the medial fenestrations, the skin should be marked to coincide with the location of the lateral fenestration of the implant. This procedure can be done by first removing the implants and placing them on top of the midface. The implants then are positioned to coincide with the desired contour and preoperative markings. The second skin mark is applied to match the location of the lateral fenestration of the implant. After passing double-armed 3-0 silk sutures through the medial and lateral fenestrations with the loop around the deep surface of the implant, the needles are placed into the wound pocket and passed perpendicularly through the skin

C

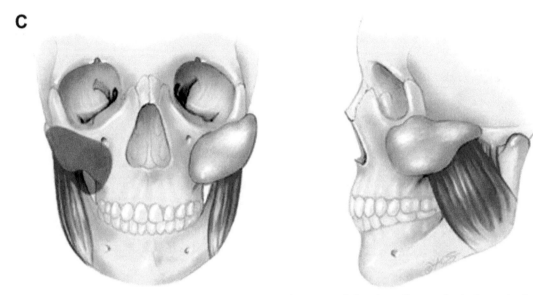

Fig. 14. (*continued*) Combined malar-submalar implants for type 3 deformity will cover both the malar bony eminence and the submalar triangle (*C*). (*From* Binder WJ, Kim BP, Azizzadeh B. Aesthetic midface implants. In: Azizzadeh B, Murphy MR, Johnson CM, editors. Master techniques in facial rejuvenation. Philadelphia: Saunders; 2007. p. 197–215; with permission.)

markings corresponding to each fenestration. The implant is then delivered into the pocket, ensuring proper position and symmetry. Finally, the sutures are tied gently over cotton roll bolsters overlying the anterior cheek. These bolsters aid in compressing the midface, reduce any potential dead space, and prevent fluid from collecting in the subperiosteal pockets. The external sutures and bolsters may be removed 24 to 48 hours postoperatively.[9]

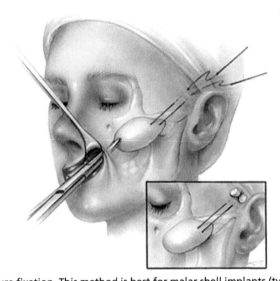

Fig. 15. Indirect lateral suture fixation. This method is best for malar shell implants (type I deformity) by applying a superolateral tension on the implants and maintaining their position over the bony malar-zygomatic eminence. Long (10 in [25.4 cm]) double-armed Keith needles on 0-0 silk suture are passed through the lateral end of the implant directed posterolaterally, exiting the temporal region behind the hairline. The implant is then placed into the final position, and the sutures are tied over a cotton roll bolster. (*From* Binder WJ, Kim BP, Azizzadeh B. Aesthetic midface implants. In: Azizzadeh B, Murphy MR, Johnson CM, editors. Master techniques in facial rejuvenation. Philadelphia: Saunders; 2007. p. 197–215; with permission.)

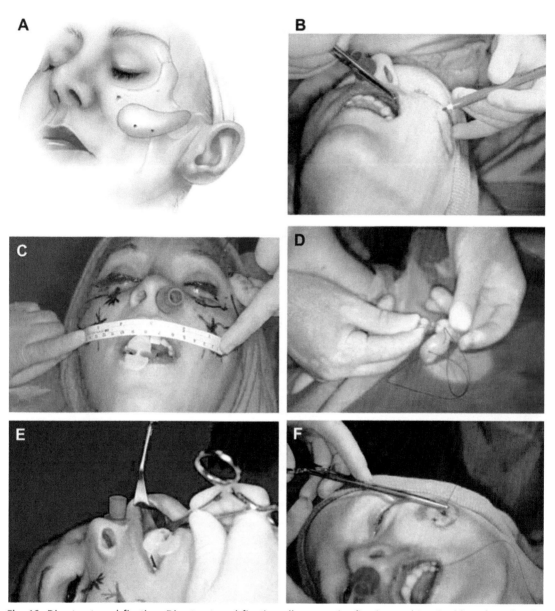

Fig. 16. Direct external fixation. Direct external fixation allows precise fixation and is suited best for submalar and combined implants in type II and type III patients. (*A*) The implant is adjusted in the pocket to obtain the exact desired location. (*B*) A right-angle clamp is used to mark the location of the implant fenestrations by pressing behind the fenestration outward through the facial skin and marking the area of protuberance. A second fenestration mark is placed to ensure adequate orientation. (*C*) Symmetric placement of marking is checked. (*D–F*) The suture needles are passed through the fenestration points and passed perpendicular through the skin markings corresponding to each fenestration.

Implants can also be secured using internal suture fixation and by attaching the medial aspect of the implant to the periosteum and soft tissues. In addition, screws can be used to fix the implant, but only in those cases where it is in an acceptable position to accept the screw over the lateral buttress and not in the canine fossa. If the implant is placed before rhytidectomy, the oral incision is reopened to fix the implant with external sutures. Intraoral Penrose drains may be placed if necessary.[9]

Wound Closure and Dressing

Intraoral incisions are irrigated copiously with antibiotic solution before closing them in one layer using chromic sutures. The external suture

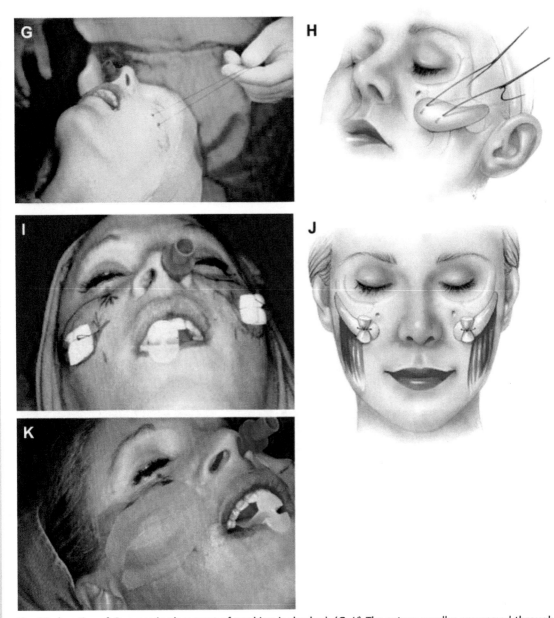

Fig. 16. (*continued*) Symmetric placement of marking is checked. (*G, H*) The suture needles are passed through the fenestration points and passed perpendicular through the skin markings corresponding to each fenestration. (*I, J*) After ensuring precise location and adequate fixation of the midface implants, the sutures are tied over a cotton roll bolster. (*K*) Benzoin and a flexible band aid then can be placed over the bolster. (*From* Binder WJ, Kim BP, Azizzadeh B. Aesthetic midface implants. In: Azizzadeh B, Murphy MR, Johnson CM, editors. Master techniques in facial rejuvenation. Philadelphia: Saunders; 2007. p. 197–215; with permission.)

bolsters are covered with bandages, and an elastic facial dressing is applied and left in place for 24 hours. A full elastic garment dressing that allows even compression of the midface is preferred (**Fig. 17**). As the elastic dressing applies adequate pressure to obliterate the pocket posterior to the implant, the suture bolster closes the midface pocket anterior to the implant. Patients are encouraged to use this elastic dressing after the bolsters are removed for an additional 24 to 48 hours. If a concomitant rhytidectomy is performed and the bolsters are in place, a lighter neck and facial dressing (which also mildly compresses the midface) comprised of cotton

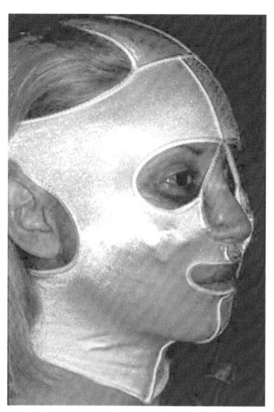

Fig. 17. Elastic facial dressing. A full-face compression garment can help reduce postoperative edema and fluid collection. (*From* Binder WJ, Kim BP, Azizzadeh B. Aesthetic midface implants. In: Azizzadeh B, Murphy MR, Johnson CM, editors. Master techniques in facial rejuvenation. Philadelphia: Saunders; 2007. p. 197–215; with permission.)

and cling is placed rather than the elastic compression dressing.[9]

Postoperative Care

Patients may recover at home or in an aftercare facility. Patients are recommended to use ice packs for 3 to 4 days and sleep with the head in an elevated position. Antibiotics, analgesics, and antiemetic medications are prescribed to all patients. The first follow-up visit occurs on postoperative day 1 at which time the facial dressings, bolsters, and any drains are removed. The mask may be reapplied and worn for another 24 to 48 hours, which helps reduce postoperative edema and overall recovery time. Patients are typically able to resume nonstrenuous routine activity 3 to 5 days postoperatively. In general, approximately 80% to 85% of the edema resolves within 3 to 4 weeks, and the remaining 15% to 20% subsides over the following 6 months.[9]

Complications

Malposition and errors in implant selection are the most frequent complications of facial implant augmentation.[9,14,20] Incorrect positioning, insufficient pocket size, or inadequate fixation of the implant can lead to postoperative displacement. During the immediate postoperative period, patients should be assessed within 48 to 72 hours after surgery to ensure against significant facial asymmetry. Implant extrusion is extremely rare, and usually occurs through the intraoperative incision because of inadequate dissection of the posterolateral pocket.[9,20]

Augmentation using alloplastic silicone implants has an estimated infection rate of approximately 1%.[9,20] Tactics to minimize the risk of infection include soaking the implant in antibiotic solution, irrigating the wound, and avoiding blood and fluid accumulation in the surgical pocket. Other complications include bleeding, hematoma, and seroma. Placement of drains can help in preventing fluid collections, especially when concomitant rhytidectomy is performed or when there is excessive bleeding intraoperatively. Injury to the infraorbital nerve can occur, and may result in infraorbital numbness lasting from days to weeks postoperatively; this is rarely permanent. Other potential risks include injury to the frontal branch of the

---

Box 1
Pearls and pitfalls

1. Have the patient smile broadly to assist in determining the most inferomedial position of the implants and to ensure that there is no interference with facial mimetic function.
2. A 3-mm stab incision is made over the lateral canine fossa in the gingival-buccal sulcus with compression of the mucosa to minimize bleeding.
3. The subperiosteal elevation is initiated with a Joseph elevator, which is changed quickly to a broader 10-mm Tessier elevator to avoid excessive dissection, stretching, and traction in the area of the infraorbital nerve. The nerve should be carefully identified if the implant is large or has a large medial component, to prevent placing the implant over the foramen.
4. The subperiosteal plane must be maintained over the zygomatic arch by using gentle blunt dissection with the Tessier elevator over the mid-arch to avoid injury to the temporal branch of the facial nerve.
5. The soft tissue over the masseter must be elevated gently without dividing the muscle or its tendinous attachments to avoid injury to the buccal branches of the facial nerve and to preserve the platform for the inferior part of the implant.
6. The dissected pocket should always be sufficiently larger than the implant, and the surgeon should be able to move it at least 3 to 5 mm in all directions.
7. It is preferable to "undercorrect" or choose an implant that is marginally smaller than the desired volume changes to account for the formation of the fibrous capsule and the bulk of the overlying tissue.
8. For larger malar implants an external, indirect, lateral suspension suture technique is preferable to apply superolateral tension on the implants and maintain their position over the bony malar-zygomatic eminence.
9. For submalar or combined malar-submalar implants, excessive mobility of the implants, or when asymmetrical placement of implants is necessary, the direct external fixation method is preferable.
10. The medial fenestration should be marked on the skin while the implant resides in the pocket. Symmetry between the 2 sides can be confirmed by comparing and measuring the distance of each marking to the midline. The lateral marking is then made with implants placed on top of the midface in the desired position.

facial nerve during dissection of the zygomatic arch and injury to the buccal branch with overly aggressive masseter dissection.

SUMMARY

Alloplastic midface implantation in the Asian and Latino patient presents various challenges and opportunities for the facial plastic surgeon. Their thicker skin, increased facial adipose tissue, and decreased facial skeletal support make them ideal candidates for anterior projection and support using midface implants. Cultural factors must also be considered in patients for whom prominent malar eminences are aesthetically displeasing. Therefore, critical analysis of the patient's face along with open and precise communication between patient and surgeon can lead to optimal patient satisfaction using this powerful modality to enhance the midface (**Box 1**).

REFERENCES

1. US Census Bureau. Census 2000 Modified Race Data. 2002.
2. Lam SM. Aesthetic facial surgery for the Asian male. Facial Plast Surg 2005;21(4):317–23.
3. Shirakabe Y, Suzuki Y, Lam SM. A new paradigm for the aging Asian face. Aesthetic Plast Surg 2003;27(5):397–402.
4. Sykes JM. Management of the aging face in the Asian patient. Facial Plast Surg Clin North Am 2007;15(3):353–60, vi–vii.
5. Lam SM. Aesthetic strategies for the aging Asian face. Facial Plast Surg Clin North Am 2007;15(3):283–91, v.
6. Cobo R. Facial aesthetic surgery with emphasis on rhinoplasty in the Hispanic patient. Curr Opin Otolaryngol Head Neck Surg 2008;16(4):369–75.
7. Molina F. Aesthetic facial osteotomies in Latin Americans. Clin Plast Surg 2007;34(3):e31–6.
8. Shire JR. Preface in "Facial Implants". Facial Plast Surg Clin North Am 2008;16(1):ix–x.
9. Binder WJ, Azizzadeh B. Malar and submalar augmentation. Facial Plast Surg Clin North Am 2008;16(1):11–32, v.
10. Binder WJ, Schoenrock LD, Terino EO. Augmentation of the malar-submalar/midface. Facial Plast Surg Clin North Am 1994;2(3):265–83.
11. Psillakis JM, Rumley TO, Carmagos A. Subperiosteal approach as an improved concept for correction of the aging face. Plast Reconstr Surg 1988;82(3):383–94.

12. Binder WJ. A comprehensive approach for aesthetic contouring of the midface in rhytidectomy. Facial Plast Surg Clin North Am 1993;1(2):231–55.

13. Binder WJ. Custom-designed facial implants. Facial Plast Surg Clin North Am 2008;16(1):133–46, vii.

14. Wilkinson TS. Complications in aesthetic malar augmentation. Plast Reconstr Surg 1983;71(5):643–9.

15. Silver WE. The use of alloplast material in contouring the face. Facial Plast Surg 1986;3:81–98.

16. Whitaker LA. Aesthetic augmentation of the malar-midface structures. Plast Reconstr Surg 1987;80(3):337–46.

17. Prendergast M, Schoenrock LD. Malar augmentation. Patient classification and placement. Arch Otolaryngol Head Neck Surg 1989;115(8):964–9.

18. Binder WJ. Submalar augmentation. An alternative to face-lift surgery. Arch Otolaryngol Head Neck Surg 1989;115(7):797–801.

19. Terino EO. Alloplastic facial contouring by zonal principles of skeletal anatomy. Clin Plast Surg 1992;19(2):487–510.

20. Rubin PJ, Yaremchuk MJ. Complications and toxicities of implantable biomaterials used in facial reconstructive and aesthetic surgery: a comprehensive review of the literature. Plast Reconstr Surg 1997;100(5):1336–53.

Forehead Augmentation with Alloplastic Implants

Joseph K. Wong, MD, FRCS(C)

KEYWORDS

• Forehead • Augmentation • Alloplastic • Implant

Very little has been reported regarding forehead augmentation with alloplastic implants. The literature has a large number of reports on autogenous grafting and repair in cranioplasties.[1–3] The use of bioabsorbable devices,[4,5] metallic devices,[6] and acrylic devices[7] has been reported. The author has reported forehead augmentation with silicone implants.[8]

Various methods have been described in augmentation of the forehead and temporal region. Most of these have been temporary measures. These methods have ranged from injection of various fillers and fat. Permanent alloplastic materials that are popular for forehead augmentation vary from expanded polytetrafluoroethylene (ePTFE) implants, to acrylic implants and silicone implants.

The author favors the use of ePTFE soft sheets or soft silicone as implant materials for forehead augmentation. The advantages of soft ePTFE sheets are the simplicity of the operation and lack of capsule formation. The disadvantages of ePTFE implants are the limited amount of augmentation achievable and the slightly higher chance of infection. Even though the disadvantages of silicone implants are the higher chance of capsule formation and possibility of mobility of the implant, the advantage of an overall better result, greater degree of augmentation, and less risk of infection would put silicone implants as the choice for patients who desire a large degree of forehead silhouette enhancement. The properly prepared forehead silicone implant with corrugated edges and central perforations will allow for a more smooth contour and fixation of the implant, with minimal capsule contraction. The proper preparation of the implant is therefore of critical importance to the success of the operation. The following is the author's personal technique.

PREOPERATIVE CONSULTATION

During the preoperative consultation, a computer imaging scan of the side profile of the forehead is important to understand the contour and degree of the patient's desirable forehead augmentation. The surgeon then decides if the simpler ePTFE augmentation is sufficient to achieve the desirable result. If silicone implant augmentation is chosen, the proper fabrication of the implant is of critical importance as there will not be much leeway for error. The template will then be put on to the patient's forehead after a digital photo is taken, and compared with the computerized imaging photo with the patient's critique and consent, before it is sent for manufacture of the actual silicone implant. The following is a step-by-step outline of the author's technique in silicone implant forehead augmentation.

TEMPLATE FABRICATION AND SILICONE IMPLANT CREATION

Fabrication of a template is a multistep process, and can be undertaken using simple materials found in a dental office (dental alginate, dental plaster, and dental wax). In overview, a negative template is created using fast-setting dental alginate, which is then used to create a positive template plaster mold of the patient's forehead. A wax template is then sculpted onto the plaster template that will be used to create the silicone implant.

Advanced Aesthetic Plastic Surgery Centre, 54 Redlea Avenue, Toronto, ON M1V 4S3, Canada
E-mail address: drjosephwong@bellnet.ca

Facial Plast Surg Clin N Am 18 (2010) 71–77
doi:10.1016/j.fsc.2009.11.006
1064-7406/10/$ – see front matter © 2010 Elsevier Inc. All rights reserved.

facialplastic.theclinics.com

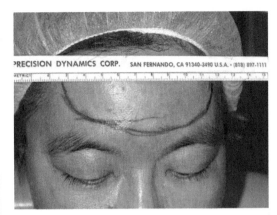

Fig. 1. Horizontal measurement for dimensions of forehead implant.

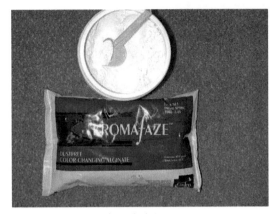

Fig. 3. Fast-setting dental alginate.

1. First, the area of the patient's forehead that requires augmentation is outlined with a surgical marking pen, and the measurements of the horizontal and vertical dimensions are recorded (**Figs. 1** and **2**).
2. A fast-setting dental alginate is combined with water in a mixing bowl to form the negative template of the forehead. Before the alginate completely dries, the paste is applied directly to the patient's forehead and sculpted to encompass the entire area that requires augmentation (**Figs. 3** and **4**).
3. A firm base plate is affixed to the backside of the alginate template as a backing material. After the alginate fully hardens in several minutes, it is gently removed from the patient's forehead (**Fig. 5**). The remainder of the process can be performed at a later time without the patient being present (**Fig. 6**).
4. A dental plaster mold is formed by pouring the plaster carefully onto the negative alginate template. A cardboard backing can be affixed

to the plaster before it dries to provide a flat surface that will aid in the next step of fabricating the wax template (**Figs. 7–9**).
5. Using digital imaging analysis as a guide, the surgeon can estimate approximately how large the wax template (and ultimately the silicone implant) should be. A dental base plate wax can be heated in hot water until it softens and then placed onto the set plaster mold to sculpt the precise dimensions of the template that will serve as a guide for the silicone implant. A thickness of 3 to 4 mm will typically be necessary to accomplish the task, and no greater than a 5-mm thick implant has been clinically necessary. The template should be designed with a thicker central region that tapers laterally in the temporal areas. Inferiorly, the implant should taper toward the superior aspect of the suprabrow ridge, or bony prominence, which typically begins several centimeters above the orbital rim. The base plate wax is packaged in sheets, which can be layered and sculpted

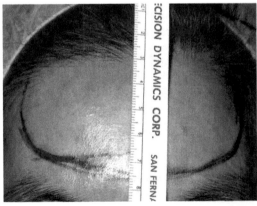

Fig. 2. Vertical measurement for dimensions of forehead implant.

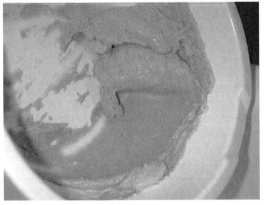

Fig. 4. Dental alginate is mixed with water until a thick, uniform paste develops.

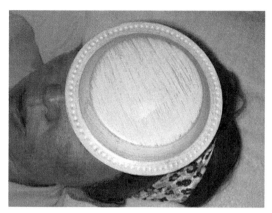

Fig. 5. Paste is applied directly to the patient's forehead.

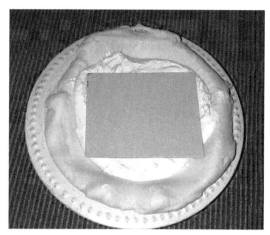

Fig. 7. Plaster is poured carefully onto the negative alginate template.

when soft until the desired size and shape have been attained according to the desired specifications (**Figs. 10** and **11**).

6. With 1 or 2 wax templates created, the patient can then return for a second visit and at that time don the wax template to see if the dimensions conform to his or her aesthetic expectations. After the template has been applied to the patient's forehead, the patient can be asked to view his or her brow obliquely using a hand-held mirror, to confirm the suitability of the design. Digital imaging of the profile view with the template in place can help the patient better appreciate whether the implant will meet the patient's aesthetic criteria. The wax template can be further refined during this session by heating it again or sculpting it more until the patient expresses satisfaction.

7. The silicone implant is carved from a standard solid rectangular block (usually 15 × 8 cm of soft silicone) that matches as precisely as possible the dimensions of the carved wax

template. (The surgeon may elect to have the carved wax template and plaster mold forwarded to a silicone manufacturer for fabrication and returned, to obviate the burden of carving the implant himself or herself. Nevertheless, acquired proficiency will often permit carving the implant within 30 minutes.) A no. 10 or 15 Bard-Parker blade can be used to refine the silicone block until the shape and size conform to the proposed wax template design. The very nature of carving the silicone block will lead to an imprecise and rough-hewn contour, which not only is acceptable but leads to better protection from site dislodgement after implantation. The general shape of the implant should approximate a crescent on profile view, with the thickest section in the midforehead that tapers gradually toward the temporal edges, as described for

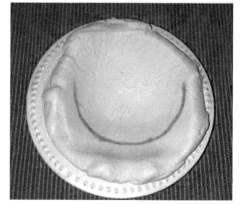

Fig. 6. Hardened alginate forms an impression of the forehead and outline of the proposed implant.

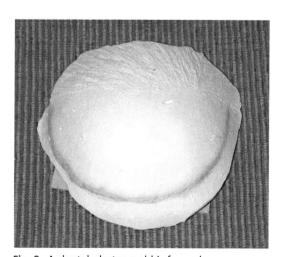

Fig. 8. A dental plaster mold is formed.

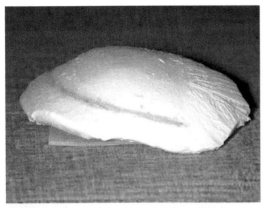

Fig. 9. A cardboard backing can be affixed to the plaster before it dries to provide a flat surface that will aid in the next step of fabricating the wax template.

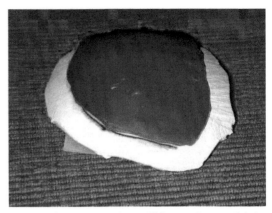

Fig. 11. The wax template will be used to model the final silicone implant.

the wax template. This crescentic shape permits a smooth transition from the augmented to the nonaugmented regions. Because of the aforementioned surface irregularities that arise after carving, it is not recommended to show the patient the carved implant for fear that he or she might misinterpret the accuracy of the design. Eight to 10 holes are then created in a uniform distribution across the implant that will facilitate tissue ingrowth and add to implant stability; a 3- or 4-mm round punch biopsy instrument can expedite creation of these holes. In addition, V-shaped wedges should be removed along the entire perimeter of the implant: the triangular excisions can measure approximately 3 to 4 mm in size and be distributed roughly every centimeter across the entire perimeter. These V-shaped excisions permit the edges of the

implant to conform to the rounded contour of the forehead more easily, and minimize the risk of buckling that may otherwise occur. After carving, the implant can be autoclaved in preparation for surgical implantation (**Figs. 12** and **13**).

SURGICAL TECHNIQUE

1. In the preoperative surgical room, the patient has 3 incisions marked out that closely match 3 of the 5 standard incisions for an endoscopic, or minimal-incision, brow lift: one vertical incision that measures about 2 cm is placed centrally immediately behind the hairline, and 2 temporal incisions are designed that extend about 4 cm in length behind the hairline. The hair can be secured with paper tape to expose the proposed incision lines to facilitate surgery. Note that a minimal-incision brow lift can be undertaken concurrently with a forehead implant in a patient who would

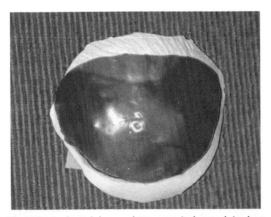

Fig. 10. A dental base plate wax is heated in hot water until it becomes soft. Wax is sculpted onto the plaster mold to the precise dimensions that will match the patient's wishes for forehead augmentation.

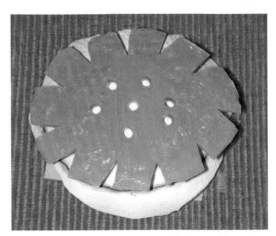

Fig. 12. The silicone implant was fashioned based on the prescribed dimensions.

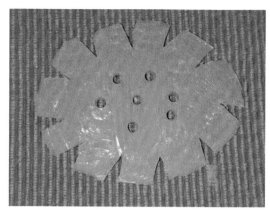

Fig. 13. Corrugated edges and central perforations on the soft silicone implant are made before surgery to minimize mobility and enhance fixation.

benefit from this rejuvenative procedure. The implant would be inserted and secured into proper position before brow-suspension sutures would be placed.

2. The patient is administered intravenous sedation or general anesthesia, and 1% lidocaine with 1:100,000 epinephrine is infiltrated into the incisions directly and along the arcus marginalis.
3. A no. 15 Bard-Parker blade is used to incise the central incision down through the periosteum, and a brow elevator is used to dissect downward to release the arcus marginalis along the orbital rim, carefully avoiding the supraorbital neurovascular bundles. A "smart

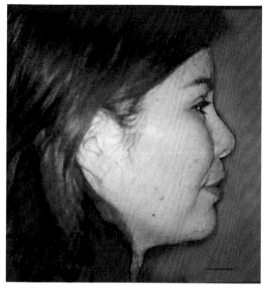

Fig. 15. 35-year-old Asian woman 3 months postoperatively.

hand" dissection or endoscopic guidance can be used. The arcus marginalis should be completely released for implants that extend to the immediate suprabrow position so that the implant can freely rest in the intended position without buckling inferiorly or being restricted from proper positioning.

4. The 2 temporal incisions are then made, and dissection is performed in the subtemporoparietal fascia plane as undertaken in a standard endoscopic, or minimal-incision, brow lift. The conjoined tendons that separate the lateral temporal from the medial subperiosteal pockets are completely severed from a lateral

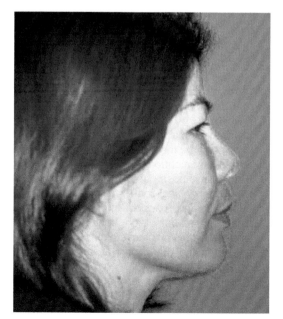

Fig. 14. 35-year-old Asian woman before surgery.

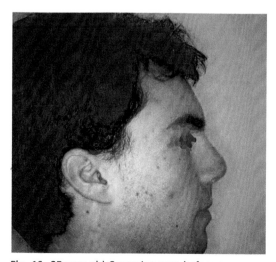

Fig. 16. 25-year-old Caucasian man before surgery.

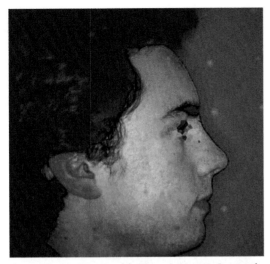

Fig. 17. ame 25-year-old Caucasian man 3 months postoperatively.

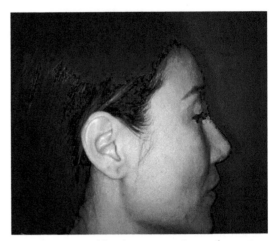

Fig. 19. 40-year-old Asian woman 3 months postoperatively.

to medial direction, as per routine for a brow lift.

5. A surgical marking pen is used to mark out 2 dots that are separated a distance of 1.0 to 1.5 cm and that are located along the central aspect of the forehead. The clear implant is then laid over the forehead where the surgeon would like it to be placed, and 2 dots are drawn onto the implant exactly over the 2 dots that were made on the skin below.

6. A 3-0 nylon suture is passed through one of the marked dots on the skin, and the needle is pulled out through one of the temporal incisions.

7. The same needle is placed through one of the marked dots on the silicone implant (the dot that corresponds with the outer skin dot that was pierced initially) from the superficial to

deep surface, and passed back through the other dot on the implant from deep to superficial.

8. The needle is driven back through the remaining dot on the skin, and the suture is gently pulled through.

9. A hemostat can be placed on both ends of the suture to prevent one end of the suture from falling through the skin inadvertently.

10. The implant is inserted into the subperiosteal pocket via 1 of the 2 temporal pockets, using the 3-0 nylon suture as a guide. The implant can be rolled for ease of insertion, as the implant often will be larger than the temporal incision length.

11. The implant is then unfurled in situ, and the edges are inspected carefully to ensure that there is no buckling or folding. The implant can be palpated carefully through the skin to ensure that it is properly positioned, and endoscopic confirmation can also be beneficial.

12. After the implant resides in perfect orientation and position, the 3-0 nylon suture can be tied down over a cotton bolster, which remains for 3 to 4 days postoperatively.

13. A 15-French Jackson-Pratt-style drain can be inserted and passed through a separate temporal stab incision behind the hairline, which is left in place overnight to be removed the following day if only a small amount of drainage is present.

14. The skin incisions are approximated with surgical staples, which can be removed on the seventh postoperative day. No compressive dressing is necessary.

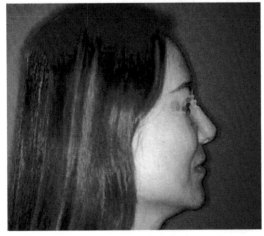

Fig. 18. 40-year-old Asian woman before surgery.

A preoperative and 3-month postoperative comparison of 3 patients is illustrated in **Figs. 14–19.**

SUMMARY

A simple, reliable, and safe technique using a soft silicone implant is described for a large degree of forehead silhouette augmentation.

REFERENCES

1. Ballin M. A method of cranioplasty. Surg Gynecol Obstet 1921;33:79.
2. Dufresne CR, Carson BS. Craniomaxillofacial deformities. In: Papel ID, Nachlas NE, editors. Facial plastic and reconstructive surgery. St. Louis (MO): Mosby Year Book; 1992. p. 520–31.
3. Shermak MA, Carson BS, Dufresne CR. Issues in craniofacial surgery. In: Dufresne CR, Carson BS, Zinreich SJ, editors. Complex craniofacial problems. New York: Churchill Livingstone; 1992. p. 137–50.
4. Pietrzak WS, Sarver DR, Verstynen ML. Bioabsorbable polymer science for the practicing surgeon. J Craniofac Surg 1997;8:87–91.
5. Pietrzak WS, Verstynen ML, Sarver DR. Bioabsorbable fixation devices: status for the craniomaxillofacial surgeon. J Craniofac Surg 1997;8:92–6.
6. Scott M, Wycis HT. Experimental observations on the use of stainless steel for cranioplasty. J Neurosurg 1946;3:310.
7. Small JM, Graham MP. Acrylic resin for the closure of skull defects. Br J Surg 1945;33:106.
8. Wong JK. Forehead augmentation. In: McCurdy JA Jr, Lam SM, editors. Cosmetic surgery of the Asian face. 2nd edition. New York: Thieme; 2005. p. 190–5.

Lip Reduction Surgery (Reduction Cheiloplasty)

Joe Niamtu III, DMD

KEYWORDS

- Lip reduction • Cheiloplasty • Reduction cheiloplasty
- Cosmetic lip surgery • Lip surgery • Double lip surgery

Lip enhancement has been a popular custom, especially in females, in most societies since the dawn of recorded history. Lip enhancement is the mainstay of the minimally invasive portion of most cosmetic facial surgery practices, but not all patients seeking cosmetic lip enhancement desire bigger lips. A certain percentage of the population seeks cosmetic consultation for lip reduction, and the cosmetic facial surgeon should be versed in this treatment option as well. In the author's personal experience, most patients presenting for lip reduction are of African American heritage but the author has performed this procedure on patients from other ethnic groups, including multiple Caucasians (**Fig. 1**).

DIAGNOSIS AND CONSULTATION

Macrocheilia defines a larger than normal lip. Various ethnic groups share the characteristic of larger lips including African American, Asian, and other groups (**Figs. 2 and 3**). For the remainder of this article racial lip differences with larger lip anatomy are referred to as "ethnic" lips. This term would apply to racial groups that commonly have lips that are larger than the Caucasoid lip and more frequently seek cosmetic lip reduction.

In the Caucasian patient the upper lip constitutes one-third of the total lip volume while the lower lip constitutes about two-thirds of the total lip volume, with a ratio of about 1:1.6 (**Fig. 4**).[1,2] African American lips are generally larger in all dimensions, and the upper and lower lip volumes are frequently nearly the same in many patients. Ethnic lips are also more protrusive, in part due to having more soft tissue mass. The normal chin and lip soft tissue thickness is approximately 12 mm in Caucasians and 15 mm in African Americans.[3] Vermilion height norms vary in different ethnicities; for example, on average, African American males have 13.3-mm upper lips and 13.2-mm lower lips, and African American females have 13.6-mm upper lips and 13.8-mm lower lips. North American Caucasian vermilion height norms of upper and lower lip for males and females are 8.0 and 8.7 mm and 9.3 and 9.4 mm, respectively.[4,5] In the normal situation there is a 0- to 3-mm intralabial gap between the lips in repose. Patients with larger intralabial space may not be good surgical candidates. The importance of ruling out dentofacial deformities as contributing factors to macrocheilia cannot be overstressed, and orthodontic, oral, and maxillofacial consultation and lateral cephalogram may be of assistance.

An additional contributing factor is fact that many African American patients exhibit a skeletal bimaxillary protrusion whereby the angulation of maxillary and mandibular alveolar bone and teeth protrude anteriorly, which influences the lip posture (**Fig. 5**). If dentofacial abnormalities are not recognized, lip reduction may be contraindicated and may worsen the cosmetic deformity by overly reducing lip size and exposing the dentofacial deformity. Finally, microgenia can frequently accompany a bimaxillary protrusive profile, and the lack of chin prominence can make the lower lip appear larger (**Fig. 6**).

A patient's self image of his or her lips, like other body parts, is relative. Some ethnic groups have

Cosmetic Facial Surgery, 10230 Cherokee Road, Richmond, VA 23235, USA
E-mail address: niamtu@niamtu.com

Facial Plast Surg Clin N Am 18 (2010) 79–97
doi:10.1016/j.fsc.2009.11.007
1064-7406/10/$ – see front matter © 2010 Elsevier Inc. All rights reserved

facialplastic.theclinics.com

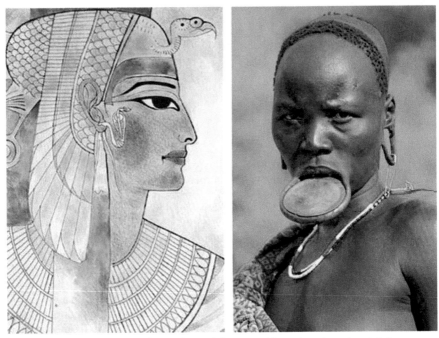

Fig. 1. Enhancing the lips is timeless and is performed for courtship, cultural, and societal purposes in women, men, and children in almost every society (*Courtesy of* Dr. Briar Diggs, Missoula, MT).

large lips and this is normal (and attractive) in that context. A subgroup of individuals in a given ethnic group may have bigger than normal lips (even for their ethnic type) and desire them smaller (**Fig. 7**).

Unusually large lips (like any body part) aesthetically can make a person appear or feel unattractive. In addition, adverse stereotypical characterizations amplify this characteristic (especially a "dangling" lower lip) and associate it with being dumb or mentally slow (reminiscent of "Bubba" in the movie Forrest Gump). Function can also be affected by very large lips as it can make speaking or eating difficult in some cases, and promote drooling in the case of abnormal orbicularis oris muscle tone.

Other ethnic patients presenting for lip reduction do not have abnormally large lips for their race, but want to look more "international." This desire falls into the same category as Asians altering their eyelids, African Americans straightening their hair, or Caucasians tanning their skin or getting lip filler. The author refers to this as the cosmetic paradox in that people with small features want

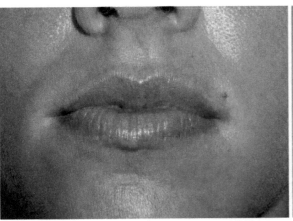
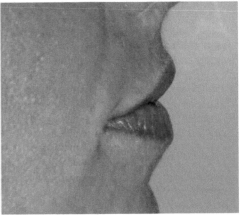

Fig. 2. This image shows what most Caucasian women would consider attractive lips.

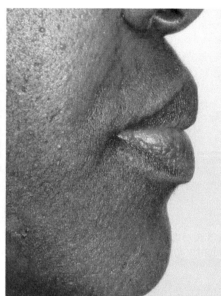
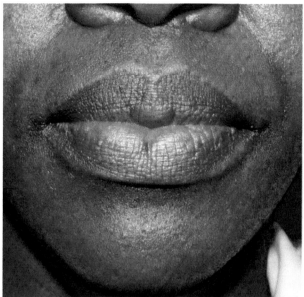

Fig. 3. Typical lip size of a patient seeking lip reduction.

big ones and people with big features want small ones. Beauty is truly in the eye of the beholder. Some people may say that "ethnic" patients have larger lips, whereas to "ethnic" patients Caucasians can be said to have small lips.

In a most eloquent dissertation on this subject Harold E. Pierce, a noted African American plastic surgeon from Howard University, states the following on the topic of race. "To the physician, as well as the public, there is confusion about the meaning of the word 'race' as applied to man. The biologist, however, who studies insects, plants, and other kinds of organisms about which there is on reason for emotional controversy, is not confused. To him a race is a collection, basically a group of individuals of both sexes definitely associated with a place of origin, habitually interbreeding and possessing a historical continuity in the reproduction of the general type. These individuals tend not only to look alike but to behave similarly. The concept of race includes differences in observable external characters, in behavior, in growth time and in other variables, all of which are genetically determined. In the long run, these variations serve to suit races to different environments or to different phases of a single environment. Near the Arctic Circle people are uniformly short; people native to areas of the greatest heat and sunlight tend to have dark skin and eye colors. The nose of an Arab would probably freeze were he to spend a day outdoors in Siberia, while flat faced Tungas are able to withstand extreme cold."[6]

Regardless of the desire, as for all cosmetic facial procedures, the surgeon must be certain that the patient is undergoing the procedure for the correct reasons and has reasonable expectations for the outcome.

DIFFERENTIAL DIAGNOSIS

Macrocheilia can be due to ethnic variation, a result of dentofacial deformities (pseudomacrocheilia), from pathology such as lymphatic

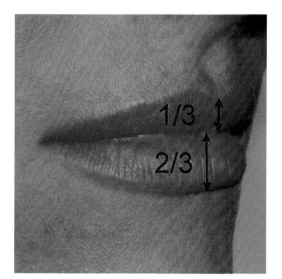

Fig. 4. The individual lip volume relative to the total lip mass in a Caucasian female.

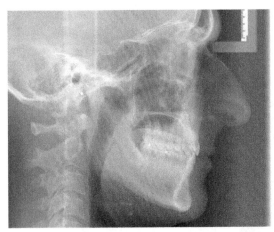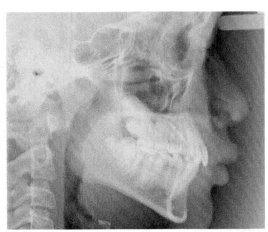

Fig. 5. (*Left*) A lateral cephalogram of a Caucasian male with a typical dentoskeletal relationship. (*Right*) A lateral cephalogram of an African American male with bimaxillary protrusion. Note the differences in alveolar, tooth, and lip relationships.

disorders or hemangiomas, and medical causes. Medical causes include Melkersson-Rosenthal syndrome, a rare neurologic disorder characterized by recurring facial paralysis, swelling of the face and lips (usually the upper lip), and the development of folds and furrows in the tongue.[7] Ascher syndrome is a rare disease first described in 1920 by an ophthalmologist of the same name. The disease is characterized by a double upper lip, blepharochalasis, and nontoxic thyroid enlargement.[8] These 2 medical entities often go undiagnosed, and the astute surgeon should always consider systemic disease as a contributing factor. In addition, some patients have lower lip ptosis due to orbicularis oris dysfunction or central nervous system problems, and orbicularis oris function should always be evaluated. Patients that cannot retract their lower lip or those with lip

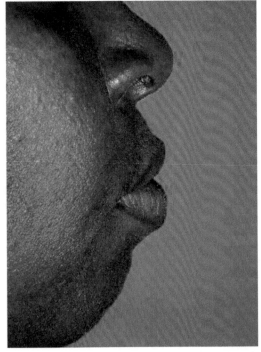

Fig. 6. Many African American patients with bimaxillary protrusion also exhibit microgenia, and the lack of chin balance further accentuates the lip protrusion.

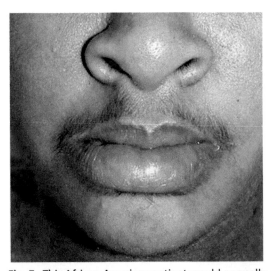

Fig. 7. This African American patient would normally have larger lips consistent with her racial characteristics but has an asymmetrically large and unbalanced lower lip, even for her ethnicity, as opposed to the patient pictured in **Fig. 3**, who has symmetrically large and balanced lips.

incompetence from poor muscle tone or other causes are not candidates for reduction cheiloplasty. Continual drooling may be a sign of poor muscle tone of the lower lip. These patients may benefit from a midline resection of lip and skin to shorten the width of the lower lip, which causes a sling effect in tightening the lip.

LIP ANATOMY AND HISTOLOGY

The lips serve many functions including eating, drinking, speaking, mimetic animation, kissing, and serving as a valve for the terminal oral airway.

The lips are among the most vascular structures on the face, and are supplied by the superior and inferior labial branches of the facial artery as it branches from the external carotid artery (**Fig. 8**). The labial artery lies in the posterior one-third of the lip at about the incisor level (**Fig. 9**). The depth of this artery is an important landmark to keep in mind, but fortunately is deep to most lip reduction procedures.

The anatomy of the lip is unique in that there is a triple transition from hair-bearing skin to vermilion tissue to oral mucosa. The hair-bearing skin terminates at the cutaneous/vermilion junction.

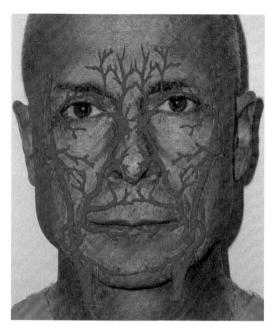

Fig. 8. The lips are supplied by the superior and inferior labial branches from the facial artery as it comes off the external carotid artery.

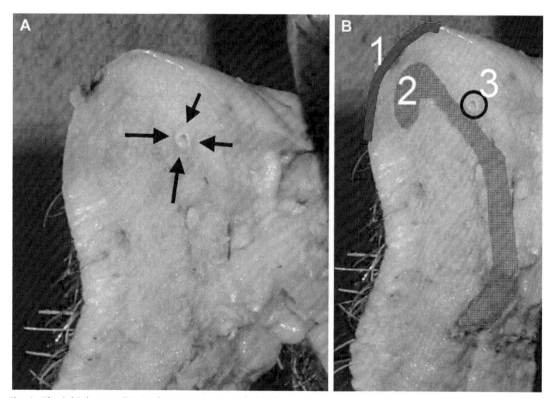

Fig. 9. The labial artery lies in the posterior one-third of the lip and is generally well out of the way in lip reduction procedures. (*A*) The labial artery; (*B*) relation of labial artery to the vermilion and orbicularis oris muscle.

The vermilion tissue consists of a very thin keratinized stratified squamous epithelium with extensive interdigitations with the underlying dermis (**Fig. 10**).

The vermilion is devoid of hair follicles, sweat glands, and sebaceous glands (although they may be sparsely present). It is the lack of sebaceous glands that causes the vermilion to dry and crack and, hence, they must remain moistened with saliva. Anecdotally (because this statement cannot be scientifically qualified), people with naturally larger lips seem to moisten them with their tongue with much greater frequency than people with smaller lips.

The vermilion derives its color from the rich vascular plexus in the underlying dermis. This area is also highly sensitive due to its rich sensory innervation.

The thin keratinized stratified squamous epithelium of the exposed vermilion transitions into a thick, nonkeratinized, stratified squamous epithelium, and becomes the intraoral mucosa (**Fig. 11**). Under this thicker epithelium lies a submucosa containing numerous accessory

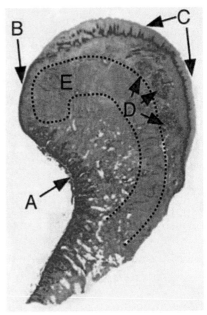

Fig. 11. The lip skin similar to surrounding facial skin contains hair follicles, and sweat and sebaceous glands (A). The vermilion portion of the lip consists of thin keratinized stratified squamous epithelium (B) and transitions to a thick non keratinized stratified squamous epithelium of the oral mucosa (C). The submucosa of the intraoral mucosa contains numerous minor salivary glands (D). The orbicularis oris muscle is seen underlying these structures and constitutes the bulk of the lip (E). The vermilion is almost in contact with the orbicularis oris muscle anteriorly. (*From* Applebaum E, Lamme A, Moss-Salentijn L. Orofacial histology and embryology: A visual integration. Philadelphia: FA Davis, 1972; with permission.)

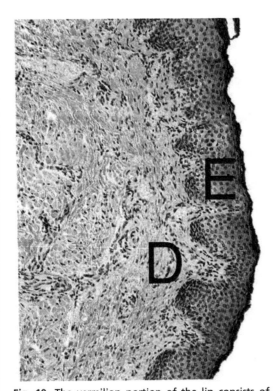

Fig. 10. The vermilion portion of the lip consists of a thin keratinized stratified squamous epithelium (E) which extensively interdigitates with the underlying dermis (D). (*From* Applebaum E, Lamme A, Moss-Salentijn L. Orofacial histology and embryology: A visual integration. Philadelphia: FA Davis, 1972; with permission.)

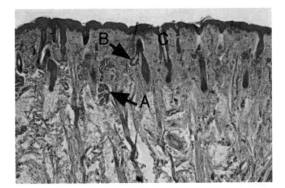

Fig. 12. The skin below the vermilion (or above in the upper lip) contains hair follicles, and sweat and sebaceous glands. The sebaceous glands open into the hair follicle while the sweat glands open to the skin. (*From* Applebaum E, Lamme A, Moss-Salentijn L. Orofacial histology and embryology: A visual integration. Philadelphia: FA Davis, 1972; with permission.)

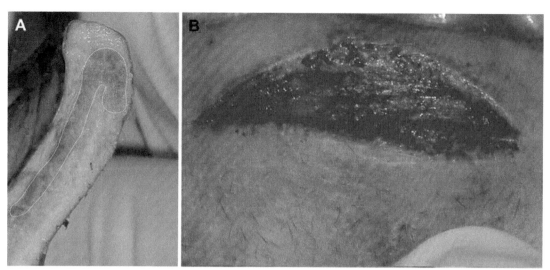

Fig. 13. The orbicularis oris muscle has circular fibers that travel circumorally, and is shown in transverse section (*A*) and exposed anteriorly (*B*).

salivary glands including serous, mucous, and mixed seromucous glands. As the anterior vermilion surface meets the skin, hair follicles, sweat glands, and sebaceous glands are present (**Fig. 12**).

The bulk of the lip volume is made up of the circumoral orbicularis oris muscle that blends laterally into the complex modiolus, which is a convergence of the perioral mimetic muscles (**Figs. 13** and **14**). Contrary to the reality of many surgeons, the orbicularis oris muscle is primarily on the intraoral surface of the lip and anteriorly only extends to the vermilion cutaneous border (**Fig. 15**).

LIP REDUCTION PROCEDURE
Preoperative

Preoperative evaluation involves discussing the procedure and anesthesia, and completing the informed consent process. Patients must understand that the recovery process can last from 1 to 3 weeks depending on swelling. The patients must further understand that sensation will be temporarily affected, as will normal function. It is also imperative to explain the need for conservative surgery, in that more tissue can be removed but it is difficult to put it back, much the same as blepharoplasty.

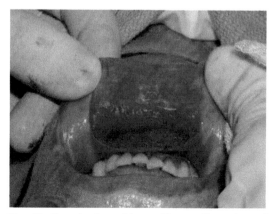

Fig. 14. The circular sphincter like configuration of the orbicularis oris fibers can be seen in this genioplasty incision.

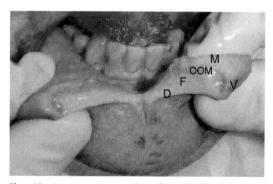

Fig. 15. A transverse section through the lower lip shows the dermis (D), fat (F), orbicularis oris muscle (OOM), vermilion (V), and oral mucosa (M). Note the orbicularis muscle is situated closer to the oral surface of the lip than the facial surface and also terminates as it curves around the vermilion cutaneous junction.

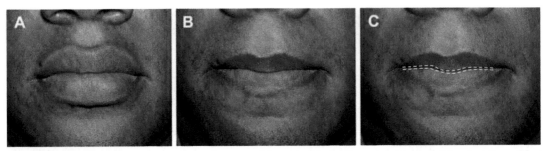

Fig. 16. This preoperative patient is shown in repose (A), and with the lips pursed to a position that the patient would like the final result to simulate (B). (C) Anterior incision markings that will be drawn in this "preview" position.

Patients are given a prescription for Cephalexin, 500 mg to be taken the day before surgery and for the first 5 days post operatively. Those with a history of frequent herpetic perioral outbreaks would also be placed on antivirals.

Anesthesia

Lip reduction can be effectively performed with local anesthesia alone, but because it can be a bloody procedure with significant manipulation, most patients and surgeons fare better with intravenous sedation.

Procedure

Reduction cheiloplasty has been described over the last 50 years by numerous investigators from multiple countries.[9–19] Like any procedure, many nuisances exist from surgeon to surgeon but, in reviewing the literature, the bases of the described procedures are very similar, and involve removing a fusiform or elliptical shaped section of tissue and closing the defect to change the posture of the lip.

When the patient arrives for surgery, all makeup is removed and a preoperative photographic series is taken with a minimum of frontal, three-quarter, and lateral views. Taking additional images of smiling and puckering can also be helpful in the future if a patient has complaints.

Similar to blepharoplasty surgery, marking the patient is very important. The lips should first be dried and wiped with alcohol to allow better ink adherence, and kept dry after marking with gauze between the lips so the saliva does not dilute the surgical markings. If the markings are lost or obscured, the result can be jeopardized. The patient should be marked in the upright position and before local anesthetic injection, as lying supine and anesthetic engorgement will distort the markings.

Marking the lips to discern the excess to be removed is more art than science. The basic premise is to make markings at or posterior to the wet/dry line as this will be the anterior extent of the incision, as well as the position of the suture line and final scar. Placing this too far forward can

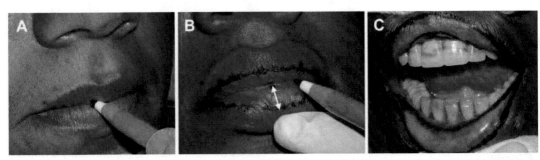

Fig. 17. Preoperative marking of the posterior extent of the excision. After the patient has been marked with the lips pursed, the patient is relaxed and a second (posterior) mark is made (A). A series of dots are marked in the relaxed position and connected with a solid line (B). (C) Final preoperative markings indicating the excess tissue to be removed. The anterior incision line should not be anterior to the wet/dry line so the scar can be hidden.

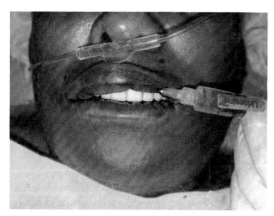

Fig. 18. Several milliliters of local anesthetic with vasoconstrictor are infiltrated into both lips.

make a visible scar and remove excessive vermilion. Placing the incision too far posteriorly can have less effect in "rolling" the lip back.

The author's personal marking technique is as follows. The patient is asked to lick his or her lips and relax them. Most patients will do this without occluding their teeth, which places the jaw and hence lip posture in a neutral position. Next, the patient is asked to purse his or her lips (pulling the lips toward the teeth), which will reduce the amount of protrusion and vermilion showing (Fig. 16).

The patient is given a mirror and asked to repeat this pursing maneuver to a point at which he or she would optimally like the amount of vermilion show and posture. This delineation is marked by making a series of dots from the commissure on one side to the commissure on the opposite side, which is then connected by a solid line.

To estimate the posterior extent of the incision, the patient relaxes the pursed lips and another series of marking dots are made, which are posterior to the first series as the lips are now relaxed and not pursed (Fig. 17).

This distance is measured, and the anterior markings are always kept at or close to the wet/dry line so the scar will not be visible. In cases of extreme vermilion hypertrophy, the incision can be carried into the "dry" vermilion. This marking method gives an approximation of conservative removal and is a reasonable guide for the novice surgeon. The experienced surgeon will find that several millimeters can be safely added without fear of overtreatment, and some clinicians advocate removing 2 to 2.5 times the measured amount, but this should be reserved for those surgeons with significant experience in treating macrocheilia. The lip midlines are also marked with a vertical hash mark to assist in symmetric wound closure at the end of the procedure.

The configuration of the marked area to be excised is a curved ellipse or "smiley face" that is larger in the center and tapers sharply toward the commissure. The width of the curved ellipse is commensurate with the amount of tissue excess to be removed. The edges of the curved ellipse gently taper into the commissure so as not to leave a "dog ear" deformity. The incision does go into the "corner of the mouth."

The author sedates all lip reduction patients, then infiltrates the lips with several milliliters of 2% lidocaine with 1:100,000 epinephrine (Fig. 18). This sedation is important for hemostasis, pain control, and hydrodissection. A vagolytic drug such as atropine or glycopyrrolate aids in reducing salivation.

Because the lips are so vascular, a scalpel or scissors are not used to dissect but, similar to the author's eyelid surgery, radiowave microneedle or CO_2 laser is used (Fig. 19). Both of these modalities provide simultaneous incision and hemostasis. Less bleeding translates into better

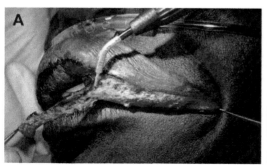
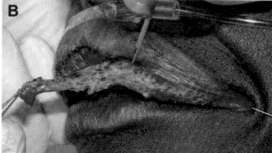

Fig. 19. The initial lip incision being performed with radiofrequency microneedle (A) and CO_2 laser (B).

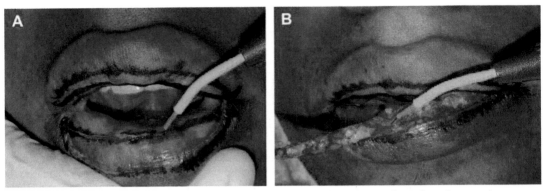

Fig. 20. The radiowave microneedle incision (*A*) and the excision of the mucosa from the submucosal structures (*B*).

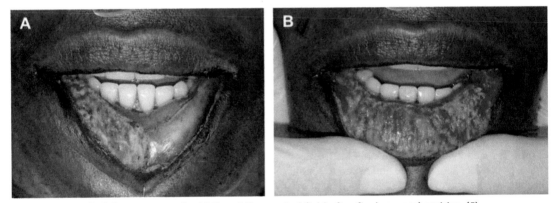

Fig. 21. One half of the mucosa excised (*A*) and the surgical field after final mucosal excision (*B*).

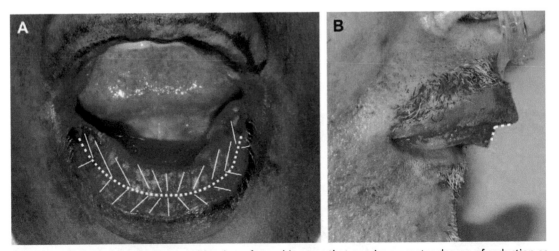

Fig. 22. A "V"-shaped deeper tissue excision is performed in cases that require a greater degree of reduction as only so much decrease in protrusion can be achieved by pulling skin alone. (*A*) An example of a case in which a wedge reduction is performed in the frontal view. (*B*) A similar case in the lateral view.

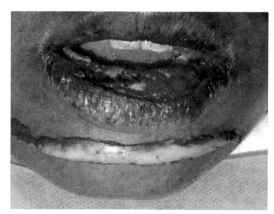

Fig. 23. Typical excess skin excised from a lip reduction procedure. The specimen is actually larger but contracts after removal.

surgery, less swelling, less pain and bruising, and faster recovery.

Dissecting the mucosa from the submucosa is very similar to peeling a grape or dissecting the skin from the orbicularis oculi muscle in blepharoplasty surgery (**Fig. 20**). The layer immediately under the mucosa consists of submucosa with abundant minor salivary glands, and occasionally the orbicularis oris muscle may be visible (**Fig. 21**).

An additional technique to control bleeding and simultaneously approximate a semblance of surgical result is to clamp the marked mucosa with a curved hemostat and crush the tissue together. This action creates a ridge whose base is easily excised, similar to a "skin pinch" blepharoplasty. When the tissues are pinched, the lip everts and the surgeon can visualize, in part, the result.

No undermining of the wound edges is performed or it would defeat the process of pulling back the lip. For minor reduction procedures removing the mucosa only may suffice to retract the lip back into a more retrusive position. For

very large reductions it may be necessary to remove some of the deeper tissue (namely submucosa, minor salivary glands and, rarely, orbicularis oris muscle) in a "V" or wedge-shaped excision to reduce some of the lip volume (**Fig. 22**). This reduction also takes tension off of the incision. Every attempt is made to not disrupt the orbicularis oris muscle so as not to affect its function. It is also important that the elliptical excision does not alter the cupid's bow or the central lip tubercle. The idea of this procedure is to remove enough tissue to roll the lip posteriorly without altering the normal anatomy. **Fig. 23** shows a typical excision specimen removed from the lip.

Hemostasis is important from the onset of the first incision, as the lips are so vascular that the surgical field can be obstructed. Final hemostasis is also important to prevent hematoma or increased swelling. A small tipped radiowave bipolar forceps is convenient for this surgery (**Fig. 24**).

After suitable tissue is removed, the wound margins can be temporarily approximated with tissue forceps to grossly anticipate the surgical result. This measurement is not entirely accurate, due to the effects of injected local anesthesia and surgical edema. Although more tissue can be removed and the result adjusted, it is always better to err on the conservative side, especially for the novice surgeon.

The surgical site is again checked for hemostasis and then closed. The author prefers to begin closure with a series of "key" sutures. First, the midline is determined and the first suture is placed. The "rule of halves" is followed by placing another suture one-half the distance to the end of the incision until 5 to 6 sutures are placed (**Fig. 25**). 4-0 gut, silk, or braided nylon is preferred for these sutures, which give strength to the wound. Finally a smaller 5-0 suture is used to close the remaining tissue (**Fig. 26**). If a continuous running suture is used, it should not be placed too tightly as to

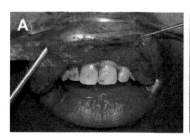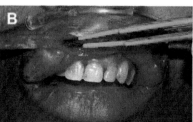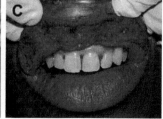

Fig. 24. Due to its extreme vascularity, lip surgery produces generous bleeding (*A*). (*B*) Areas of bleeding being cauterized with small tipped radiofrequency bipolar forceps. (*C*) The surgical site after hemostasis.

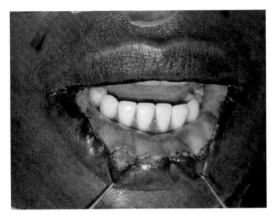

Fig. 25. 4-0 gut "key" sutures placed along the incision line to stabilize the repair.

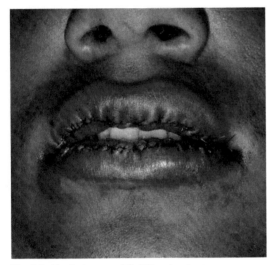

Fig. 26. Final closure with 5-0 gut suture.

prevent drainage. In addition, postsurgical edema can be significant and tight sutures can cause necrosis.

Initially, the suture line is visible due to edema and the patient must be made aware that, as healing progresses and the edema resolves, the lip will settle and the suture line will be hidden.

Subtotal Lip Reduction

Although most lip reduction cases involve removing a contiguous band of excess mucosa, some cases do not. In particular, some patients present with a "double lip" deformity where excess tissue is bilateral but not in the midline region (**Fig. 27**). These patients may show a significant amount of oral mucosa in addition to increased vermilion.

The surgical procedure is the same as previously described, and the midline is not resected (**Fig. 28**). In some cases the excision must encompasses the entire length of the lip to prevent "dog ear" deformities or maintain symmetry of the resection. Although, not in an ethnic patient, **Fig. 29** shows a case of a patient who presented for only midline lip excess reduction.

Traumatic Lip Excess

Although not an ethnic consideration, traumatic lip excess deformities are commonly seen in the cosmetic facial surgery practice (**Fig. 30**). Lip lacerations are frequently treated without proper closure and a hypertrophic scar can result, manifested by increased vermilion or mucosa show. This problem can also occur with proper closure, and can indicate retained foreign body. If these patients present shortly after injury, heat, massage, and intralesional steroid injection is first

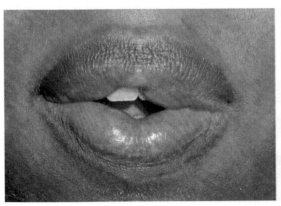

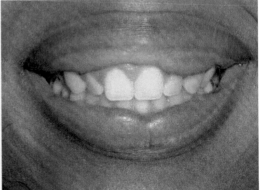

Fig. 27. A "double lip" deformity in repose and smiling. Patients can present with this situation from large lips, or sometimes with normal lip size, but pleated and pendulous oral mucosa that hangs down into view.

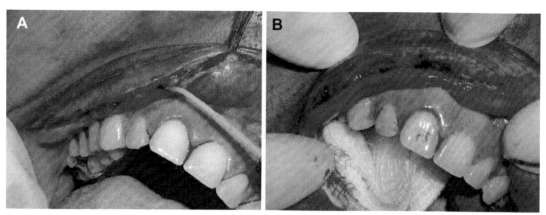

Fig. 28. Some patients present with unilateral or in this case bilateral lateral lip excess. Some of these cases can be treated singularly without crossing the midline, whereas other scenarios require midline incision to prevent "dog ear" deformities when closing. (*A*) Radiowave microneedle excision of excess lateral lip excess. (*B*) The surgical site.

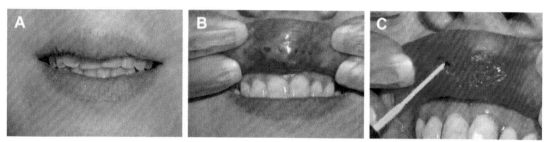

Fig. 29. (*A*) A Caucasian patient who presented with the chief complaint of midline upper lip excess. (*B*) The proposed surgical outline. (*C*) The excision site.

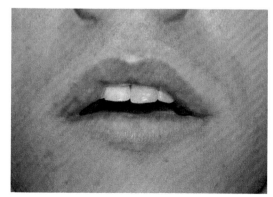

Fig. 30. Isolated posttraumatic lip excess deformities are commonly seen in the cosmetic facial surgery practice, and are treated in a similar manner as previously detailed.

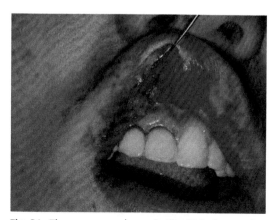

Fig. 31. The same case shown in **Fig. 30** is shown after excess mucosal resection. The dense scar tissue is evident and was removed with primary closure.

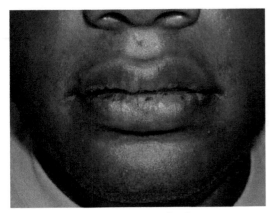

Fig. 32. A typical patient 1 week after surgery presenting for suture removal.

attempted. Resistant or long-standing traumatic lip excess lesions are surgically excised in a similar manner as previously described to excise excess mucosa and scar tissue (**Fig. 31**).

Postoperative Care

No distinct dressing is used for lip reduction cases, but the author occasionally tapes lips at the vermilion from cheek to cheek for 24 hours to restrict swelling. This dressing may be effective, but is very cumbersome to the patient. Intraoperative steroids are used, and the patient may be placed on postoperative oral steroids. Ice is applied immediately postoperatively and used for the next 2 to 3 days, and patients are asked to

sleep with their head elevated. Patients are asked to follow a liquid or soft diet for the first 72 hours, to refrain from excessive animation, and to use care while brushing the teeth. Wound care includes hydrogen peroxide and antibiotic ointment. Sutures are removed at 1 week postoperatively (**Fig. 32**).

Complications

Significant complications are rare with lip reduction surgery, and can be subjective in the case of under-resection. In this case a revision procedure may be necessary. Similar to blepharoplasty, over-resection is more problematic, and overly aggressive resections should be avoided, especially by novice surgeons. In the case of over-resection, a mucosal graft maybe required. In this situation, the incision is opened in the midline and the anterior and posterior tissue margins are undermined to create a gap, which should allow the lip to roll out anteriorly. This defect is then grafted with a mucosal graft harvested from the intraoral cheek mucosa.

Due to the extreme vascularity of the lips, some patients may experience alarming but harmless edema, and the patients should be forewarned (**Fig. 33**). The author has experienced several patients for whom this level of edema took 2 to 3 weeks to resolve. Head elevation, heat, and prednisone, 60 mg per day for 5 days is used to control postsurgical edema.

Due to the vascularity of the lips, postoperative lip reduction surgery infection is uncommon; for patients underoing lip reduction surgery, the author uses Cephalexin, 500 mg every 6 hours beginning the day before surgery and for the next 5 days.

As stated earlier, patients must be aware that sensation and movement of the lip will be affected for the first several weeks; these are considered sequelae and not complications.

Suture lines may be visible until the swelling resolves, and patients should be advised that they will feel irregularities along the suture line during the healing process. The extreme sensory sensitivity of the lips causes patients to take notice of these small irregularities more so than on other facial surfaces. Mucous retention "cysts" can develop and are simply ablated, but this has been a rare finding.

In the author's experience, most patients are happy after 4 to 8 weeks, and the biggest complaint is usually "I really like the result but I wish a tiny bit more could have been removed." Similar to eyelid surgery, this "last little bit" can

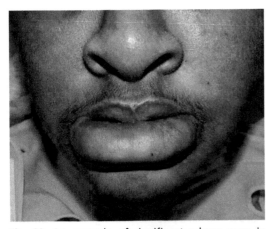

Fig. 33. An example of significant edema seen in some patients after lip reduction surgery.

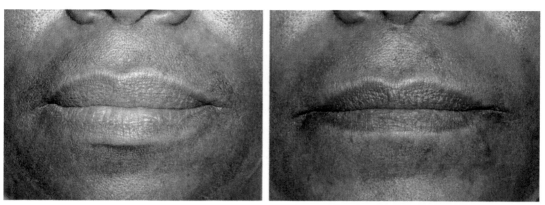

Fig. 34. This patient is shown 10 weeks after upper and lower lip reduction surgery.

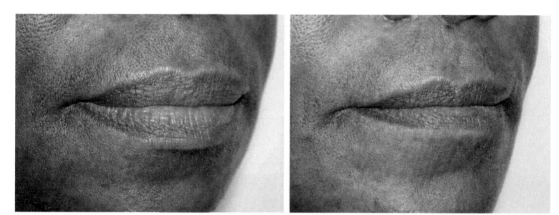

Fig. 35. The patient shown in **Fig. 34** is shown in the oblique view.

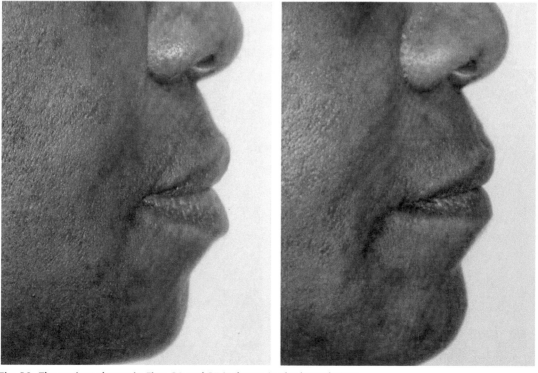

Fig. 36. The patient shown in **Figs. 34 and 35** is shown in the lateral view.

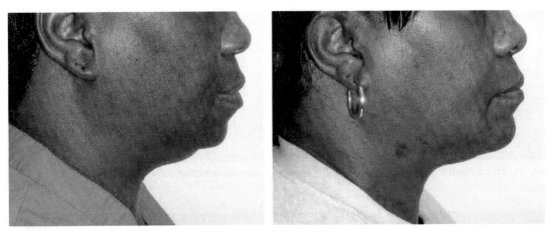

Fig. 37. The patient shown in **Figs. 34–36** is shown in the lateral facial view. A chin implant was simultaneously performed with the lip reduction surgery, and enhanced the overall perioral aesthetics.

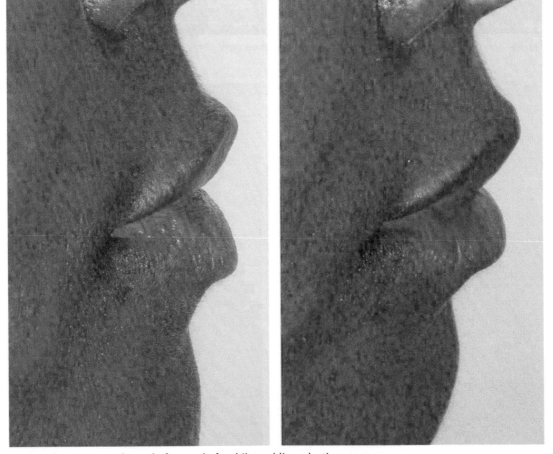

Fig. 38. This patient is shown before and after bilateral lip reduction surgery.

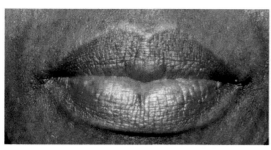
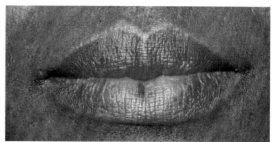

Fig. 39. This patient is shown after a conservative bilateral lip reduction.

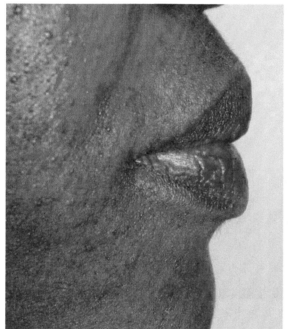
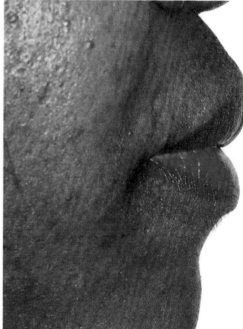

Fig. 40. The patient shown in **Fig. 39** is shown in the lateral view.

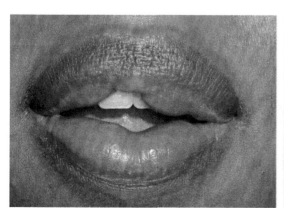
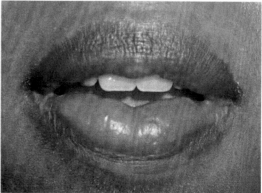

Fig. 41. This patient is shown in repose before and after upper lip only lateral excess reduction.

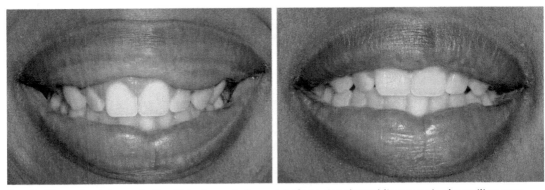

Fig. 42. The patient shown in **Fig. 41** is shown before and after upper lateral lip excess in the smiling pose.

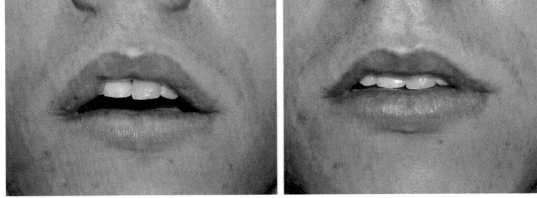

Fig. 43. This patient is shown before and after resection of posttraumatic lip hypertrophy on the upper right lip.

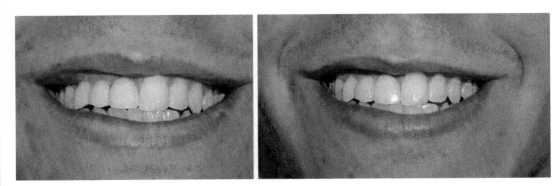

Fig. 44. The patient shown in **Fig. 43** is shown in the smiling pose.

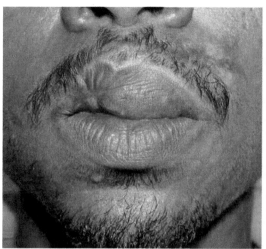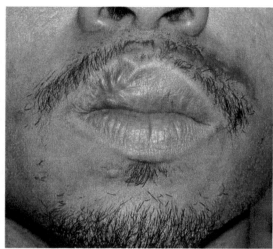

Fig. 45. This patient sustained a gunshot wound to the upper lip and is shown after the first stage of reconstruction, which involved reducing the hypertrophic lip scar excess. A secondary reconstruction is planned.

be the difference between a successful case and an overtreated case (**Figs. 34–45**).

REFERENCES

1. Niamtu J. The use of restylane in cosmetic facial surgery. J Oral Maxillofac Surg 2006;64:317–25.

2. Niamtu J, editor. New lip and wrinkle fillers. In: Minimally invasive cosmetic surgery oral and maxillofacial surgery clinics of North America, vol. 17. Philadelphia: Saunders; 2005. p. 17–27, 1.

3. Epker BN, Wolford LM. Reduction cheiloplasty: its role in the correction of dentofacial deformities. J Maxillofac Surg 1977;5(2):134–41.

4. Dev VR, Wang P. Lip reduction. Available at: http://emedicine.medscape.com/article/1288624-overview. Accessed June 15, 2009.

5. Farkas LG. Anthropometry of the head and face in medicine. New York: Elsevier Science; 1981.

6. Pierce HE. Cosmetic head and face surgery. In: Pierce HE, editor. Cosmetic plastic surgery in nonwhite patients. New York: Grune and Stratton; 1982.

7. El-Hakim M, Chauvin P. Orofacial granulomatosis presenting as persistent lip swelling: review of 6 new cases. J Oral Maxillofac Surg 2004;62(9):1114–7.

8. Ali K. Ascher syndrome: a case report and review of the literature. Oral Surg Oral Med Oral Pathol 2007; 103:e26–8.

9. Fanous N, Brousseau VJ, Yoskovitch A. The "bikini" lip reduction: an approach to oversized lips. Plast Reconstr Surg 2008;122(1):23e–5e.

10. Hoffman S. A simple technique for mucosal irregularities of the lip. Plast Reconstr Surg 1999;103(1):328.

11. Manstein CH. Vermilionectomy and mucosal advancement. Plast Reconstr Surg 1997;100(5): 1363. No abstract available.

12. O'Sullivan ST, O'Shaughnessy M. A simple technique for correction of mucosal irregularities of the lip. Plast Reconstr Surg 1998;101(4):1146–7.

13. Cortés-Aroche S. [Double lip treated with "midmoon" incision. Report of a case]. Rev Med Inst Mex Seguro Soc 2007;45(3):277–80 [in Spanish].

14. Pinto Rdos S, Marzola C. [Double lips–surgical technic]. Rev Assoc Paul Cir Dent 1966;20(5): 203–6 [in Portuguese].

15. Kruse-Lösler B, Presser D, Metze D, et al. Surgical treatment of persistent macrocheilia in patients with Melkersson-Rosenthal syndrome and cheilitis granulomatosa. Arch Dermatol 2005; 141(9):1085–91.

16. Rey R, Carreau JP, Gola R, et al. [Melkersson-Rosenthal syndrome. Value of reduction cheiloplasty]. Ann Dermatol Venereol 1996;123(5):325–7 [in French].

17. Stucker FJ. Reduction cheiloplasty. An adjunctive procedure in the black rhinoplasty patient. Arch Otolaryngol Head Neck Surg 1988;114(7):779–80.

18. Pierce HE. Cheiloplasty for redundant lips. J Natl Med Assoc 1976;68(3):211–2.

19. Calnan J. Congenital double lip: record of a case with a note on the embryology. Br J Plast Surg 1952;5(3):197–202.

The New "Genetico-Racial" Skin Classification: Maximizing the Safety of Skin Treatments for Asians

Valérie Côté, MD[a], Nabil Fanous, MD, FRCS(C)[a,b,c],*

KEYWORDS

• Skin • Classification • Racial • Asian • Peel • Laser

Current skin classifications, such as the "Fitzpatrick" or the "Obagi" ones, are mostly based on the skin color of patients contemplating whether to undergo a skin treatment.[1–5] These classifications also take into consideration other characteristics of lesser importance, such as the ease of acquiring sunburn, skin oiliness and thickness, and so forth. Predicting the outcome of a peel or a laser treatment is supposedly tied to the depth of the skin color, escalating from very white, to white, to olive, to yellow, to brown, to black.

According to these traditional classifications, Asians are all lumped into the "yellow" category; this vaguely means that they are better candidates than the darker "brown" and "black" ones, but less so than the lighter "white" and "olive" ones. Asians are thus considered somewhat "below average" on the scale of candidate idealism while the very white are supposedly the best, and the black the worst.

The new skin classification presented herein, first suggested by Fanous and colleagues,[6–11] is based on the patients' hereditary baggage: their race with its accompanying particular genetic composition. This "genetico-racial" classification proposes that patients' susceptibility and reaction to any skin treatment, whether it is a peel, a laser, a photo rejuvenation, and so forth, follow their genetic programming. Each race, therefore, comes with its genetic predisposition to any skin treatment.

THE RACES AND THEIR ORIGINS

Our earliest ancestors are believed to have appeared in Africa, the primary ancient continent, around 4 million years ago. Only a million or so years ago, they wandered out of Africa and into the other 2 ancient continents: Europe and Asia. Later, the human race ventured out of those 3 ancient continents and into the relatively younger ones.

Most anthropologists agree that the different populations spread across the planet all come from the same African origins. Yet, if one examines the inhabitants of the 3 ancient continents (the "Blacks" in Africa, the "Whites" in Europe, and the "Asians" in Asia), one cannot help but wonder at the amazing variations between those 3 races in their skin colors, and especially in their features in terms of shape, size, and contour.

[a] Department of Otolaryngology – Head and Neck Surgery, McGill University, Montreal, QC, Canada
[b] Department of Surgery, Sherbrooke University, Sherbrooke, QC, Canada
[c] The Canadian Institute of Cosmetic Surgery, 1, Westmount Square, Suite 1380, Montreal, QC H3Z 2P9, Canada
* Corresponding author. The Canadian Institute of Cosmetic Surgery, 1, Westmount Square, Suite 1380, Montreal, Quebec H3Z 2P9, Canada.
E-mail address: cosmeticsurgery123@videotron.ca (N. Fanous).

Facial Plast Surg Clin N Am 18 (2010) 99–104
doi:10.1016/j.fsc.2009.11.008
1064-7406/10/$ – see front matter Crown Copyright © 2010 Published by Elsevier Inc. All rights reserved

At this point, some intriguing questions come to mind: Why did the original African race metamorphose into 3 very dissimilar races? Furthermore, why does each one of these 3 races seem to be confined to mostly one continent? And, to further complicate the picture, why are the skin color and features lighter and finer respectively in the Northern parts of each continent, but gradually become darker and coarser as one moves more southward on each of those 3 continents?

The genetico-racial classification advances that the answer to the previous 3 puzzles is not a coincidence, but rather the product of evolutionary mechanisms.[12–15] According to Darwin, Nature enhances the survival of species by retaining their valuable physical characteristics suited to a specific environment. Nature does so by favoring the procreation of the individuals carrying those characteristics, while at the same time eliminating the undesirable ones with unsuitable physical traits.

In other words, it is most likely that over the course of many hundreds of thousands of years, each of the 3 races underwent evolutionary physical changes in response to their new habitat. These slow changes explain why Africans maintained their dark, thick skin as a protective shield against the intense ultraviolet sun radiation, as well as their large nasal cavities as an air-cooling mechanism. On the other hand, the Northern Europeans developed the opposite characteristics in the form of a light, thin skin and narrow nasal airways to accommodate the cloudy, cold weather.

THE GENETICO-RACIAL CATEGORIES

For the sake of simplicity, and for practical reasons, the 3 founding races, mainly the African, Caucasian, and Asian, are subdivided into 6 categories.

As one proceeds from north to south across the 3 ancient continents (Africa, Europe, and Asia), both the skin color and features change gradually and predictably, from lighter skin and finer features in the North to darker skin and coarser features in the South. As shown in **Fig. 1**, the racial categories run in a North-to-South manner, vertically across Europe and Africa, and in a parallel vertical manner across Asia.

The characteristics of the 6 categories may be summarized as follows.

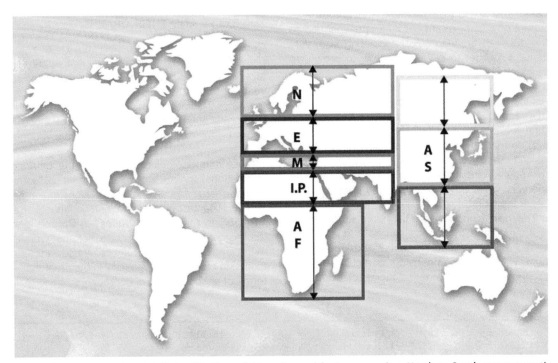

Fig. 1. The new "genetico-racial" classification of skin color and features runs in a North-to-South manner, vertically across Europe and Africa, and in a parallel vertical manner across Asia. In Europe and Africa, one finds the roots of: N = Nordic (*pink*), E = European (*red*), M = Mediterranean (*green*), I.P. = Indo-Pakistani (*brown*), AF = African (*gray*). In Asia, one finds the roots of: Northern Asian (*yellow*), Central Asian (*light orange*), Southern Asian (*dark orange*).

The Nordics (**Fig. 2A**) are individuals with Northern European roots (eg, Scandinavian, Irish). Nordics have thin pale white skin, fair hair, and fine features. Eyes are light brown, green, or blue.

The Europeans (**Fig. 2B**) are individuals with Central European roots (eg, France, Germany). The skin of Europeans is white with a slight tan, and their features are medium, neither too refined nor too coarse. Eyes are mostly brown, black, or gray.

The Mediterraneans (**Fig. 2C**) are individuals with Southern European (eg, Southern Italian, Greek) or Western Asian (eg, Turkish, Lebanese) roots. Mediterraneans are slightly darker than the Europeans, and their features are slightly coarser.

The Indo-Pakistanis (**Fig. 2D**) are individuals with Northern African (eg, Egyptian, Libyan, Tunisian) and Southern Asian (eg, Indian, Sri Lankan, Afghan) roots. Indo-Pakistanis have thick medium to deep brown skin and moderately coarse features.

The Africans (**Fig. 2E**) are individuals with Central African (eg, Sudanese, Ethiopian, Nigerian) or Southern African (eg, South African) roots. The skin of Africans is very thick and black, and their features are very coarse.

The Asians (**Fig. 3**) are individuals with Eastern Asian roots. Asians form a separate North-to-South classification across the Eastern section of Asia.

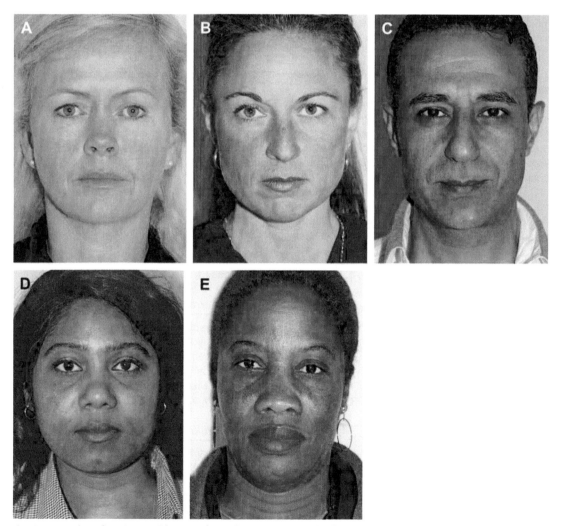

Fig. 2. Examples of patients with roots from the European and African continents. (*A*) Nordic: thin pale white skin, fine features. (*B*) European: white or slightly tanned skin, medium features. (*C*) Mediterranean: darker tanned skin, mildly coarse features. (*D*) Indo-Pakistani: thick medium to deep brown skin, moderately coarse features. (*E*) Africans: thick black skin, very coarse features.

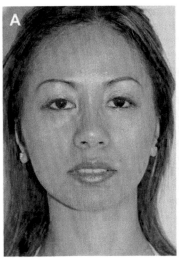
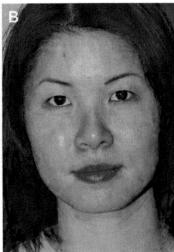
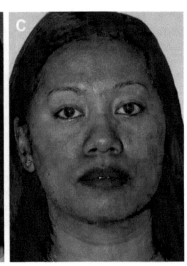

Fig. 3. Examples of patients with roots from the Asian continent. (*A*) Northern Asian: white or mildly tanned skin, mildly coarse features. (*B*) Central Asian: medium tanned skin, moderately coarse features. (*C*) Southern Asian: medium to dark brown skin, coarse to very coarse features.

Asians may be further subdivided into 3 subcategories.

Northern Asians (**Fig.** 3A), with roots in the northern part of Eastern Asia (eg, Mongolian, Northern Chinese, Northern Korean). The skin color of Northern Asians varies from white to one with a mild tan, and their features are mildly coarse.

Central Asians (**Fig.** 3B), with roots in the central part of Eastern Asia (eg, Japanese, Southern Chinese, Southern Korean). The skin of Central Asians has a medium tanned color, and their features are moderately coarse.

Southern Asians (**Fig.** 3C), with roots in the southern part of Eastern Asia (eg, Thai, Filipino, Vietnamese, Malaysian, Indonesian). The skin of Southern Asians is dark, varying from medium to dark brown; their features are coarse to very coarse.

RESPONSE OF THE GENETICO-RACIAL CATEGORIES TO PEELS AND LASERS
The Nordics

The main reaction is transient erythema. However, deep redness that persists beyond 3 or 4 weeks is possibly an early sign of potential complications, such as permanent erythema, telangiectasia, or even scarring.

Because of their lightly colored skin, Nordics rarely develop hyperpigmentation. Many physicians perceive the lack of pigmentation as a desirable reaction. Inflammatory hyperpigmentation is rarely permanent and almost always reversible.

Therefore, contrary to the classic skin classifications, the new genetico-racial classification considers the Nordic skin as a "good" candidate for peels and lasers, yet a potentially dangerous one because of being too thin. Nordics who are exposed to deep peels or aggressive laser resurfacing may develop one of the most dreaded complications of any skin treatment: scarring.

The Europeans

The main reaction is usually minimal erythema or minimal hyperpigmentation.

Therefore, Europeans are considered the ideal candidates for all skin treatments.

The Mediterraneans

The main reaction is mild to moderate erythema, which quickly turns into mild to moderate inflammatory hyperpigmentation. Because hyperpigmentation is almost always reversible and temporary, Mediterraneans are considered to be good to very good candidates for skin treatments.

The Indo-Pakistanis

The main reaction is moderate to deep hyperpigmentation, with possibly mild hypopigmentation in cases of aggressive skin procedures. Hypopigmentation, contrary to hyperpigmentation, often stays permanently, which makes it one of the two most feared complications of peels and lasers (the other one being scarring). Therefore, Indo-Pakistanis are passably good candidates, as long as skin treatments are moderate. As a general rule, they are more vulnerable to laser resurfacing than to peels.

The Africans

The main reaction, like the Indo-Pakistanis, is hyperpigmentation, but they exhibit a greater tendency toward hypopigmentation. Therefore, Africans are passable candidates, on the condition that their treatments do not exceed mild to moderate peels or very mild laser procedures.

The Asians

The main reaction of the Northern and Central Asians is a moderate to severe erythema and hyperpigmentation (Table 1). It is the hyperpigmentation response that scares physicians not accustomed to treating Asian skin.

As for the Southern Asians, they also share the same combined reaction of erythema and hyperpigmentation, in addition to being somewhat vulnerable to hypopigmentation because of their darker skin.

Therefore, Asians in general are very good candidates for medium or medium-to-deep peels, as well as for conservative laser resurfacing. The only exception is the Southern Asians, who are still good candidates but require gentler treatments.

POST PEEL/POST LASER CARE FOR ASIAN PATIENTS

There are 5 steps that are valuable regarding the care for Asians following their skin treatments (peels, lasers), with the aim of controlling side effects and enhancing results.

Wet Treatment

Showers, with only lukewarm water, should be started 24 to 48 hours following the skin treatment. After each shower, a very light layer of petroleum-based jelly (eg, Vaseline) is used to cover the skin.

Avoiding the Daylight and Sun

Nothing is more crucial to control post-treatment hyperpigmentation than to avoid sun rays. Avoiding the sun means not being exposed to the sun at all, period! Patients are instructed to stay indoors. Although sun blocks have a beneficial but limited effect, some of them may actually exacerbate the inflammatory hyperpigmentation if they irritate the skin. Patients are instructed to use a heavy make-up foundation (as a physical block) even while being indoors during the day, because the indoor daylight is nothing less than some indirect sunlight that has found its way through the doors and windows (UVAs have in fact been shown to be well transmitted through glass).

Steroid Creams

Inflammatory hyperpigmentation responds well to mild or moderately strong steroid creams, applied in small amounts on dark skin areas nightly.

The regimen is adjusted depending on the response of the skin, and often lasts a few weeks to a few months. This regimen is satisfactory as long as the mildest strength of steroid is used, with the least possible frequency.

Topical Tretinoin (Retin-A)

The application of tretinoin, in concentration of 0.025% to 0.1% nightly, is an excellent antihyperpigmentation agent. One rule to remember is not

---

Table 1
Summary of the response of Asians to peels and lasers

Asian Category	Geographic Origin	Skin Reaction to Peels/Laser	Candidate Rating
Northern Asian	Mongolia, Northern China, Northern Korea	Moderate to severe erythema and hyperpigmentation	Very good
Central Asian	Japan, Southern China, Southern Korea	Moderate to severe erythema and hyperpigmentation	Very good
Southern Asian	Thailand, Philippines, Vietnam, Malaysia, Indonesia	Moderate to severe erythema and hyperpigmentation Susceptibility to hypopigmentation	Very good (if gentle treatments)

to start it before 2 or 3 weeks after the skin treatment, to make sure the initial healing has taken place. Another rule to observe is to interrupt the tretinoin treatment if it irritates the skin too much (if the skin feels itchy and sensitive, or it peels), then resume it when the skin recovers.

Hydroquinone

Contrary to popular convictions, the authors believe the role of hydroquinone in hyperpigmentation is helpful, but limited and very slow acting. The authors still use it, but only as a secondary line of treatment.

SUMMARY

The geneticoracial classification introduces a "paradigm shift" in the way one sees skin prior to, during, and after any peel or laser treatments:

- Genetic programming of the different races controls the patients' response to skin treatments and their susceptibility to complications.
- Three criteria allow one to determine the patient's geneticoracial category: (1) features; (2) skin color; and (3) the country of origin of the patient's two parents.
- Patients belonging to the most Northern category (Nordics) as well as those belonging to the most southern categories (Indo-Pakistanis and Africans) are potentially dangerous candidates, because they are susceptible to "irreversible" complications, mainly scarring and hypopigmentation, respectively.
- Asians are very good candidates if one understands their characteristic skin response, if the ideal depth of treatment is used, and if the proper postoperative care guidelines are followed.

ACKNOWLEDGMENTS

The authors express their thanks to Michael Fanous for the literature research and for organizing the manuscript; to Ildiko Horvath, medical artist, Montreal General Hospital, for her assistance in preparing the artwork; to Catherine Dalal, administrative assistant, for the typing of the manuscript; to Minerva Khalife and Annick Laporte for their photographic contribution; and to Barbara Armbruster, MA, for the editing.

REFERENCES

1. Fitzpatrick TB. The validity and practicality of sun-reactive skin types 1 through V1. Arch Dermatol 1988;124:869–71.
2. Brody H. Chemical peeling. St-Louis (MO): Mosby; 1992. p. 35–41.
3. Monheit G. Advances in chemical peeling. Facial Plast Surg Clin North Am 1994;2:5–9.
4. McCollough G, Langston P. Dermabrasion and chemical peeling. A guide for facial plastic surgeons. New York: Thieme Medical Publishers; 1998.
5. Obagi Z. Obagi Symposium manual; 1992.
6. Fanous N, Hopping S. TCA peel course, annual meeting of the American Academy of Cosmetic Surgery. Los Angeles (CA), 1995.
7. Fanous N. TCA for Asians. Facial Plast Surg Clin 1996;4:1195–200.
8. Fanous N, Prinja N, Sawaf M. Laser resurfacing of the neck. Aesthetic Plast Surg 1998;22:159–65.
9. Fanous N, Bassas AE, Ghamdi WA. Co2 laser resurfacing of the neck and face: 10 golden rules for predicting results and preventing complications. vol. 8, n 2: Facial Plast Surg Clin 2000. p. 405–13.
10. Fanous N. A new patient classification for laser resurfacing and peels: predicting responses, risks and results. Aesthetic Plast Surg 2002;26:99–104.
11. McCurdy JA, Lam SM. Cosmetic surgery of the Asian face. New York: THIEME Medical Publishers; 2005. p. 253–54.
12. Darwin C. The origin of species. London: John Murray; 1859.
13. Friedrichs HF. Neuer untersuchen zeitschrift fur anatomie und entwicklungsgeschchichte. Schodel und Unterkiefer: von Piltdown 1932 [in German].
14. Wolpoff M, Caspari R. Race and human evolution. New York: Simon and Schuster; 1997.
15. Blumenbach JF. De generis humani varietate nativa. 1775.

Laser Treatment for Ethnic Skin

Paul J. Carniol, MD[a,b,]*, Heather Woolery-Lloyd, MD[c], Alice S. Zhao, BA[a], Kim Murray, MD[a]

KEYWORDS

- Ethnic skin • Laser treatment • Fitzpatrick skin types
- Complications

Over the past 10 years, there has been a paradigm shift in facial rejuvenation. With the growth of new technology and products, there has been an increased ability to improve a patient's appearance with procedures that can be performed in an office setting, including laser procedures. Demand for these procedures has grown among all ethnic groups. Therefore, it is important to understand the issues related to laser and light therapy for patients with all skin types.

There are several issues related to treating patients with ethnic skin. Depending on multiple factors, patients with ethnic skin can have varying response to lasers. This factor should be considered when planning their treatment.

Patients with ethnic skin are at greater risk for post-treatment pigment-related issues through at least 3 mechanisms. The first mechanism is the increased unanticipated laser energy absorption by melanin, or incidental absorption laser energy by melanin as a competing chromophore. The second is greater risk for problems with postinflammatory hyperpigmentation. The third is loss of pigment due to laser effects on melanin production or the melanocyte population, leading to hypopigmentation.

Considering this, any laser therapy should be planned carefully, especially in the treatment of patients with darker skin types as there are increased associated risks. In addition to this edition of the *Clinics*, further information can be found in other publications.[1]

COMPETING CHROMOPHORES

Substances that absorb laser/light energy are called chromophores. For any laser treatment there are target chromophores and competing chromophores. The target chromophore is the molecule or tissue component at which the laser is being directed to obtain the desired effect. A competing chromophore is a molecule or tissue component that is incidentally affected by the light energy. When performing laser/light treatments, melanin will frequently act as a competing chromophore. Darker skin has more melanin than lighter skin; therefore, potential issues caused by incidental melanin absorption as a competing chromophore is more significant in patients with darker skin. Whenever planning a laser treatment, it is important to consider the effects on both the target and competing chromophores.

SKIN TYPES

There is more than one classification of skin types. Skin types can be identified according to base hue, sensitivity to sun exposure, and propensity for photodamage or photoaging. The most common classification of skin is the Fitzpatrick grading system,[2] based on response to UV exposure. This system is very useful clinically as it has some correlation with pigmentation issues post laser treatment, and is summarized in **Table 1**. Individual members of an ethnic group can fall into different Fitzpatrick groups, and patients

[a] New Jersey Medical School - University of Medicine and Dentistry, New Jersey, NJ, USA
[b] PJC Laser, 33 Overlook Road, Suite 202, Summit, NJ 07901, USA
[c] University of Miami School of Medicine, Miami, FL, USA
* Corresponding Author. PJC Laser, 33 Overlook Road, Suite 202, Summit, NJ 07901.
E-mail address: PJCLaser@aol.com

Facial Plast Surg Clin N Am 18 (2010) 105–110
doi:10.1016/j.fsc.2009.11.009
1064-7406/10/$ – see front matter © 2010 Elsevier Inc. All rights reserved.

Table 1
Fitzpatrick skin types

Skin Type	Skin Tone/Hair/Eye Color	Skin Reaction to Sun Exposure
I	Lightest skin/light hair/light eyes	Always burns, never tans
II	Light skin/fair to dark hair/light eyes	Always burns, minimal tan
III	Medium tone skin/brown hair/dark hazel-brown eyes	Burns minimally, tans gradually
IV	Tan skin/dark hair/brown eyes	Burns minimally, tans well
V	Brown skin/dark hair/brown eyes	Rarely burns, tans profusely
VI	Dark brown/dark hair/dark eyes	Never burns, tans deeply

should not immediately be assigned to a Fitzpatrick group based solely on their ethnicity.

DYSCHROMIA

When evaluating patients who present for laser treatment, it is important to note if they have any dyschromia. Many patients have some baseline dyschromia or melasma. Depending on the laser and the conditions being treated this can improve, remain the same, or increase with laser/light treatments. Furthermore, laser procedures can cause dyschromia.

In general, the greater the amount of melanin in a patient's skin the greater the tendency toward dyschromia or other pigmentation issues, so for patients with darker skin this should be taken into consideration. The risk of pigment alterations can also correlate with the depth of laser injury as well as dermal bulk heating effects. This correlation can vary with laser wavelength, pulse duration, fluence, or number of pulses/passes to the same region. Increased depth of laser penetration or energy dispersion can be associated with longer term hypopigmentation.

Hypopigmentation secondary to laser resurfacing can be separated into 2 types.[3] The first type is relative hypopigmentation of the resurfaced skin, in which photodamage has been reduced compared with the untreated adjacent skin. Relative hypopigmentation can be minimized by treating the entire face, or a specific unit or blending into the surrounding skin.[3] Hypopigmentation occurs less frequently in skin rejuvenation procedures when more superficial or fractionated lasers are used. It is important to take this into consideration when planning laser treatments. The second type is delayed hypopigmentation, which is loss of pigment occurring 6 to 12 months after treatment.[3] Several studies have examined the incidence of delayed hypopigmentation in treatment of

various conditions using different laser procedures.

POSTINFLAMMATORY HYPERPIGMENTATION

Often in association with the response to a procedure, there is an inflammatory reaction as part of the healing process. Some patients develop hyperpigmentation in relation to this inflammatory reaction, which has been called postinflammatory hyperpigmentation (PIH). Furthermore, there is a correlation between the quantity of melanin in the skin and the tendency to develop PIH. PIH is associated with injury extending into the papillary dermis.[4] After laser skin resurfacing, PIH is the most common adverse effect among patients with higher Fitzpatrick skin types.[3] This is also an issue after fractional laser treatments. In the experience of the first 2 authors, PIH is rare after treatment with an infrared skin-tightening device (Titan; Cutera, Brisbane, CA, USA).

SKIN REJUVENATION

Laser skin rejuvenation procedures are challenging in patients with higher Fitzpatrick skin types due to potential dyschromia. In a retrospective review of fractional laser treatments, Graber and colleagues[5] reported on the incidence of hyperpigmentation. These investigators used a 1550-nm erbium-doped laser (Fraxel, Reliant Technologies Inc, Hayward, CA, USA) for the treatment of photodamaged skin and scars in 961 patients. Posttreatment hyperpigmentation increased with Fitzpatrick skin type. For patients with skin type II, the incidence of PIH was 0.26%, but in skin types III, IV, and V the incidence was 2.6%, 11.6%, and 33%, respectively. In addition, in evaluating the overall complication rate by Fitzpatrick skin type, it was noted that the complication rate increased proportionate to higher skin types.[5] Considering the increased incidence of hyperpigmentation, the authors do not favor these lasers for skin rejuvenation in patients with Fitzpatrick type V or VI skin. Therefore, most physicians will only treat these patients with nonablative technology.

For patients with Fitzpatrick skin types V and VI, Battle and Hobbs[6] and others have stated that patients with darker skin types have less risk of problems with nonablative laser treatments. Nonablative lasers for skin rejuvenation induce collagen remodeling by thermally stimulating the dermis. By a variety of techniques, these lasers minimize their effect on the epidermis. These lasers can also affect the vascular endothelial cells,[7] which leads to the induction of an inflammatory response in the dermis, inducing neocollagen formation. A series of treatments is usually necessary. As these lasers induce neocollagen formation, improvement occurs gradually post treatment. Patients should be advised about this before starting treatment.

Nonablative lasers include 1064 nm (LightPod Neo, Aerolase, Valhalla, NY, USA; Laser Genesis, Cutera, Brisbane, CA, USA), 1450 nm, and 1540 nm lasers. Even with these lasers test spots should be considered before initiating a full treatment. In using these types of lasers the patient and surgeon are accepting an often less dramatic result than can be obtained with more invasive lasers in exchange for a lower risk of complications.

In nonablative lasers that use a coolant spray, the spray can induce PIH. If one of these lasers is being considered, it is important to appropriately adjust the coolant spray and fluence. For these lasers the authors recommend the use of test spots and allowing adequate time for a healing inflammatory response before initiating treatment in darker skinned patients.

The nonablative 1064-nm Nd:YAG laser has also been used in the treatment of atrophic facial acne scars, and for facial skin rejuvenation. This laser targets oxyhemoglobin within the dermal vasculature to induce new collagen formation. The short-pulsed 1064 nm nonablative Nd:YAG laser pulse is designed to match the thermal relaxation time of the capillaries.

Keller and colleagues[8] evaluated the histology, patient satisfaction, and effect on scars over 6 months post treatment with a 1064-nm laser. The 12 patients in this study had skin types II to V with mild to moderate atrophic facial scars. There was a significant increase histologically in dermal collagen after treatment. Based on pre- and post-treatment photographs, clinically there was at least moderate improvement in at least 50% of the patients. One patient with dark skin experienced PIH; however, it resolved within 4 months. The patient in **Fig. 1**, who was not part of this study, has facial acne scars that were treated with a 1064-nm laser.

In another study, Lipper and Perez[9] examined the use of the short-pulsed, low-fluence 1064-nm Nd:YAG laser (Vantage, Cutera) for the treatment of moderate to severe facial acne scarring in skin types I to V. Evaluation of before and after photographs by physicians showed improvement of facial acne scars in all 9 patients and a mean improvement of 29.36%. Eight of 9 patients reported improvement of 10% to 50%. One patient reported scar improvement of less than 10%. Eight of 9 patients reported no discomfort to minimal discomfort during treatment. The only adverse effects were transient and mild erythema, lasting up to 2 hours post treatment.

At 6- to 12-month follow-up, only 5 of the 9 patients were available for follow-up. Moderate scar improvement in the 26% to 50% range was reported. The 5 patients also reported no changes in skin pigmentation, erythema, or worsening of scar. The investigators concluded that this laser offered effective treatment of facial acne scarring.

Further, the microsecond 1064-nm Nd:YAG laser (CoolGlide Vantage, Cutera) has been reported to be effective in treating erythema and fine lines. Schmults and colleagues[10] found that the laser treatment produces new collagen formation in the papillary dermis. Collagen formation was determined by decrease in collagen fiber diameter. Younger patients with less photoaging have the greatest improvement with nonablative laser treatment.

NONABLATIVE FRACTIONAL LASERS

Asian patients have been reported to do well with fractional nonablative lasers. In a series reported by Kono and colleagues,[11] 30 Asian patients with type III or IV skin were treated with a 1550-nm fractional laser (Fraxel SR 750; Reliant Technologies, Hayward, CA, USA). Different halves of the face were treated with different fluence or density. Pain, erythema, and swelling were significantly higher or persisted longer in patients treated with higher densities and higher energy settings. Increased density was more likely to produce swelling, redness, and hyperpigmentation when compared with increased energy. These investigators also reported that double density was associated with an increased risk of dyspigmentation. Lower densities that minimized the disruption of the epidermal-dermal junction had the lowest the incidence of PIH.

Chan and colleagues[4] similarly completed a retrospective study investigating the incidence of PIH with fractional resurfacing in Asians using

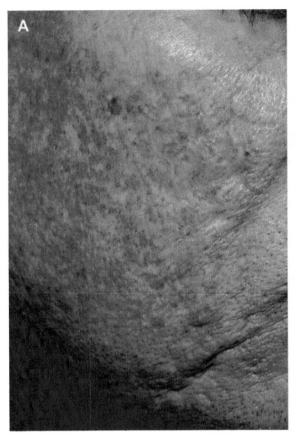
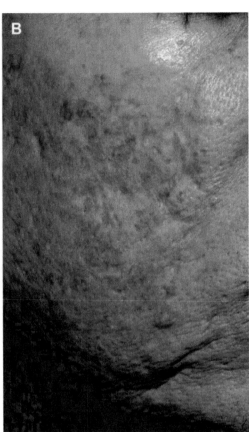

Fig. 1. (*A, B*) This patient, who has a Fitzpatrick IV skin type, was unhappy with facial acne scars. After a series of treatments with a nonablative 1064-nm laser there was noticeable improvement in the appearance of the scars.

a 1540-nm Erbium glass laser (Fraxel SR; Reliant Technologies, Palo Alto, CA, USA). One hundred and nineteen treatment sessions were observed with a high energy and low density, being 7 to 20 mJ and 1000 MTZ, and low energy and high density, being 6 to 12 mJ and 2000 MTZ. Patients who underwent high-energy, low-density treatment were associated with a lower prevalence of generalized PIH. Of note, perioral PIH developed in patients who did not receive air cooling. Chan and colleagues also noted that small anatomic treatment sites and inadequate epidermal cooling are 2 of the factors associated with development of PIH. It was their opinion that small areas are at risk of bulk tissue heating with repeated passes if cooling is not applied. To reduce the prevalence of PIH in dark-skinned patients, they suggested reducing the fractional density by half, extending the treatment interval, and using skin cooling.

In another study, Lee and colleagues[12] found marked improvement in the appearance of acne scars at 3 months post treatment in 27 patients with skin types IV and V using the 1550-nm erbium-doped fractional photothermolysis laser (Fraxel Laser; Reliant Technologies, Hayward,

CA, USA). Thirty percent of patients self-assessed their condition as excellent improvement, 59% as significant improvement, and 11% as moderate improvement. Sequelae included transient pain, mild erythema, edema, and minimal downtime. Pigment changes, crusting, scarring, and infection were not observed in any of the patients.

FRACTIONAL ABLATIVE RESURFACING

Currently there are 3 types of ablative fractional lasers: CO_2, YSGG, and erbium:YAG. Of these 3 types of lasers, erbium:YAG fractionated lasers have been reported on more frequently in patients with darker skin.

Lapidoth and colleagues[13] reported on a series of 28 women, skin types II, III, and IV, who underwent treatments for mild to moderate actinic damage. Each patient received 1 to 4 treatments at 4-week intervals using the 2940-nm Er:YAG laser (Pixel; Alma Lasers Ltd, Caesarea, Israel). Two months after the last session, 75% of patients rated the results as excellent (75%–100% clearance), 25% as good (50%–75% improvement), and no cases of fair, poor, or worse. There was minimal pain, erythema that lasted 2 to 10 days, minimal downtime, and no permanent side effects noted 6 to 9 months post treatment.

Tay and Kwok[14] also used a low-fluence minimally ablative 2940-nm erbium:YAG laser (Laser Peel; Medical Laser Technologies, Homewood, AL, USA) for treatment of facial atrophic acne scars in 9 Asian patients with Fitzpatrick skin types IV and V. The parameters were 6 mm spot size, fluence 400 mJ, pulse duration 300 μs, and depth of 20 μm of tissue per pass. Two physicians evaluated photographs 2 months after the last treatment, with results of mild (≤25% improvement) to moderate (26%–50% improvement) in all patients. The procedure complications included moderate discomfort, transient posttreatment erythema, peeling, and crusting, which all resolved in 2 weeks. The study by Lapidoth and colleagues[13] uses the same laser; however, the parameters are set at a higher fluence of 1400 mJ as compared with this study by Tay and Kwok using a fluence of 400 mJ. The former study using a higher fluence showed better results at the 2-month evaluation with the 2940-nm laser.

SKIN TIGHTENING

The infrared device (Titan, Cutera) used for skin tightening emits light at wavelengths of 1100 to 1800 nm and targets water as the chromophore. In a recent study, Carniol and colleagues[15] evaluated 9 patients after skin tightening and found the greatest tightening over the malar region, the upper neck, and the body of the mandible, with an overall average of 10%, 10%, and 12%, respectively. On self-assessment, the patients reported a 32% improvement in the appearance of their cheeks and a 20% improvement in neck laxity. Based on photographic demonstration, skin tightening continued to progress for up to 3 months after the second treatment. As compared with carbon dioxide resurfacing, nonablative skin tightening does not have a prolonged recovery time and provides effective but limited benefit.

In another study by Alexiades-Armenakas,[16] 22 female patients, of Caucasian and Asian ancestry, were treated with 1 to 3 treatments of infrared light (Titan, Cutera) for treatment of skin laxity. Based on a 4-point grading scale from photographs, there was statistically significant difference between before and after measurements. Treatment discomfort was graded on a scale of 1 to 10, with a mean of 0.7 based on patient questionnaire. None of the patients reported pain or heat-related pain sensation during the treatment. There was minimal erythema that resolved within 1 to 3 hours, but no crusting, dyspigmentation, or scarring was observed.

In an evaluation of 13 Chinese women (Fitzpatrick skin types I–III) who underwent infrared treatment with contact cooling (Titan, Cutera) on one side of the face, using the contralateral side as control, Chan and colleagues[17] reported mild improvement in 23%, moderate improvement in 15%, and significant improvement in 54% 3 months after their second treatment. Blistering occurred in one patient; however, this resolved completely by the 3-month follow-up. The infrared device uses gradual heating of the collagen over a prolonged period of time at low temperature, allowing for minimal recovery time. Based on this split-face study, the infrared device with contact cooling is an effective and safe treatment for skin laxity.

Goldberg and colleagues[18] also evaluated the infrared light device (Titan, Cutera) in the treatment of skin laxity and soft tissue ptosis of the lower face and neck in patients in the sixth decade of life. These investigators found improvement in the patients, with loose skin that appears separated from the deeper tissue. There was improved mandibular definition, cervicomental angularity, and slimming of the neck contour. This study demonstrated the effectiveness of infrared light devices in neck and jowl skin tightening for patients in their sixth decade.

In these studies, nonablative skin tightening with an infrared laser device provided efficacious treatment with minimal downtime and adverse effects.

SUMMARY

Recent innovations in laser/light technologies have increased the ability to treat patients with ethnic skin. Even with these new technologies, treatment of these patients should be carefully planned. Such planning should include selection of technology as well as the way the technology is used.

REFERENCES

1. Carniol PJ, Monheit G, editors. Aesthetic rejuvenation challenges and solutions: a world perspective. London: Informa HealthCare; 2009.
2. Freedberg IM, Eisen AZ, Wolff K, et al. Fitzpatrick's dermatology in general medicine. 5th edition. McGraw-Hill Professional Publishing; 1999.
3. Alexiades-Armenakas MR, Dover JS, Arndt KA. The spectrum of laser skin resurfacing: nonablative, fractional, and ablative laser resurfacing. J Am Acad Dermatol 2008;58(5):719–37.

4. Chan HHL, Manstein D, Yu CS, et al. The prevalence and risk factors of post-inflammatory hyperpigmentation after fractional resurfacing in Asians. Lasers Surg Med 2007;39:381–5.

5. Graber EM, Tanzi EL, Alster TS. Side effects and complications of fractional laser photothermolysis: experience with 961 treatments. Dermatol Surg 2008;34(3):301–7.

6. Battle EF Jr, Hobbs LM. Laser therapy on darker ethnic skin. Dermatol Clin 2003;21:713–23.

7. Nikolaou VA, Stratigos AJ, Dover JS. Nonablative skin rejuvenation. J Cosmet Dermatol 2005;4:301–7.

8. Keller R, Belda Junior W, Valente NY, et al. Nonablative 1,064-nm Nd:YAG laser for treating atrophic facial acne scars: histologic and clinical analysis. Dermatol Surg 2007;33(12):1470–6.

9. Lipper GM, Perez M. Nonablative acne scar reduction after a series of treatments with a short-pulsed 1,064-nm Neodymium: YAG laser. Dermatol Surg 2006;32:998–1006.

10. Schmults CD, Phelps M, Goldberg DJ. Non-ablative facial remodeling: erythema reduction and histologic evidence of new collagen formation using a new 300–microsecond, 1064-nm Nd:YAG laser. Arch Dermatol 2004;140:1373–6.

11. Kono T, Chan HH, Groff WF, et al. Prospective direct comparison study of fractional resurfacing using different fluencies and densities for skin rejuvenation in Asians. Lasers Surg Med 2007;39:311–4.

12. Lee HS, Lee JH, Ahn GY, et al. Fractional photothermolysis for the treatment of acne scars: a report of 27 Korean patients. J Dermatolog Treat 2008;19(1): 45–9.

13. Lapidoth M, Yagima Odo ME, Mayumi Odo L. Novel use of erbium:YAG (2,940-nm) laser for fractional ablative photothermolysis in the treatment of photodamaged facial skin: a pilot study. Dermatol Surg 2008;34(8):1048–53.

14. Tay YK, Kwok C. Minimally ablative erbium:YAG laser resurfacing of facial atrophic acne scars in Asian skin: a pilot study. Dermatol Surg 2008; 34(5):681–5.

15. Carniol PJ, Dzopa N, Fernandes N, et al. Facial skin tightening with an 1100-1800 nm infrared device. J Cosmet Laser Ther 2008;10:67–71.

16. Alexiades-Armenakas M. Assessment of the mobile delivery of infrared light (1100-1800 nm) for the treatment of facial and neck skin laxity. J Drugs Dermatol 2009;8(3):221–6.

17. Chan HH, Yu CS, Shek S, et al. A prospective, split face, single-blinded study looking at the use of an infrared device with contact cooling in the treatment of skin laxity in Asians. Lasers in Surgery and Medicine 2008;40:146–52.

18. Goldberg DJ, Hussain M, Fazeli A, et al. Treatment of skin laxity of the lower face and neck in older individuals with a broad-spectrum infrared light device. J Cosmet Laser Ther 2007;9:35–40.

Chemical Peels for Darker Skin Types

Peter Rullan, MD[a],*, Amir M. Karam, MD[b,c]

KEYWORDS

- Chemical peel • Acne scars
- Postinflammatory hyperpigmentation
- Chemabrasion • Multimodal treatment

This article focuses on chemical peels for darker skin types. All races comprise a range of Fitzpatrick skin color types (**Table 1**)[1]: light skin types III and IV in African Americans, Asians, Middle Easterners, and Latinos and dark skin type IV in whites. With the focus on Fitzgerald skin types IV to VI, the article discusses chemical peels, providing current information on types of peels, detailed techniques, preoperative and postoperative care, complications, hazards, and nuances of management. When evaluating a patient for a skin-resurfacing procedure, it is often inaccurately assumed that race and ethnicity equate with skin color. This rainbow of skin tones within any race erodes the notion that all nonwhites are dark skinned, or that all whites are light skinned.

In addition to the wide intraracial variation in skin color, the global population is becoming increasingly mixed. Although categorization of race and ethnicity is useful in demographic or socioeconomic evaluation, it has poor predictive value for skin-resurfacing outcomes. The American melting pot (the result of migration, wars, and inter-race relationships) shows why classification systems based on original geographic distributions have become archaic. Although the scientific literature is sparse on this topic, clinicians practicing aesthetic facial surgery and medicine should be aware of the nuances of evaluating and managing patients across the spectrum of Fitzpatrick skin types. This awareness is accentuated by the results of the 2000 US Census, which showed

that Latinos are the fastest increasing minority in the United States and Filipino Americans are the fastest increasing group of Asian Americans.

International census reports illustrate similar observations. Mixed race (2 or more races in the heritage) and darker skin types (IV–VI) constitute most of the global population and one-third of the US population.[2] Terms like mestizo, mulato, trigueno, moreno, pardo, Chindian, and Eurasian reflect how widespread and varied the mixed race has become all around the world. Celebrities like Alicia Keys (African American, Irish, Italian) and President Barak Obama (English, Cherokee, Irish, Kenyan, Scottish) reflect this phenomenon.

HISTOLOGY AND FUNCTION

Skin types and races have key differences other than tone. The darker tone is caused by a higher melanin content within keratinocytes (the number of melanocytes is the same as in lighter skin).[3] Dark skin contains eumelanin, a highly cross-linked dark brown to black pigment. Melanin is synthesized in melanosomes in a pathway controlled by the enzyme tyrosinase. The skin of blacks has a high content of large, singly dispersed melanosomes (stage IV) within melanocytes and keratinocytes.[4–6] In contrast, pale white skin has few melanosomes in the epidermis. However, the skin of darker-skinned whites, on sun exposure, can temporarily produce melanosomes similar to black skin.[7] Likewise, blacks

[a] Dermatology Institute, 256 Landis Avenue, Chula Vista, CA 91910, USA
[b] Carmel Valley Facial Plastic Surgery, San Diego, CA, USA
[c] Division of Otolaryngology-Head and Neck Surgery, Department of Surgery, University of California, San Diego, CA, USA
* Corresponding author.
E-mail address: prullan@yahoo.com (P. Rullan).

Facial Plast Surg Clin N Am 18 (2010) 111–131
doi:10.1016/j.fsc.2009.11.010
1064-7406/10/$ – see front matter © 2010 Elsevier Inc. All rights reserved.

Table 1
Fitzpatrick skin classification

Type	Color	Reaction to Sun Exposure
I	Very white or freckled	Always burn
II	White	Usually burn
III	White to olive	Sometimes burn
IV	Brown	Rarely burn
V	Dark brown	Very rarely burn
VI	Black	Never burn

Data from Fitzpatrick TB. The validity and practicality of sun-reactive skin types I through VI. Arch Dermatol 1988;124(6):869–71.

with a lighter complexion have a combination of large dispersed and smaller aggregated melanosomes like whites. In Asians, skin that has not been exposed to sun has aggregated melanosomes like whites, whereas areas that have been exposed to the sun have predominantly dispersed melanosomes. These similarities and differences suggest significant intraracial and inter-racial variation in pigmentation. Recent work suggests that the activity of the protease-activated receptor-2 correlates with skin color and may influence ethnic skin color phenotypes.[8,9]

The stratum corneum in skin of color has more layers and more phospholipids than white skin. The dermis tends to be thicker because of the increased number and size of fibroblasts.[10] Because of the photoprotective nature of melanin, aging in dark-skinned individuals is associated with soft tissue and gravitational changes rather than wrinkles. Whereas whites and Asians undergo significant epidermal changes with photodamage,[11] blacks have only marginal changes. Fibroblasts, elastic fibers, mast cells, blood vessels, hair follicles, and other dermal structures also differ in quantity and function between races.

Melanocytes are labile in darker skin, resulting in a high incidence of dyschromia, such aspostinflammatory hyperpigmentation (PIH) following injury or cutaneous surgery.[12] Similarly, melasma is more prevalent in blacks, Hispanics, and Asians, and is attributed to hormonal factors, ultraviolet (UV) and infrared radiation exposure, and lability of melanocytes.

INDICATIONS, NUANCES, AND HAZARDS FOR CHEMICAL PEELING IN SKIN TYPES IV TO VI

Individuals with darker skin typically request correction of conditions such as PIH, melasma, acne vulgaris and scarring, textural changes (fine wrinkles), lentigos, dermatosis papulosa nigra, and seborrheic keratosis (SK). Diagnostic mistakes commonly occur in the initial evaluation of patients of dark skin. Brown lesions are lumped together as pigmented instead of hyperkeratotic-like (eg, SK). This misclassification leads to ineffective ablative treatments that may actually worsen the complexion, whether these peels are from light sources or chemicals. Chung and colleagues[13] assessed Korean patients and found that pigmentary changes are common features of photoaging in Asians, with SK being the major pigmentary lesion in men and lentigo in women. Physicians therefore need to individualize their treatments to different types of lesions. For example, careful electrocautery of individual SK lesions is not only more effective than chemical or laser ablation, it is also safer (associated with lower risk of PIH). Long-pulsed 532-nm neodymium:yttrium-aluminum-garnet laser treatment was similarly found to be more effective and have a lower incidence of PIH for lentigines in darker-skinned patients than other modalities.[14] Intense pulsed light has also been studied extensively in Asians for the treatment of lentigines and freckles[15] but would be ineffective in patients with a misdiagnosis of SK. The novel use of modified phenol formulas for spot peels of lentigines (eg, with Hetter VL) had been routinely practiced for years by 1 of the authors (PPR) (**Fig. 1**). Benign dermal tumors, such as syringomas, must be

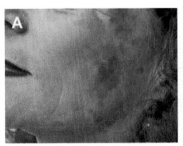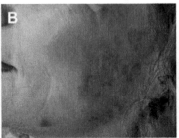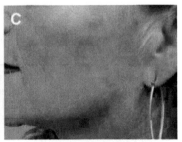

Fig. 1. Lentigines on the cheek of a Latina woman with skin type IV to V. (*A*) Before treatment; (*B*) with spot treatment with Hetter VL (medium depth) showing frost; (*C*) 1 month after treatment with normal skin tones.

identified and treated with techniques that cause less PIH and scarring, such as fine-needle tipped electrocautery.[16]

A common mistake is to treat with only 1 modality (eg, chemical peel), and then respond with a stronger peel when the results are unsatisfactory. Melasma and acne scar management are good examples. Melasma is a dysfunction of the pigmentary system, and cannot be cured with any type of peel[17]; it is commonly worsened by unimodal aggressive peels. These conditions require a multimodal approach. For melasma, prescription creams are recommended that address the existing melanophages, the lability of the melanocytes, the synthesis of melanin, and that promote attempts to increase cellular turnover. Protective measures require blocking of UV-B, UV-A, and infrared (heat) radiation, using physical sunblocks (oxides), cooling measures, and protective clothing and hats. The significance of inflammation as a cofactor in melasma is documented by the effectiveness of applying 0.01% fluocinolone cream twice a day, along with sun and heat protection, in achieving notable improvement (**Fig. 2**). All resurfacing modalities should be superficial, so as to minimize the risk of PIH or hypopigmentation,[2] because even superficial peels can cause PIH (**Fig. 3**) if the patient is retinized. Another common condition, macular PIH, is better treated with intralesional injections of dilute triamcinolone (2 mg/mL) or fluocinolone rather than with peels.

Acne scars are categorized as ice-pick, box scar, rolling scar, atrophic, or hypertrophic types.[18] In pigmented skin, correction of ice-pick scars, for example, is better accomplished with precise intralesional injury, which results in negligible PIH.[19] This is achieved with chemical reconstruction of skin scars (CROSS) using a pointed toothpick or paintbrush to apply the acid (**Fig. 4**).[19,20] Shallow lesions (eg, box scars)

respond to more superficial peels. Rolling scars (eg, atrophic scars with adhesions) require subcision and possible dermal fillers. Hypertrophic scars require treatment with intralesional steroids, occlusion, and pulsed-dye laser therapy.

When performing an ablative procedure on skin of color, deeper ablation, greater thermal effect, and greater inflammation of the injury all increase the risk of PIH.[21] One of the authors (PPR) has performed more than 40,000 chemical peels in a Southern California city 10 miles north of Tijuana, Mexico, where more than 50% of the population is of Hispanic, black, Filipino, or mixed race. In this referral center for correction of acne scars, superficial, medium, and deep chemical peels are frequently combined in the same patient. For example, a stronger solution can be applied for individual ice-pick scars using the CROSS method, medium-depth peels are useful for scarred sebaceous areas, and superficial agents can be used on thinner skin overlying bony prominences (**Fig. 5**).

As noted by Grimes, retinoids, hydroquinones (HQ), steroids, azelaic acid, and antioxidants (alone or in combinations) are used in the treatment of PIH.[2] When used for 2 to 6 weeks before a peel, these agents provide benefit. However, when PIH occurs as a complication of other treatments, it is usually more responsive to conservative measures (within 2–3 months) (see section on Complications).[22] Correction of PIH is easier than correction of melasma in the same patient.

TYPES OF CHEMICAL PEELS AND FORMULAS

Each chemical formula or component has specific effects, and can be categorized by the depth of the peel or by the mechanism of the action. Superficial peels target the stratum corneum to the papillary dermis (100 μm); medium peels penetrate to the

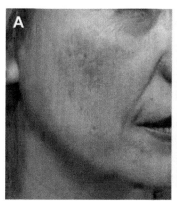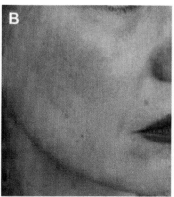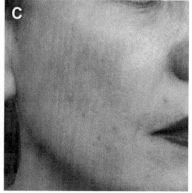

Fig. 2. Latina woman with melasma. (*A*) Starting a regimen with strict heat and sun avoidance plus fluocinolone cream twice daily; (*B*) 3 weeks later showing significant improvement; (*C*) 7 weeks later.

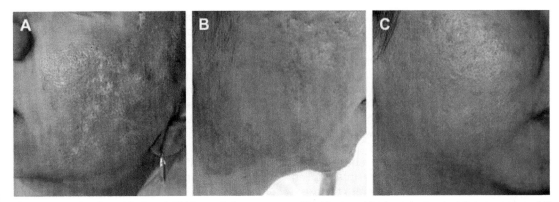

Fig. 3. Example of peel-induced PIH in an Asian woman with skin type V who was treated for acne scars. (*A*) Patient is undergoing a Jessner peel (2+ frost with edema); (*B*) appearance of PIH soon after healing; (*C*) correction of PIH by fluocinolone cream, HQ, and microdermabrasions.

upper reticular dermis (200 µm); and deep peels penetrate to the midreticular dermis (400 µm) (**Table 2**). Variables such as pH, concentration, quantity applied, and concomitant use (and duration) of other chemicals modify wounding ability. In general, peels consist of α-hydroxy acids (AHA), β-hydroxy acids (BHA), trichloroacetic acid (TCA), tretinoin, or various phenolic compounds (HQ, resorcinol, and carbolic acid).

AHA Peels

AHA peels, particularly glycolic acid (GA) peels, function by promoting epidermolysis (corneocyte detachment), dispersing basal cell melanin, thinning the epidermis, and increasing collagen synthesis in the dermis. Unbuffered GA with a low pH has the potential to induce greater epidermal and dermal damage. GA peels are available in concentrations ranging from 20% to 99%.

BHA Peels

BHA peels, particularly salicylic acid (SA) peels, are lipophilic compounds that remove intercellular lipids that are covalently linked to the cornified envelope surrounding the epithelial cells. Studies have shown that BHA peels activate basal cells

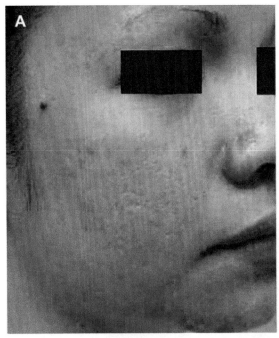
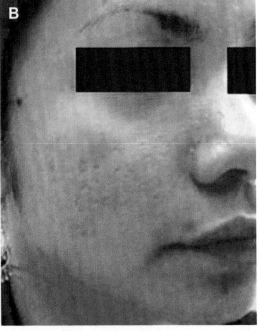

Fig. 4. Filipina-Asian woman with skin type IV to V treated for acne scars. (*A*) Before treatment with lesional CROSS using Stone phenol chemabrasion; (*B*) 1 month post peel with normal skin tones, using a protective skin care regimen.

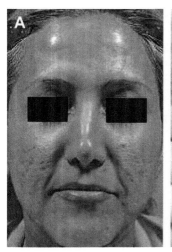 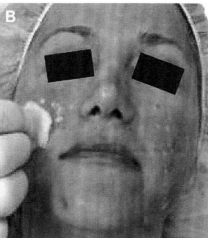 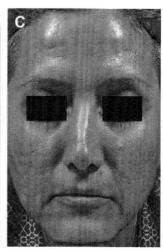

Fig. 5. Middle Eastern woman with skin type IV treated for acne scars. (*A*) Before subcision and Stone phenol CROSS; (*B*) application of a Vi Peel; (*C*) 1 month post peel with visible correction of scars and no PIH.

and underlying fibroblasts without directly wounding the dermis or causing inflammation.[23] They also have antiinflammatory and antimicrobial properties. The common formulations have concentrations of 20% and 30% in ethanol.

Jessner Peel

Jessner peel is a keratolytic, which combines SA (14 g), resorcinol (14 g), and lactic acid 85% (14 g) mixed in ethanol for a final volume of 100 mL. Lactic acid is an AHA that causes epidermolysis. Resorcinol is structurally similar to phenol, and disrupts the weak hydrogen bonds of keratin.

TCA

TCA is a protein denaturant that precipitates epidermal proteins, causing sloughing and necrosis, and dermal inflammation. These processes appear as white frosting (coagulation of epidermal keratinocyte proteins) on the skin surface. Common applications combine an AHA, a BHA, or a Jessner peel, followed by TCA. The Blue Peel (Obagi Medical Products, Long Beach, CA, USA) contains a blue-dye indicator that helps the physician recognize the depth of the peel penetration (**Fig. 6**). The recommended strength of TCA is 20% to 35%. TCA is formulated commercially or in the office as a weight-volume preparation from 10% to 100%. This versatile peel can be used to achieve superficial, medium, or deep peels, depending on the skin conditioning, the strength of the acid, and the number of coats applied. Multiple studies in the past 40 years have shown that TCA can be safely used in nonwhite dark skin types (**Fig. 7**).[24] Safe use of TCA requires longer preconditioning of the skin, use of the lowest effective strength of TCA, and strategies for dealing with any occurrences of PIH. As shown in the Korean study by Lee and Kim,[25] applying TCA in a smaller area, for example inside an ice-pick scar, significantly reduces the risk of PIH and facilitates correction of PIH when it occurs.

Table 2 Types of peels by depth		
Peel Type	**Depth (μm)**	**Examples**
Superficial	100	Glycolic acid (buffered); salicylic acid; Jessner (1 to 2 coats, nonretinized); TCA 10% to 15% (1 coat); combination peels: TCA + salicylic acid; Jessner + salicylic acid; Vi Peel/ApothePeel; Nomelan fenol kh; Melanage
Medium	200	Glycolic acid unbuffered (time dependent); Jessner (multiple coats on retinized skin); Jessner + 20% to 35% TCA; Hetter VL (phenol)
Deep	≥400	Hetter all around; Stone 100 (Grade 2); Exoderm-Lift; Baker-Gordon (not recommended)

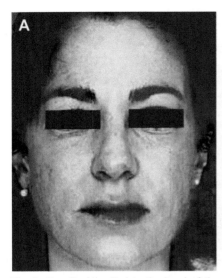
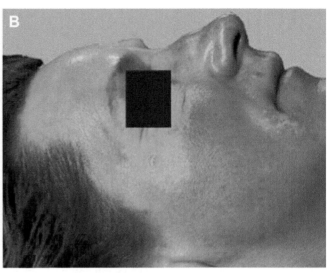

Fig. 6. Blue Peel applied to the level of the (A) papillary dermis and (B) immediate reticular dermis.

Phenol

Phenol formulas typically consist of 88% phenol (carbolic acid), croton oil, hexachlorophene, olive oil, or distilled water (**Table 3**). Phenol disrupts sulfide bonds, resulting in keratolysis and protein coagulation. Phenol is also melanotoxic. Hexachlorophene is an antiseptic with surfactant properties, which allows a more uniform penetration by decreasing surface tension. Croton oil is a vesicant (and therefore epidermolytic) that greatly enhances the absorption of phenol. Olive oil is added to slow the cutaneous absorption rate of these agents to reduce any systemic toxicity. Commonly used phenol formulas (**Fig. 8**) include Hetter VL (**Fig. 9**), Hetter all around, Stone (**Fig. 10**),[26,27] Exoderm,[28,29] and Baker-Gordon.

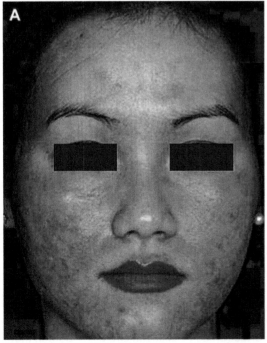
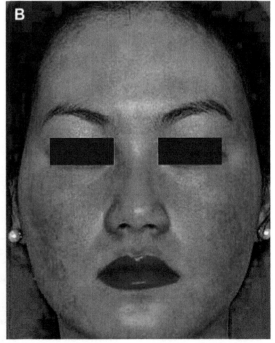

Fig. 7. Asian woman with skin type III treated for acne scars. (A) Before treatment with a Blue Peel; (B) post peel showing normal skin tones and good scar correction.

Table 3 Phenol formulas		
Formula[a]	Croton Oil Content (%)	Phenol Content (%)
Hetter VL neck/eyelid	0.1	30
Stone-2 (Stone 100/Grade II)	0.2	60
Hetter all around	0.4	35
Hetter (range 0.1%–1.0%)	0.7	50
Exoderm-Lift	0.6–0.7	64
Baker-Gordon	2.1	50

[a] Some commercially available formulas contain additional ingredients.

Phenol peels have the potential to cause cardiotoxicity and renal toxicity. Patients should be hydrated during the peripeel period and monitored for cardiac arrhythmias. To avoid these side effects, the peels should be administered slowly in a subunit approach. Typically, peel administration should span 60 to 90 minutes.

Tretinoin Peels

Tretinoin is the acid form of vitamin A, also known as all-*trans* retinoic acid. A tretinoin peel (1%–5%) produces effects that are similar to commercially available creams, resulting in increased epidermal thickness, decreased stratum corneum, and decreased melanin content (**Fig. 11**).

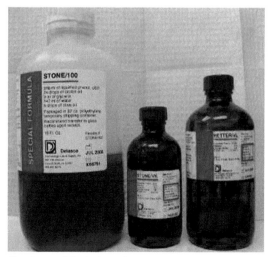

Fig. 8. Modified phenols Stone 100, Stone VK, and Hetter VL.

Vi Peel

The Vi Peel (a variation of the ApothePeel) is a premixed formula containing TCA (10%–12% in alcohol), phenol (10%–12%), SA (10%–12%), and tretinoin (0.4%) (see **Fig. 11**). The home regimen consists of 2 nightly applications of a pad containing tretinoin oil and vitamin C.

Nomelan Fenol kh (SeSDERMA)

This peel contains TCA, phenol, HQ, kojic acid, GA, α-arbutin, ascorbic acid, SA, phytic acid, mandelic acid, and retinoic acid mixed in an alcohol base. The mixture is applied for 3 to 5 minutes, followed by application of a 10% retinol/1% retinyl propionate cream for 6 to 8 hours. The home regimen consists of 10% vitamin C/5% niacinamide and a cream with 15% lactic acid, 4% retinol, and 1% retinyl propionate.

Melanage Peel

The Melanage Peel (a commercial version of the Krulig Amelan Peel) comes as a kit (**Fig. 12**) that includes a 1% tretinoin solution, a powder formulation of HQ, which is freshly mixed with 10% azelaic acid, 10% lactic acid, and 10% phytic acid, and applied as a mask. Physicians can make up to a 14% HQ peel, which is left for up to 8 hours on the skin (**Fig. 13**). The home regimen consists of freshly mixed cream of 4% HQ and 0.75% tretinoin with an optional 0.7% hydrocortisone for possible irritation. The key features of this peel are that it is weakly acidic, noncorrosive, minimally inflammatory, and causes no protein precipitation; it is designed for dark skin types with melasma or PIH (**Fig. 14**). It can be performed once yearly, with the option of a series of 3 to 4 minipeels during the year.

INDICATIONS AND APPLICATION TECHNIQUES

All patients require a full personal, family, and medical history. Special consideration should be focused on history of cutaneous malignancy, history of acne scarring or PIH, herpes simplex outbreaks, and use of isotretinoin in the last 12 months. Performing a chemical peel on a patient on isotretinoin, or within 6 months of discontinuation of isotretinoin, is contraindicated, and the skin must have regained its normal sebaceous activity.

Patients preparing to have a phenol-based peel require a full laboratory work-up, including hepatic, renal, and cardiac testing. During the initial evaluation, the physician should assess parameters that can help predict healing, such as the presence of a suntan, the level of exercise

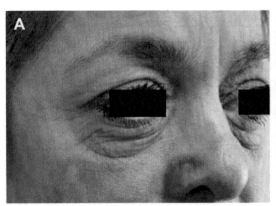
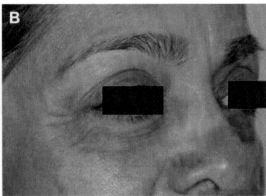

Fig. 9. Latina woman with skin type IV to V treated to correct lower eyelid wrinkling. (*A*) Before upper blepharoplasty and 2 Hetter VL phenol peels; (*B*) postoperative appearance with normal skin tones and good color match between cosmetic units.

(or other temperature-increasing activities), use of make-up, tendency to heal with PIH, parents' skin color, and available downtime. Guidance for peel selection is shown in **Table 4**.

Preconditioning the Skin

To reduce the risk of PIH and to improve the efficacy of the peel outcome, preparation of the skin for chemical peels requires preconditioning of the skin[30,31] for 2 to 12 weeks (**Table 5**). Topical agents are used to help reduce the seborrhea and thin the epidermis. These products allow rapid penetration of the peel, accelerate re-epithelization and wound healing, and decrease the risk of PIH caused by the bleaching effect that results from dispersion of melanin granules. Bacterial infections and flares of herpes simplex must be prevented during healing with the use of antibacterial and antiviral prophylaxis. In contrast with laser ablation, the status of the skin on the day of the peel is critical. If the skin is dry, has an abrasion, or is retinized, the peel will be much stronger than expected, which can be an advantage (in patients with thick, sebaceous, scarred skin) or detrimental (in patients with melasma or PIH, especially over thin skin).

The Obagi Nu-Derm (or the similar Dermesse line), Triluma (or EpiQuin with 0.01% fluocinolone cream for the more sensitive skin), or a glycolic-HQ combination cream (Lustra) is used for 2 to 12 weeks before the peel. Treating active acne before the peel gives better cosmetic results and may require the use of retinoid creams, acne surgery, and isotretinoin pills. The peel should be delayed until the patient has discontinued

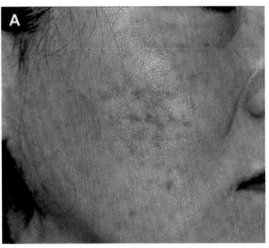
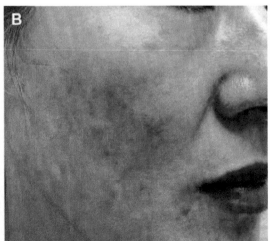

Fig. 10. Korean American woman with skin type IV treated for acne scars. (*A*) Before full-face Stone phenol and 1 regional touch-up; (*B*) 2.5 years after the first peel.

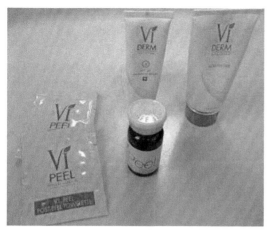

Fig. 11. Vi Peel system.

isotretinoin for 6 months or until the skin has regained its normal sebaceous activity and thus its healing capacity.

Complications

Many of the same complications that can affect patients with lighter skin types can occur in patients with darker skin types, including herpes simplex infection, bacterial infection, prolonged erythema, contact dermatitis, scarring, PIH, and hypopigmentation. The early recognition and management of these complications is essential for a successful resolution.

PIH remains the most common complication in patients with darker skin types and occurs with

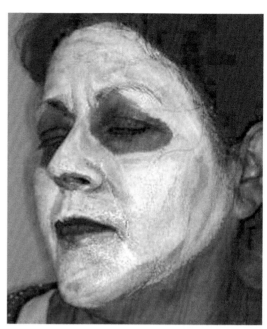

Fig. 13. Latina woman with skin type IV to V treated for melasma with 14% HQ and 1% tretinoin applied for 5 to 10 hours, demonstrating white paste appearance of the peel.

most types of peels, especially deep ones (**Fig. 15**). Regional deep peels on dark skin types outside a cosmetic unit should be avoided because of this risk (**Fig. 16**). PIH generally develops when the pink stage begins to fade. In addition to the use of sunblocks (eg, Colore Science products) and heat avoidance, the early use of class V or VI steroid creams (eg, 0.01% fluocinolone twice a day) can be effective in reversing the first signs of PIH. As the redness fades, the use of the steroid cream can be discontinued and replaced with barrier-repair creams (CeraVe, Cetaphil). If the pigmentation progresses, the use of HQ alone or in combination with a glycolic cream (eg, Lustra) or a retinol (eg, Epiquin) can be used twice a day or at bedtime depending on the level of irritation. Tretinoin is not recommended, as it can irritate the skin and worsen the PIH in sunny or hot conditions. Persistent redness, either from the peel or from the creams, should not be allowed to continue untreated.

Postpeel Regimen

With most superficial peels, the postoperative care is simple: wash and lubricate with a gentle, soap-free product (eg, CeraVe, Cetaphil) twice a day and avoid irritating the skin with sun, sweat, or acidic creams. Medium-depth peels require some analgesia and antiinflammatory therapy. Burning sensations are treated with white vinegar

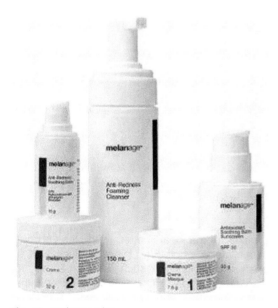

Fig. 12. Melanage kit.

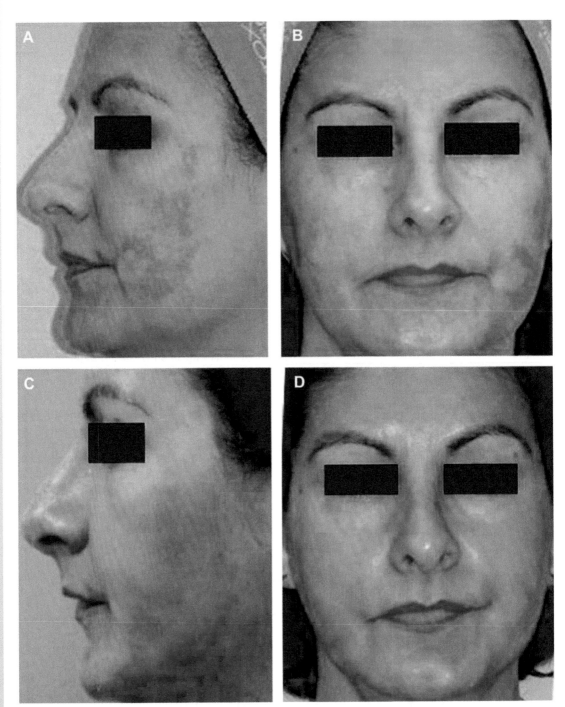

Fig. 14. Latina woman with skin type IV to V with melasma. (*A, B*) Before Melanage Peel, followed by an additional bleaching skin care regimen for 2 months; (*C, D*) 28 days post peel.

(1 tablespoon in 1 cup of water) compresses twice to 4 times daily and application of ointment (eg, Aquaphor) until the skin peels and recovers a strong epithelial layer (usually 5–7 days). Finally, soothing gentle barrier-repair cream systems (eg, aloe vera hydrocortisone balm [Topix]) are used.

Deeper peels heal better with the bismuth subgallate powder (**Fig. 17**) mask than with an open-wound system such as that used for medium-depth peels. Once the skin has re-epithelialized following a deep peel, the regimen of Cetaphil plus sunblocks is used.

Table 4
Peel selection

Indication	Peel	Key Features
PIH, melasma	SA 20%–30% (series of 3–6 peels)	Low cost, safe, good for acne-prone patients, somewhat effective
	GA buffered (series of 3–6 peels)	Low cost, safe, good for dry skin types, somewhat effective
	Vi Peel (series of 1–3 peels)	Brand name, safe, good for all skin types, more effective
	Melanage Peel (1–2 peels per year)	Brand name, safe, good for all skin types, most effective
Acne scars (box and ice-pick scars)	CROSS with 30% TCA plus a full-face Jessner or Vi Peel	Good for scars of mild severity, little downtime
	CROSS with Stone phenol chemabrasion + Jessner (full-face) or Vi Peel	Good for more severe scars, little downtime
	Stone phenol (full-face) 2-day chemabrasion (with 1 regional touch-up) Obagi Blue Peel Jessner + 20%–35% TCA	Good for more severe scars, 10–14 days of downtime, must avoid sun exposure for 1–3 months
Photoaging	Jessner Vi Peel GA series SA series SA + 15% TCA Jessner + 15% TCA GA unbuffered (35%–70%)	For mild cases For moderate cases
	Stone phenol 2-day chemabrasion Obagi Blue Peel + 20%–35% TCA Jessner + 20%–35% TCA	For moderate to severe cases, 2 weeks of downtime, must avoid sun exposure for 1–3 months

GA PEEL TECHNIQUE

Multiple studies[32] in dark-skinned patients have confirmed the efficacy of a series of GA peels (every 2 weeks for 3 to 6 times) to help improve PIH and melasma, as measured by the melasma area severity index score in all skin types and races, especially when combined with topical regimens.[33–37] The topical regimens vary from a modified Kligman formula (5% HQ, 1% hydocortisone

Table 5
Preconditioning treatments

Indication	Drug and Dose
Antiviral	Famciclovir (500 mg twice a day), valacyclovir (500 mg twice a day), or acyclovir (400 mg twice a day) for 7–10 days starting 1–2 days before peel
Prevention of PIH and enhanced peel quality	Retinoid creams applied for up to 12 weeks for medium-depth peels,[a] to be restarted after skin peeling and irritation subsides; discontinue 1–2 days before peel if photodamage is evident and 1–2 weeks before peel if treating melasma or PIH
If weather is sunny or patient is sensitive to retinoids, use of a glycolic cream for 2–4 weeks is suggested	Retinoid and glycolic creams can be used with 2%–8% HQ at bedtime
Pre-existing PIH	Fluocinolone cream (0.01%–0.025%) twice a day for 2–12 weeks
PIH, acne scars	Tazarotene cream (0.05%) at bedtime
UV radiation protection	Physical sunblocks, eg, zinc or titanium oxide creams, ColoreScience or mineral make-up, visors

[a] Including Epiquin, Triluma, Obagi Nu-Derm, or Dermesse systems.

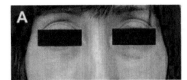
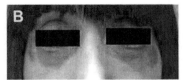
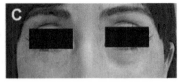

Fig. 15. Latina woman with skin type IV treated for lower eyelid crepiness and laxity. (*A*) Before treatment with a Hetter VL phenol regional peel; (*B*) appearance of severe PIH 3 weeks post peel; (*C*) 3 months post peel after a regimen of retinol, HQ, and fluocinolone cream with complete resolution and noticeable cosmetic improvement.

cream, 0.05% tretinoin), to a mixture of an AHA with HQ mixture (especially in Asian patients), such as 2% HQ with a 10% GA twice daily and 0.05% tretinoin cream at bedtime. Retinoids must be discontinued at least 2 days before the peel.

Before starting a series of GA peels, the status of the skin should be assessed for dry, scaly, oily, open sores that may have been acidified from using GA/tretinoin creams. Required materials include a fan, a small cup with 10 mL of 10% sodium bicarbonate, another small cup with 3 to 4 mL of the GA peel (usually 70% buffered), Q-tips, gauze (for drying the peel), and a stopwatch. The GA peel is stopped with sodium bicarbonate; this can be done at 2 minutes, 10 minutes, or once an end point is reached. End points such as pink edema (mildest), perifollicular edema, and vesiculation (the maximum safe end point, which can lead to crusting and possible PIH) are most easily assessed using a magnifier visor. The next peel in the series is chosen based on the results of the previous peel. Grimes[2] recommends free, unbuffered GA (pH 0.6–1.7) as a solo agent for medium-depth peels in pigmented skin because of a lower incidence of PIH than with other peels at that depth. However, erosive blisters can occur with the use of unbuffered GA

(especially in the central porous face regions) and can cause scarring.

SA PEEL TECHNIQUE

This is an inexpensive, simple, and safe peel to perform on pigmented skin with acne, PIH, or melasma. A 20% or 30% formulation is applied after thoroughly cleansing the area to be treated. One of the authors (PPR) routinely applies it on patients receiving low-dose isotretinoin (0.25–0.5 mg/kg) to accelerate the correction of active acne lesions or PIH. Each layer is applied with regular Q-tips from a plastic cup holding around 5 mL of solution. A white pseudofrost precipitate forms immediately, which can be wiped off. Two to three coats are usually applied; however, if there is burning, 1 coat is sufficient. This solution can be washed off after 5 minutes or left on for several hours to achieve a more drying effect. When it is washed off, a bland moisturizing cream should be applied and continued for 2 days. In studies conducted in African American, Hispanic[38] and Asian[25] patients, only mild or transient side effects (peeling, redness) and no cases of PIH were observed. Garg and colleagues[39] compared GA with an SA-mandelic combination to treat acne, scars, and PIH, and showed that although both

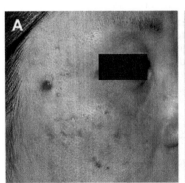
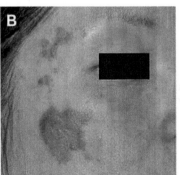
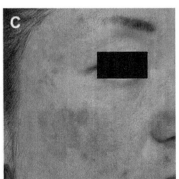

Fig. 16. Example of peel-induced PIH in a Japanese woman with skin type IV who was treated for acne. (*A*) Before a regional Exoderm phenol peel; (*B*) 3 weeks post peel with PIH and redness; (*C*) 7 months post peel after treatment with retinoids, HQ, and steroid creams.

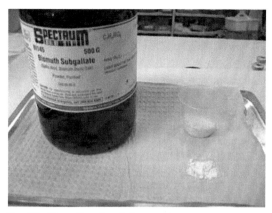

Fig. 17. Bismuth subgallate powder.

peels worked well, the SA-mandelic peel was superior overall. This result was attributed to the lipophilic and comedolytic superiority of SA to GA. Salicylism has never been seen by 1 of the authors (PPR) and has been reported only rarely.[40]

JESSNER ACID PEEL TECHNIQUE

In contrast with the opinions of others,[2] one of the authors (PPR) has performed thousands of Jessner peels on skin types IV to VI (**Fig. 18**); many of those patients were also being treated with low-dose isotretinoin but to do so safely requires the use of the Obagi Skin Classification guide (**Table 6**). For example, the solution should be applied on the more sebaceous or thicker regions of the face (sparing the thin skin overlying bony prominences and the porous creases or just barely covering them with a light amount). As with most

peels, the face is first thoroughly cleansed and degreased, and the Jessner solution is placed in a small disposable plastic cup (5.0–7.5 mL). Two regular Q-tips with wooden handles are used for easier application. A portable personal fan is offered. To best avoid PIH, only 1 coat is applied (producing a slight whitish precipitate), which achieves slight drying of acne lesions. If the clinical endpoint is the improvement of acne scars or to prepare the skin for application of TCA, a deeper peel is needed, which can be accomplished by the application of multiple coats or by leaving the single application until a patchy, slightly white frost is achieved. Jessner solution can be used also for truncal acne with or without scars with PIH by using a larger (obstetrics and gynecology type) Q-tip or 2-inch × 2-inch gauze. Neutralization is not required, but one of the authors (PRR) has used 10% sodium bicarbonate successfully for this purpose. He has also used the original Retin-A 0.05% solution to calm the burning and to enhance the peel, allowing this oil to remain on the face overnight. As noted previously, dry, retinized skin that receives multiple coats of Jessner solution can reach the upper reticular dermis and cause a medium-depth injury (see **Fig. 3**).

TCA PEEL TECHNIQUE

According to the procedure described by Monheit,[42] Jessner solution is applied first to achieve a 1+ frost followed by application of 20% to 35% TCA (**Fig. 19**). The Blue Peel, which uses 20% to 30% TCA, has a color-sensitive reaction to indicate the depth of the peel. The procedure

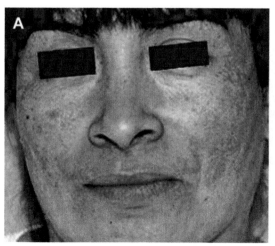
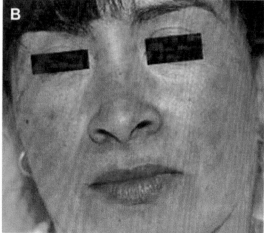

Fig. 18. Latina woman treated for recalcitrant melasma. (A) Before Jessner peels and triple bleach formula (retinol, HQ, fluocinolone); (B) follow-up with noticeable improvement requiring sun and heat protection and nightly skin-care regimen.

Table 6
Obagi skin classification

Characteristic	Key Features and Considerations for Peels
Color	Hypopigmentation versus hyperpigmentation
Oiliness	Based on time when T-zone is oily: by 10 AM = very oily; by 12:00 PM = oily; by 2:00 PM = normal
Thickness	Determined by pinching the nasolabial fold: thin = lighter procedures; medium = all procedures; thick = dermabrasion, chemical peels
Laxity	Separate skin versus muscle laxity
Fragility	Procedures should be restricted to the papillary dermis for fragile skin; correlates with scarring

Data from Obagi Z. Obagi skin health restoration and rejuvenation. New York: Springer; 1999.[41]
   Data from Halder RM, Nootheti PK. Ethnic skin disorders overview. J Am Acad Dermatol 2003;48(6 Suppl):S143–8.

used by Grimes[2] includes a superficial peel with 20% to 30% SA followed by 15% TCA for resistant melasma or mild photodamage in all skin types. If the goal is a superficial peel, a thin coat should be applied so that little or no frost appears, regardless of the combination of peels used. To achieve a medium-depth peel to the papillary dermis, 20% to 30% TCA is applied, with the goal of producing an organized white sheet with a pink background. When the peel reaches the deepest safest level (the immediate reticular dermis) the pink background gradually diminishes (because of the coagulation of blood vessels) and the sheet appears pure white.[41]

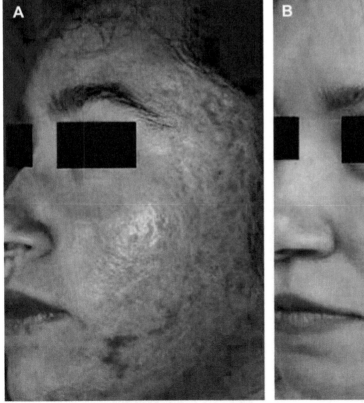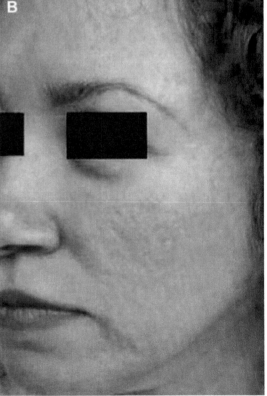

Fig. 19. Latina woman with skin type III to IV treated for acne scars. (*A*) Before treatment with Jessner solution plus 35% TCA; (*B*) 10 years after peel, using a skin-care regimen and HQ.

Sedation and analgesia are usually necessary with TCA peels. The area is thoroughly cleansed with hexachlorophene, alcohol, and acetone. If using Jessner solution, only 1 to 2 coats are applied to achieve a blotchy frosting. A 2-inch × 2-inch gauze is then dipped into a plastic or stainless-steel cup containing the TCA solution and squeezed dry before the application. The solution is first applied laterally, then slowly to the central area, and lastly to the perioral and periorbital regions. The solution should be left on for 2 to 5 minutes for complete frost formation; overcoating with more TCA should be avoided. The peel is then feathered into the hairline and the neckline just below the mandibular border. Several immediate postoperative maneuvers can be used to reduce burning, such as an ice-water compress, 10% sodium bicarbonate rinse, cold aloe vera lotion, a Zimmer cooler, or topical lidocaine ointment. Depending on the depth of the peel, exfoliation with some redness to intense redness, edema, blistering, and crusting starting within 24 hours will be observed. A 20-mg intramuscular dose of triamcinolone is useful to reduce swelling.

The standard regimen used by one of the authors (AMK) is as follows: Aquaphor is used up to day 5 or so and the skin is washed with dilute vinegar in water 4 times per day. Cetaphil lotion and cleanser (Galderma Laboratories, Fort Worth, TX, USA) are used for the next 5 days. Healing typically takes 7 to 10 days. A class II steroid cream administered twice daily is a consideration for dark-skinned patients, beginning as soon as the skin is re-epithelialized and is no longer tender. A 2% HQ cream can also be started after the second week, together with chemical-free sunblocks.

MODIFIED PHENOL PEEL TECHNIQUE

Research over the last 11 years has clearly distinguished the early Baker-Gordon phenol peel from the newer and much safer modified versions that are based on lower concentrations of croton oil. A series of articles by Hetter in 2000[43–46] characterized the active ingredients and established a major role for croton oil in peels. In those studies, nonwhites received peels safely with the lower-strength phenol formulas. Studies by Stone in 1998 and in 2001[26,27] delineated the active ingredients and refined the technique of application for the modified phenols. The Fintsi Exoderm-Lift peel[28,29] has been performed in skin type IV without producing an alabaster-white hypopigmentation, but rather a pseudohypopigmentation (the color of skin that has not been exposed to sun). In a 2004 publication by one of the authors (PPR) describing his technique for chemabrasion,[47] 44% of the 72 patients were Latinos, Afro-Caribbean, or Asian. Since then, he has treated 250 such patients, and has monitored the incidence of late-onset dyschromias. There have been no cases of depigmentation or persistent PIH using this technique (**Figs. 20** and **21**). As expected, darker skin types have 2 different skin tones between the face and neck, with the peeled facial skin being lighter than the tanned neck with an appearance similar to the skin that has not been exposed to sun. Some patients have been able to tan almost normally. One of the authors (PPR) has used the Exoderm-Lift and Stone (Grade II) formulas (**Fig. 22**), which demonstrated equivalency in the clinical and histologic studies. The stronger Hetter formulas have been used and

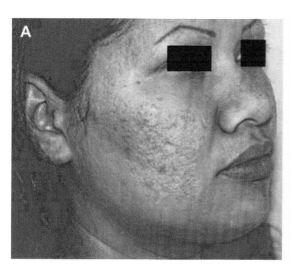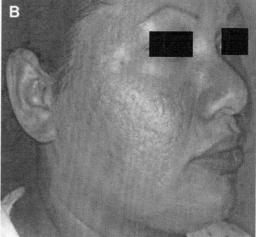

Fig. 20. An Afro-Caribbean woman with skin type VI treated with a full-face Stone phenol peel for acne scars without hypopigmentation or hyperpigmentation. (*A*) Patient before peel; (*B*) almost 3 years post peel showing lighter but normal skin tone.

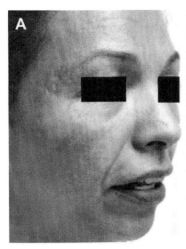
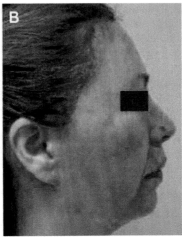
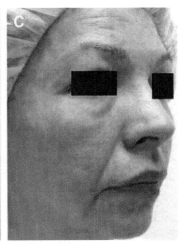

Fig. 21. Latina woman with skin type V treated for acne scars and melasma. (*A*) Before 2-day Stone phenol; (*B*) 10 days post peel with severe discordance between pink face and dark neck; (*C*) 1 year post peel, showing some PIH on forehead but overall improvement in scars and normal face-to-neck color match.

shown to be equally as effective as Stone. PRR has used the 2-day phenol chemabrasion technique described later with reliable results for 6 years (**Fig. 23**).

THE 2-DAY PHENOL CHEMABRASION TECHNIQUE FOR ACNE SCARS

As noted earlier, the best results on acne scars (because they are of different types) usually require a combination of subcision, dermal fillers, lasers, and repeated peels. If laxity or volume deficiency accompanies deep facial wrinkling, then dermal or periosteal fillers along with cosmetic surgery are also necessary to achieve optimal results, although this is less common in darker skin types. Also, full-face phenol peels are not always necessary and, as already noted, combining deeper

and lighter peels can result in sufficient improvement without the risk of dyschromias or prolonged downtime.

Patient Evaluation

If the skin type is a dark VI (black) and the neck is also dark, then a full-face phenol peel is contraindicated because of the probability of discordant tones, unless the patient agrees to strict avoidance of sun and the chronic use of skin lighteners on the neck. Types IV and V, and even a light VI, have been peeled with acceptable concordance of skin tone between face and neck. For the patient with dark skin type VI, performing 2-day chemabrasion only on individual ice-pick or box scars with the Stone formula or CROSS with 30% TCA is a safer and effective option. Subcision can be performed weeks before, during, and after

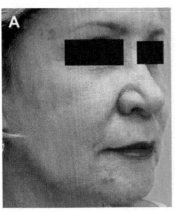
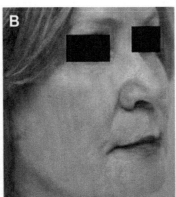
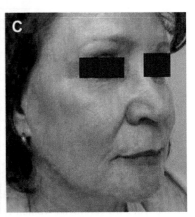

Fig. 22. Latina woman with skin type IV treated for acne scars and photoaging. (*A*) Before full-face Stone phenol; (*B*) 6 months post peel; (*C*) 3 years post peel.

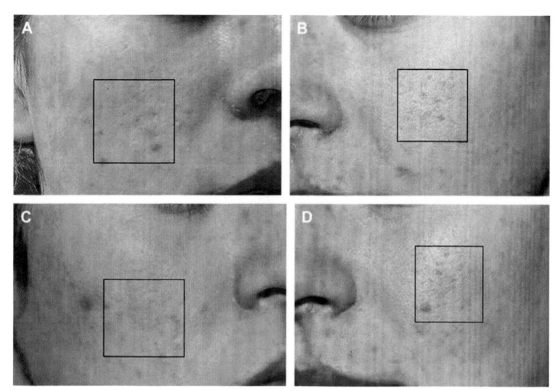

Fig. 23. Paired comparison study comparing 2-day Stone phenol chemabrasion (*A, C*) with occluded phenol (*B, D*) for the treatment of acne scars. Patient is shown (*A, B*) before peel and (*C, D*) 1 month post peel, demonstrating better scar remodeling, even in ice-pick scars (*boxed*) in cheeks treated with the chemabrasion method.

the peel (for rolling scars) and a medium peel performed on the rest of the face or neck with TCA or with fractionated CO_2 laser ablation (**Fig. 24**). Test spots and lighter peels are suggested before doing a full face. Photographic documentation should be obtained with direct lighting and shadows. A supportive family member should be recruited and trained on pre- and postoperative care along with the patient.

Preconditioning

As noted, preconditioning of the skin with creams and treatment of acne is required to improve the efficacy of the peel, reduce the risk of PIH, and promote healing.

Anesthesia and Monitoring

Intravenous (IV) access with either oral (diazepam, triazolam, hydromorphone, or fentanyl oral transmucocosal) or IV conscious sedation (midazolam, fentanyl, propofol, ketamine) is necessary. The use of facial nerve blocks is effective at reducing the need for systemic medication. The use of epinephrine has been avoided or minimized in these blocks to reduce the risk of arrhythmias. Clonidine

(1–2 mg) orally used as a preoperative medication also reduces this risk. General anesthesia is not recommended because of respiratory and pH issues. The Po_2 must be kept at more than 90% throughout the procedure, and sinus tachycardia must be brief and minimized. The patient is discharged home with diazepam, hydromorphone, and triazolam with IV access still in place, with the trained family member assisting.

Day 1

Ringer lactate (1–2 L) is infused for 2 hours. The face is thoroughly cleansed and degreased as described earlier. For a full-face peel (**Fig. 25**), preformulated Stone formula (Delasco, Council Bluffs, IA, USA) is applied with regular Q-tips, which are rolled against the edge of the stainless-steel cup to remove excess fluid. The formula is applied to 5 anatomic areas (forehead, 2 cheeks, perioral and chin, and periorbital and nose), spending 10 to 15 minutes per area so that the peel application takes approximately 60 minutes. Ice-pick scars receive an additional peel application with a fine paintbrush to ensure complete wetting of the lesion. A complete, organized frost has to be achieved in each area, and a yellowish edematous

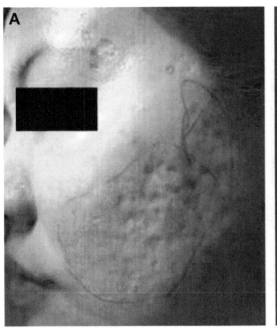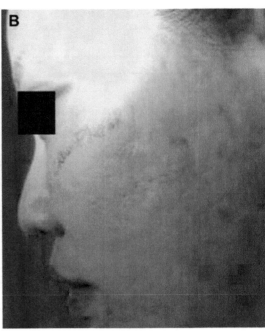

Fig. 24. Korean woman with skin type IV treated for acne scars. (*A*) Before treatment with subcision, CROSS with 2-day Stone phenol peel followed immediately by 30 W fractionated CO_2 therapy (2 sessions); (*B*) postoperative shadow photograph showing improvement in acne scars.

appearance indicating epidermolysis is noted after 15 to 30 minutes. The face is completely taped (except the upper lids) with 1-inch to 2-inch strips of waterproof Hy-Tape (Hy-Tape International, Patterson, NY, USA) (**Fig. 25C**) and covered with a surgical face net. The patient is discharged with a trained family member or nurse. Patients can only drink fluids through a straw or poured

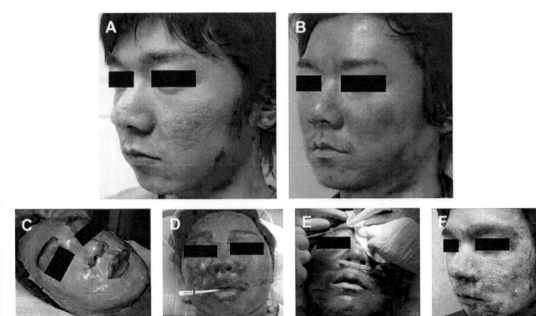

Fig. 25. Korean man with skin type IV treated for acne scars. (*A*) Before treatment with subcision and Stone phenol chemabrasion; (*B*) 10 days post peel fully re-epithelialized; (*C*) following application of the peel, the patient's face is covered with Hy-Tape on day 1; (*D*) tape is removed on day 2, revealing the coagulum of necrotic epidermis and upper reticular dermis; (*E*) the coagulum is debrided with a tongue depressor or large curette; (*F*) the bismuth subgallate powder mask is applied on day 7 and removed on day 9.

into the mouth through a long-tipped water bottle for the next 8 days.

For regional acne scars, the authors suggest applying Stone 100 phenol only on ice-pick and box scars, using a fine paintbrush to deliver it directly into the scars, whereas the rest of the face is then peeled with a lighter acid or with fractional CO_2 ablative resurfacing. Subcision can also be performed at this visit (see **Fig. 24**).

Day 2

The patient is usually groggy but pain free on returning to the clinic. The Hy-Tape is easily removed (**Fig. 25D**). Additional sedation and analgesia are sometimes given if the condition is severe and aggressive abrasion is expected. The necrotic coagulum is debrided using a tongue blade or a large Fox curette (**Fig. 25E**). Ice-pick scars and box scars (or deep wrinkles) are debrided using 1- to 2-mm chalazion-type curettes, achieving punctate bleeding inside the scars, thus ensuring de-epithelialization of these types of lesions. The goal is to create a true open wound within the lesions to induce secondary healing and wound closure. An antiseptic, antiinflammatory powder, bismuth subgallate (Delasco or Spectrum Pharmaceuticals, Irvine, CA, USA) is applied to the entire face (except the upper lid) (**Fig. 25F**) and the patient is sent home. This mask dries out and stays in place for the next 7 to 8 days. The authors call it the protective "green cocoon."

Days 3 to 8

The patient is restricted to home and should not shower until the mask is removed. On approximately the eighth day, the mask separates because the skin has re-epithelialized. Vaseline is applied all over the mask, allowed to soak in, and left overnight. The mask is gently removed the next morning by applying more Vaseline (while showering), under the slowly separating mask. Gentle creams or Aquaphor ointment (Eucerin, Beiersdorf AG, Hamburg, Germany) are then used until the skin is no longer tender or red. Nearly all patients are 99% re-epithelialized by day 9. There has been no incidence of infections following this procedure in the authors' clinic.

Touch-up

Two or three months after the peel has healed, a regional or lesional peel can be repeated, even in skin types IV to VI. These lighter skin types can tolerate a regional peel (**Fig. 26**). The intent is to recreate an open wound inside the ice-pick scars, adding new collagen to the inside of these scars so they eventually fill in almost completely.

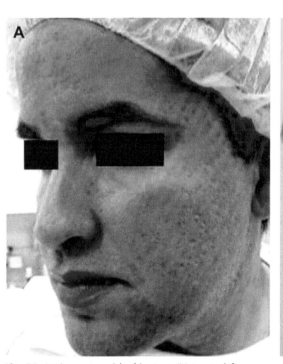
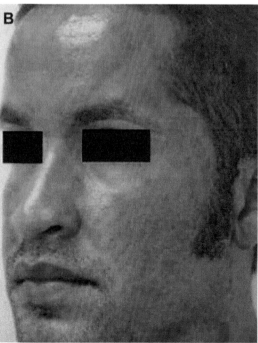

Fig. 26. Latino man with skin type IV treated for acne scars. (*A*) Before Stone phenol 2-day chemabrasion; (*B*) after a full-face peel and a regional touch-up phenol peel.

Postoperative care

With all peels, the immediate postoperative procedure is similar. Cool compresses (water or dilute white vinegar) or oral analgesics should be used for pain. A bland moisturizer should be applied and the skin should be washed with a soapless cleanser (CeraVe, Cetaphil). Sweating should be avoided until redness subsides and sunscreens applied once the skin has re-epithelialized (powder make-up is an option for coverage). Deeper-peeled areas should be treated with Aquaphor. Previous skin conditioning can be re-initiated once skin is no longer sensitive, red, and peeling. Fluocinolone 0.01% cream is started when reaction is stronger, PIH is noted, or when persistent redness is observed.

SUMMARY

Chemical peels to correct dyschromias, acne scars, and other conditions are recommended in patients with darker skin. Peel selection is determined by the depth of the peel required and the mechanism of action of the peel. Peels are commonly used in combinations, as a series, or as a component of a multimodal approach with laser ablation, electrocautery, surgery, dermal fillers, and neurotoxins to correct multiple defects. Care must be taken to reduce the risk of peel-associated PIH. Preconditioning is required for all peels and a rigorous postoperative maintenance regimen ensures long-term satisfaction.

Long-term care and commitment are required from patients who have had peels. Patients may expect peels to control or shrink pores in a lasting manner, but this does not happen. Patients, particularly those with large pores or active acne, need to control the oiliness of their skin by the use of cleansers and drying agents such as medications that are typically used to treat acne. Lifestyle changes may also be required, including avoidance of sun and the reduction of exercise-induced heat (eg, swimming rather than running). These measures will help to ensure patients' lifelong satisfaction with their appearance following a chemical peel.

ACKNOWLEDGMENTS

The authors thank Julia R Gage PhD for assistance with writing the manuscript.

REFERENCES

1. Fitzpatrick TB. The validity and practicality of sun-reactive skin types I through VI. Arch Dermatol 1988;124(6):869–71.

2. Grimes PE. Aesthetics and cosmetic procedures in darker racial ethnic groups. Philadelphia: Lippincott Williams & Wilkins; 2008.

3. Fitzpatrick TB, Ortonne JP. Normal skin color and general considerations of pigmentary disorders. In: Freedberg IM, Eisen AZ, Wolff K, et al, editors. Fitzpatrick's dermatology in general medicine, vol. 1. New York: McGraw-Hill; 2003. p. 819–25.

4. Szabo G, Gerald AB, Pathak MA, et al. Racial differences in the fate of melanosomes in human epidermis. Nature 1969;222(5198):1081–2.

5. Olson RL, Gaylor J, Everett MA. Skin color, melanin, and erythema. Arch Dermatol 1973;108(4):541–4.

6. Halder RM, Nootheti PK. Ethnic skin disorders overview. J Am Acad Dermatol 2003;48(6 Suppl): S143–8.

7. Toda K, Pathak MA, Parrish JA, et al. Alteration of racial differences in melanosome distribution in human epidermis after exposure to ultraviolet light. Nat New Biol 1972;236(66):143–5.

8. Babiarz-Magee L, Chen N, Seiberg M, et al. The expression and activation of protease-activated receptor-2 correlate with skin color. Pigment Cell Res 2004;17(3):241–51.

9. Sharlow ER, Paine CS, Babiarz L, et al. The protease-activated receptor-2 upregulates keratinocyte phagocytosis. J Cell Sci 2000;113(Pt 17): 3093–101.

10. Rawlings AV. Ethnic skin types: are there differences in skin structure and function? Int J Cosmet Sci 2006;28(2):79–93.

11. Yosipovitch G, Theng CTS. Asian skin: its architecture, function and differences from Caucasian skin. Cosmet Toiletries 2002;117(9):104–10.

12. Grimes PE, Stockton T. Pigmentary disorders in blacks. Dermatol Clin 1988;6(2):271–81.

13. Chung JH, Lee SH, Youn CS, et al. Cutaneous photodamage in Koreans: influence of sex, sun exposure, smoking, and skin color. Arch Dermatol 2001; 137(8):1043–51.

14. Chan HH, Fung WK, Ying SY, et al. An in vivo trial comparing the use of different types of 532 nm Nd:YAG lasers in the treatment of facial lentigines in oriental patients. Dermatol Surg 2000;26(8):743–9.

15. Negishi K, Wakamatsu S, Kushikata N, et al. Full-face photorejuvenation of photodamaged skin by intense pulsed light with integrated contact cooling: initial experiences in Asian patients. Lasers Surg Med 2002;30(4):298–305.

16. Karam P, Benedetto AV. Intralesional electrodesiccation of syringomas. Dermatol Surg 1997;23(10):921–4.

17. Ortonne JP, Bissett DL. Latest insights into skin hyperpigmentation. J Investig Dermatol Symp Proc 2008;13(1):10–4.

18. Jacob CI, Dover JS, Kaminer MS. Acne scarring: a classification system and review of treatment options. J Am Acad Dermatol 2001;45(1):109–17.

19. Lee JB, Chung WG, Kwahck H, et al. Focal treatment of acne scars with trichloroacetic acid: chemical reconstruction of skin scars method. Dermatol Surg 2002;28(11):1017–21.

20. Yug A, Lane JE, Howard MS, et al. Histologic study of depressed acne scars treated with serial high-concentration (95%) trichloroacetic acid. Dermatol Surg 2006;32(8):985–90.

21. Ruiz-Esparza J, Barba Gomez JM, Gomez de la Torre OL, et al. UltraPulse laser skin resurfacing in Hispanic patients. A prospective study of 36 individuals. Dermatol Surg 1998;24(1):59–62.

22. Al-Waiz MM, Al-Sharqi AI. Medium-depth chemical peels in the treatment of acne scars in dark-skinned individuals. Dermatol Surg 2002;28(5):383–7.

23. Imayama S, Ueda S, Isoda M. Histologic changes in the skin of hairless mice following peeling with salicylic acid. Arch Dermatol 2000;136(11):1390–5.

24. Brody HJ, Monheit GD, Resnik SS, et al. A history of chemical peeling. Dermatol Surg 2000;26(5):405–9.

25. Lee HS, Kim IH. Salicylic acid peels for the treatment of acne vulgaris in Asian patients. Dermatol Surg 2003;29(12):1196–9.

26. Stone PA. The use of modified phenol for chemical face peeling. Clin Plast Surg 1998;25(1):21–44.

27. Stone PA, Lefer LG. Modified phenol chemical face peels: recognizing the role of application technique. Clin Plast Surg 2001;28(1):13–36.

28. Fintsi Y. Exoderm – a novel, phenol-based peeling method resulting in improved safety. Int J Cosmet Surg 2001;1(4):40–4.

29. Fintsi Y. Exoderm chemoabrasion original method for the treatment of facial acne scars. Int J Cosmet Surg 2001;1(4):45–52.

30. Obagi S, Bridenstine JB. Lifetime skin care. Oral Maxillofac Surg Clin North Am 2000;12(4):531–40.

31. Obagi S, Bridenstine JB. Chemical skin resurfacing. Oral Maxillofac Surg Clin North Am 2000;12(4):541–53.

32. Grimes PE. Chemical peels in dark skin. In: Tosti A, Grimes PE, Pia De Padova M, editors. Color Atlas of chemical peels. Heidelberg: Springer-Verlag; 2006. p. 139–48.

33. Sarkar R, Kaur C, Bhalla M, et al. The combination of glycolic acid peels with a topical regimen in the treatment of melasma in dark-skinned patients: a comparative study. Dermatol Surg 2002;28(9):828–32.

34. Lim JT, Tham SN. Glycolic acid peels in the treatment of melasma among Asian women. Dermatol Surg 1997;23(3):177–9.

35. Wang CM, Huang CL, Hu CT, et al. The effect of glycolic acid on the treatment of acne in Asian skin. Dermatol Surg 1997;23(1):23–9.

36. Burns RL, Prevost-Blank PL, Lawry MA, et al. Glycolic acid peels for postinflammatory hyperpigmentation in black patients. A comparative study. Dermatol Surg 1997;23(3):171–4.

37. Javaheri SM, Handa S, Kaur I, et al. Safety and efficacy of glycolic acid facial peel in Indian women with melasma. Int J Dermatol 2001;40(5):354–7.

38. Grimes PE. The safety and efficacy of salicylic acid chemical peels in darker racial-ethnic groups. Dermatol Surg 1999;25(1):18–22.

39. Garg VK, Sinha S, Sarkar R. Glycolic acid peels versus salicylic-mandelic acid peels in active acne vulgaris and post-acne scarring and hyperpigmentation: a comparative study. Dermatol Surg 2009; 35(1):59–65.

40. Brubacher JR, Hoffman RS. Salicylism from topical salicylates: review of the literature. J Toxicol Clin Toxicol 1996;34(4):431–6.

41. Obagi Z. Obagi skin health restoration and rejuvenation. New York: Springer; 1999.

42. Monheit GD. The Jessner's + TCA peel: a medium-depth chemical peel. J Dermatol Surg Oncol 1989; 15(9):945–50.

43. Hetter GP. An examination of the phenol-croton oil peel: Part I. Dissecting the formula. Plast Reconstr Surg 2000;105(1):227–39.

44. Hetter GP. An examination of the phenol-croton oil peel: part IV. Face peel results with different concentrations of phenol and croton oil. Plast Reconstr Surg 2000;105(3):1061–83.

45. Hetter GP. An examination of the phenol-croton oil peel: Part III. The plastic surgeons' role. Plast Reconstr Surg 2000;105(2):752–63.

46. Hetter GP. An examination of the phenol-croton oil peel: Part II. The lay peelers and their croton oil formulas. Plast Reconstr Surg 2000;105(1):240–8.

47. Rullan P, Lemmon J, Rullan JM. The 2-day phenol chemabrasion technique for deep wrinkles and acne scars. Am J Cosmet Surg 2004; 21:199–210.

Botox Facial Slimming/Facial Sculpting: The Role of Botulinum Toxin-A in the Treatment of Hypertrophic Masseteric Muscle and Parotid Enlargement to Narrow the Lower Facial Width

Woffles T.L. Wu, MBBS, FRCS, FAMS (Plast Surg)[a,b,*]

KEYWORDS

- Facial slimming • Facial sculpting • Botox
- Lower face reduction • Jawline definition
- Masseteric reduction • Parotid gland reduction
- Microbotox

Thin, waiflike models with sculpted cheekbones and fashionable hollows under these cheekbones leap out at us from every page of a glossy magazine. Female and male consumers are increasingly influenced by these images and seek facial improvements that will bring them closer to these aesthetic ideals. With these current media perceptions, in Asia, a lady with a square-shaped face and strong jawline may not be considered beautiful and can, in fact, find herself the butt of derogatory comments. There is therefore pressure to conform to the more triangular and heart-shaped classic ideal of a face.

Botulinum toxin-A (Botox) is a useful tool for the cosmetic reduction of the bulk and volume of the masseteric muscle, thereby narrowing the width of the lower face.[1–3] Botulinum toxin-A can be administered in such a way as to control the degree of reduction and control whether the upper or lower half of the muscle is to be narrowed in accordance with the patient's wishes. Consequently, the jawline becomes more well-defined and the cheekbones take on a sculpted appearance with relative, aesthetic cheek-hollowing and "model-like" shadows under the zygomatic arch.

The result is not permanent, and injections need to be repeated at least six-monthly, after an initial start-up phase in which the botulinum toxin-A is administered monthly, until the degree of desired reduction is achieved. The technique is grounded in craniofacial principles, is safe and reversible, and has few side effects. An adjunct to this technique is the concomitant administration of botulinum toxin-A to enlarged or visible parotid

a Camden Medical Centre, 1 Orchard Boulevard, Suite 09-02, Singapore 294615
b Department of Plastic Surgery, Zhejiang Provincial Peoples Hospital, Hangzhou, China
* Camden Medical Centre, 1 Orchard Boulevard, Suite 09-02, Singapore 294615.
E-mail address: woffles@woffleswu.com

Facial Plast Surg Clin N Am 18 (2010) 133–140
doi:10.1016/j.fsc.2009.11.014
1064-7406/10/$ – see front matter © 2010 Published by Elsevier Inc.

facialplastic.theclinics.com

glands, also to achieve reduction of lower facial width and better definition of the jawline.

HISTORY

The author started this novel approach to reducing lower facial width in 1998, in response to the need for a nonsurgical and easy solution to treat patients with wide, "boxy" faces or "square jaws". These patients complained of a masculine, aggressive appearance, lack of feminine face shape, and protruding angles of the jawline. Many patients who could not articulate the problem merely felt they looked fat in pictures. Some patients, on questioning, also suffered from headaches or migraine and some had excessive wear from grinding their teeth.

At the time, the only solution for patients with prominent mandibular angles was mandibular angle ostectomy and removal of part of the masseteric muscle (usually the inner attached portion).[4–6] This was a bloody operation with significant postoperative downtime and swelling. Complications, such as nerve trauma or intraoperative fractures of the mandible, were known to happen.

Botulinum toxin-A had first been reported in 1994 as a treatment for patients with excessive grinding.[7,8] As the masseter muscle was responsible for the grinding and a widened lower face, the author decided to inject this muscle to reduce its bulk and any other symptoms arising from its malfunction. This would give the patient a cosmetic and functional benefit.

In accordance with Moss'[9–11], Rankow's[10] and Enlow's[12] theories of the bone-muscle matrix, bony growth and maintenance of volume is under the influence and related to the activity of the muscles attached to the bone. A bone responds to the activity of the attached muscles and thickens and becomes denser when there is increased muscle stimulation or when it is "force loaded". Thus, senior citizens are encouraged to exercise to strengthen their bones and increase bone density. Conversely, in the days before rigid fixation of fractured limbs, affected bones were immobilized in plaster casts for many weeks. On removing the cast, the affected bone was always much smaller (confirmed by radiographs) than the unaffected, contralateral side, mainly because of lack of muscle activity during the immobilization period. The author also observed that patients with masseteric hypertrophy invariably had flaring of the mandibular angle and vice versa, lending further weight to the validity of Moss', Rankow's and Enlow's principles. It was further reasoned that long-term changes of the bony shape could possibly be achieved if the activity of the masseter muscle could be kept to a minimum by regular and constant administration of botulinum toxin-A. Clinically, the author has seen a reduction of the protruding mandibular angle and profound changes in facial shape in many patients receiving this treatment for several years, which could not be solely due to muscle reduction.

ANATOMICAL CONSIDERATIONS

The masseter muscle arises as 3 heads from the length of the zygomatic arch, with the superficial head arising anteriorly; the intermediate head, from the middle; and the deep head, more posteriorly. The 3 heads fan downwards in reverse direction to become attached to the angle and the ascending ramus of the mandible, with the superficial head attached more posteriorly and the deep head more anteriorly (**Fig. 1**). Thus, there is an overlap zone where the 3 heads cross each other, and this represents the thickest part of the muscle that can be palpated when patients clench their teeth. The masseteric nerve and artery run between these heads but are not at risk during the treatment because the needles used are very fine.

The limits of the muscle and hence, the botulinum toxin-A injection site are determined by palpation and observation.

The upper border of the muscle corresponds to the zygomatic arch. The posterior border is the posterior border of the mandible. The inferior border corresponds to the inferior border of the mandible, and the anterior border can be palpated when patients clench their teeth; there is a distinct difference between the soft tissues anteriorly and the masseter muscle posteriorly, which becomes rock hard on clenching.

As a general guide after defining the 4 borders, a line should be drawn from the angle of the mouth to the tragus. Six to 10 injections of Botox should be administered beneath this line, to avoid unwanted diffusion through the coronoid notch to the pterygoid muscles and over-hollowing of the superior third of the muscle (**Fig. 2**).

INJECTION TECHNIQUE AND SCHEDULING

Although other types of botulinum toxin-A can be used effectively, the author prefers Botox. A dilution of 2.5 mL nonbuffered saline is used for 100 units of Botox, 1 mL thus containing 40 units of Botox. If 20 or 32 units are to be injected, 0.5 mL and 0.7 mL are drawn up, respectively, after which the syringe is topped up with the requisite amount of saline to make a 1-mL volume for ease of administration of the drug.

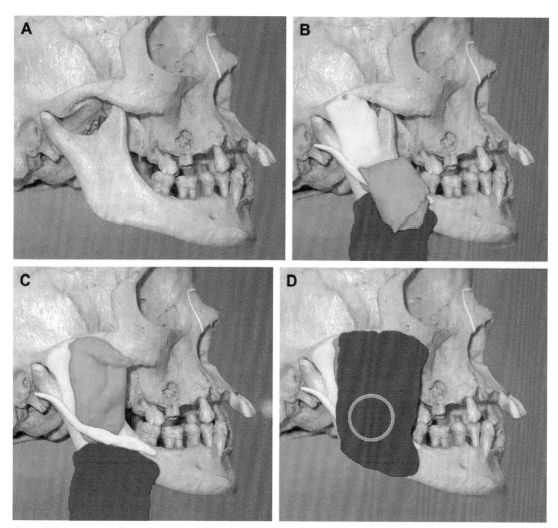

Fig. 1. (*A*) Side view of zygomatic arch and mandible. (*B*) Orientation of the 3 masseteric heads: deep (*yellow*), intermediate (*blue*), and superficial (*red*). The deep head arises from the middle one-third and part of the posterior one-third of the zygomatic arch (ZA) and runs vertically down to insert into the body of the ramus. (*C*) The intermediate head arises from the middle one-third of the ZA in continuity with the deep head. The masseteric artery (*white*) runs between the intermediate and superficial heads. (*D*) The superficial head arises from the anterior two-thirds of the ZA up to the zygomatic process of the maxilla, and the fibers slope backwards and downwards 45° to insert into the angle, the lower border of the mandible, and the lower part of the ascending ramus. The blue circle represents the overlap zone where the masseter is at its thickest on clenching.

Two factors to consider when administering botulinum toxin-A to the masseter are dosage and frequency of injections. The only finite end point is when there is no palpable masseter muscle activity and the muscle has shrunken in size such that the ramus of the mandible can be felt. Other than that, there are only variable end points to be decided by the physician or the patient, because it is a constant tug-of-war between the action of Botox weakening and shrinking the masseter and the returning function and bulk of the muscle. As function returns, so does size.

Different combinations of treatment can result in different shapes. A larger dose administered 1 month apart for 3 months does not yield the same clinical result as a smaller dose administered more frequently but at the same total dose. For example, 60 units administered monthly for 3 months (180 units in total) does not yield the same result as 30 units administered monthly for 6 months.

The shape achieved is different, as is the side-effect potential. With a larger dose over a shorter period, faster shrinkage of the masseter is seen, which may lead to more cheek or infrazygomatic

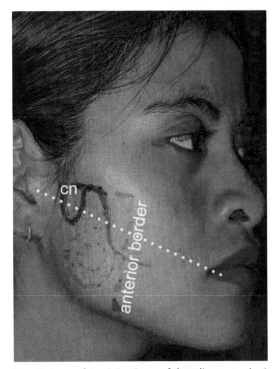

cn

anterior border

Fig. 2. For safety, injections of botulinum toxin-A should be injected below a line drawn from the angle of the mouth to the tragus and not through the easily palpated coronoid notch (cn), because this creates weakness in normal biting and chewing.

hollowing and visible jowl formation. These outcomes are caused by the muscle shrinking faster than the overlying skin can accommodate, leading to sagging of the overlying soft tissue. Over time, this sagging skin will tighten over the new shrunken volume but in the interim, patients can be distressed if they are not forewarned. With a smaller dose given more frequently, the muscle shrinks slowly, giving the skin time to accommodate and contract in tandem. A guide to dosage is presented below:

- For most patients, the initial dose in an average masseter is 40 units, repeated twice at 1-month intervals until there is no palpable movement of the muscle on clenching the teeth. This is considered the endpoint. The patient is then instructed to palpate the masseter muscle weekly until movement returns. This interval is anywhere from 5 to 9 months.
- At that point, the patient returns for follow-up. and a maintenance dose of Botox is administered varying from 20 to 40 units depending on how much masseteric activity there is and how thin and sculpted the patient wants to look. It is

essential to continue the Botox for persistent results.

- In the maintenance phase, patients return at least once or twice a year to repeat the treatment. The more complete the reduction of volume, the longer it takes for the muscle to return to its former size, which could take more than a year.
- If the muscle is very large, 60 units (1.5 mL) can be injected initially. One should wait a month before administering more. A volume of more than 1.5 mL at any one time may lead to unwanted diffusion of the botulinum toxin-A to adjacent muscles; and a common side effect is diffusion anteriorly with weakening of the risorius and levator anguli oris that are responsible for a full and wide open smile. Some patients can become very anxious about this. Care should also be taken not to inject too close to the coronoid notch, which can lead to diffusion into the lateral and medial pterygoid muscles and, in turn, to significant weakening of chewing action.

COMPLICATIONS

The most frequent complications of botulinum toxin for masseter reduction are as follows:

1. Loss of a full smile or an asymmetric smile due to diffusion of the botulinum toxin-A forward to the risorius and levator anguli oris;
2. Weakness and an aching sensation on chewing; typically, the patient finds difficulty in opening the mouth wide and initiating biting, as needed to eat a hamburger or thick, juicy steak;
3. Jowling due to overrapid volume reduction and sagging of the overlying skin envelope;
4. Overhollowing of the infrazygomatic region giving a cachectic appearance;
5. Bruising;
6. Hematoma, which is rare;
7. Visible fasciculation of the muscles;
8. Neurapraxia (never seen by the author).

RESULTS

The author has treated more than 600 patients with this technique and most patients have been extremely pleased with the results. Very few patients discontinue treatment; cost is the main reason for stopping treatment. Most patients are young and fashion conscious; some may not have the financial resources to maintain the result long-term. The longest follow-up seen was 11 years. The Botox was as efficacious in the last dose as in the first. No antibodies or resistance has been seen or demonstrated in any of these patients.

In the author's regimen,[2] the aim is to shrink the masseter muscle maximally with repeated doses of Botox and then allow the masseter volume to slowly return to approximately 20% to 30% before instituting maintenance doses. These are used to keep the facial width narrow and slim within a narrow range. Other physicians prefer to give a single large loading dose that can achieve a 20% to 50% reduction of masseter size and to wait for the patient to complain of a wide face again before giving the second dose. This typically takes 4 to 6 months. This approach produces wide fluctuation in the patient's face width.

It is not the intention of this regimen to allow the facial width to swing between normal and 50% reduction, but rather to fluctuate gently between total atrophy and 20% return of function. In this way, the slimness of the face is maintained, and a greater possibility exists of influencing bony remodeling of the mandibular angles over time.

The treatment has been effective in Asians and Caucasians, although the vast majority of patients have been of Asian descent.

There were few complaints of weakness of bite force or chewing.[13,14] Most patients experienced mild weakness and an ache on chewing in the first 1 or 2 months, but the sensation resolved spontaneously with no further complaints. All patients were comfortable by the third month. Those patients who had concomitant grinding tendencies or headaches would specifically request a maintenance dose whenever their headaches returned.

BOTOX AND THE PAROTID GLANDS

Patients who complain of a widened, lower face have also to be examined carefully for parotid hypertrophy, because this can also contribute to the impression of flared mandibular angles. The parotid gland is identified by observing and palpating a diffuse swelling that extends beyond the posterior border of the mandibular angle. The parotid also pushes the earlobe outwards giving patients a "bull necked" look. Occasionally, this may be missed in patients with thick skin and overlying soft tissue padding and only becomes obvious after the masseter muscle has been reduced and residual swellings are seen at the posterior aspect of the mandible. In such cases, 40 units of Botox can be injected into the parotid gland monthly until the swelling becomes less obvious. This usually takes 3 to 4 sessions and is very effective. There have been no complaints of dryness of mouth or decrease in saliva production.

As the masseter bulk and parotid size decrease, the lower border of the mandible becomes well defined, which patients find aesthetically pleasing. Combining this with the MicroBotox technique of the platysma muscle further serves to shape and define the jawline and allows the platysma to hug the undersurface of the neck, making it youthful and tight. This has the effect of a nonsurgical neck lift.

Case 1

A 28-year-old woman complains of a fat face that does not photograph well. She has no symptoms of grinding or headaches. Very large masseter muscles are seen on examination (**Fig. 3**A). The Botox administered in month 1 was 60 units per side and month 2 and 3, 40 units per side. She experienced rapid deflation of the lower face with mild sagging of the jowls (**Fig. 3**B). Forty units were administered every 4 to 6 months and **Fig. 3**C shows her 3 years later. Note the skin now conforming well to the new shape without any jowling. The lower face appears much thinner with better cheekbone definition.

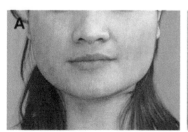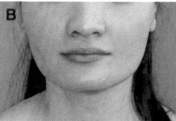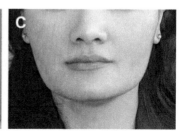

Fig. 3. Case 1. A 28-year-old woman complaining of a fat face that does not photograph well. No symptoms of grinding or headaches. Very large masseter muscles seen on examination (*A*) Botox administered in month 1 was 60 units per side and in month 2 and 3, 40 units per side. She experienced rapid deflation of the lower face with mild sagging of the jowls (*B*) Forty units were given every 4 to 6 months and (*C*) shows her 3 years later. Note the skin now conforming well to the new shape without any jowling. The lower face appears much thinner with better cheekbone definition.

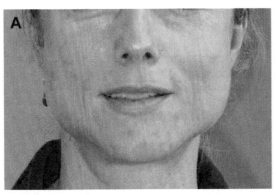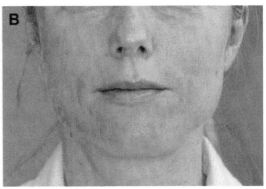

Fig. 4. Case 2. A 37-year-old Caucasian woman felt that her jawline was too masculine and that the angles protruded in an unusual and unaesthetic fashion. She had occasional headaches. Three doses of 40 units of Botox per side were administered one month apart to achieve a slimmer, more aesthetically pleasing appearance (*A* and *B*).

Case 2

A 37-year-old Caucasian woman felt that her jawline was too masculine and that the angles protruded in an unusual and unaesthetic fashion. She had occasional headaches. Three doses of 40 units of Botox per side were administered one month apart, to achieve a slimmer, more aesthetically pleasing appearance (**Fig. 4**).

Case 3

A 25-year-old woman requested extreme thinning of her face and declined any surgery. Forty units of Botox per side were administered monthly for 3 months, followed by a maintenance dose of between 32 and 40 units per side every 4 to 6 months. She is shown 2 years later with significant narrowing of the face. She feels as if her bones have shrunk and her bizygomatic distance decreased (**Fig. 5**).

Case 4

A 33-year-old man felt he was getting thick around the neck with poor definition of the lower jawline. He requested an expedient, nonsurgical technique, because he had an important photography session coming up in 2 months. He received 2 doses of 50 units of Botox per side, a month apart and 16 units of microBotox[2] into each side of his jawline and upper neck. He is seen 6 weeks after his first dose (**Fig. 6**).

Case 5

A 30-year-old woman with a broad lower face requested nonsurgical aesthetic improvement. Her masseter muscles were injected with 40 units of Botox per side monthly for 4 months and subsequently maintained with this dose every 4 months. Her parotid glands were also seen to be diffusely enlarged, contributing to the width of her lower face. These were injected with 40 units Botox per

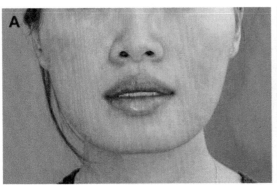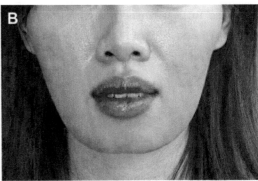

Fig. 5. Case 3. A 25-year-old woman requested extreme thinning of her face and declined any surgery. Forty units of Botox per side were given monthly for 3 months followed by a maintenance dose of between 32 to 40 units per side every 4 to 6 months. She is shown 2 years later with significant narrowing of the face. She feels as if her bones have shrunk and her bizygomatic distance decreased (*A* and *B*).

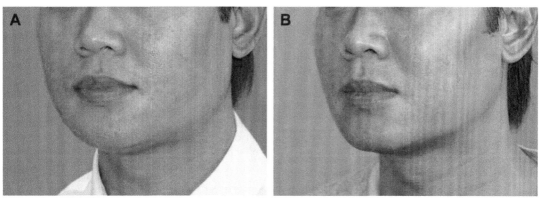

Fig. 6. Case 4. A 33-year-old man felt he was getting thick around the neck with poor definition of the lower jawline. He requested an expedient, nonsurgical technique, because he had an important photography session coming up in 2 months. He received 2 doses of 50 units of Botox per side 1 month apart and 16 units of Micro-Botox into each side of his jawline and upper neck. He is seen 6 weeks after his first dose (*A* and *B*). (*Data from* Wu Woffles. Innovative uses of BOTOX and the Woffles lift. In: D Panfilov, editor. Aesthetic surgery of the facial mosaic. Berlin, Heidelberg (Germany): Springer; 2006. Chapter 72. p. 636–49.)

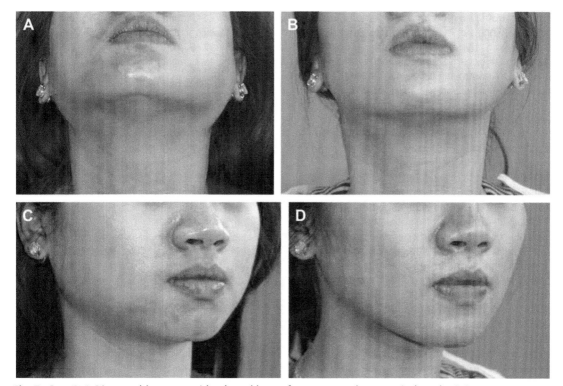

Fig. 7. Case 5. A 30-year-old woman with a broad lower face requested nonsurgical aesthetic improvement. Her masseter muscles were injected with 40 units of Botox per side monthly for 4 months and subsequently maintained with this dose every 4 months. Her parotid glands were also seen to be diffusely enlarged, contributing to the width of her lower face. These were injected with 40 units Botox per side monthly for 3 sessions commencing in the fifth month of her treatment (after the masseter size had been resolved). Every 4 to 5 months, she would return for 40 units to each masseter and 28 units to each parotid. She is shown before and after 2.5 years of treatment (*A* to *D*).

side monthly for 3 sessions commencing in the fifth month of her treatment (after the masseter size had been resolved). Every 4 to 5 months, she would return for 40 units to each masseter and 28 units to each parotid. She is shown before and after 2.5 years of treatment (**Fig. 7**).

DISCUSSION

Before the use of botulinum toxin-A to treat the "square jaw" phenomenon, surgery was the only option. The procedure was often bloody, especially if part of the masseter muscle was resected and in some cases, it was quite difficult if the mandibular angle spur projected posteriorly. Achieving symmetry always posed challenges, because most of these patients exhibit facial and jaw asymmetry to some degree. Fractures of the mandibular ramus due to unfavorable splits of the bone during the ostectomies would necessitate an open incision to fix the fracture, thus giving the patient an unwanted, visible scar.

Nonetheless, in the hands of the skilled surgeon, the results can be very pleasing and stable, although there are some reports that over time, the bony spur can recur and the mandibular width increase. This was thought to be due to persistent masseteric hyperactivity and subsequent regrowth. It became obvious to the author that the key to controlling lower facial width was to control the size and function of the masseter muscle. If the muscle could be atrophied, the facial width would reduce and there was a possibility that the muscular influence on the bone would also decrease, allowing the bones to remodel and narrow the face further.

At the time, the one paper discussing the role of Botox in treating masseteric hypertrophy concentrated only on the medical aspects. The author decided to implement this treatment on those patients primarily wanting cosmetic improvement. The initial results were impressive, and as more patients were recruited and months of follow-up turned into years, the drug's full effect over time on the muscle could be seen. The change in facial shape was even more dramatic than with mandibular angle ostectomy alone, with many patients achieving a perceived narrowing of the mandibular angle width and the bizygomatic width. This had the effect of profoundly slimming the face; hence, the 2 names "Botox Facialslimming" and "Botox Facialsculpting" were coined by the author.

Decreasing parotid size with Botox was incorporated into the author's regime after a patient whose masseter muscles had been successfully reduced displayed a persistent bulging in the vicinity of the mandibular angle.

SUMMARY

Botulinum toxin-A is a highly efficacious and cost-effective, nonsurgical option for reducing the width and shape of the lower face and jawline. The results can vary from the subtlest thinning of the face to an extremely thin, cachectic appearance. Many nuances can be achieved. The administration is simple, and the process takes barely 5 minutes in an office setting. Botulinum toxin-A can also be effectively used to reduce the bulk of an enlarged parotid gland without affecting saliva production.

REFERENCES

1. Wu WTL. Facial rejuvenation without facelifts—personal strategies. Regional conference in dermotological laser and facial cosmetic surgery 2002. Hong Kong, September 13–15, 2002.
2. Woffles Wu. Innovative uses of BOTOX and the Woffles lift. In: Panfilov D, editor. Aesthetic surgery of the facial mosaic. Berlin, Heidelberg (Germany): Springer; 2006. Chapter 72. p. 636–49.
3. Park MY, Ahn KY, Jung DS. Botulinum toxin type A treatment for contouring of lower face. Dermatol Surg 2003;29:477–83.
4. Gurney C. Chronic bilateral benign hypertrophy of the masseter muscle. Am J Surg 1947;78:137.
5. Adams W. Bilateral hypertrophy of the masseter muscle: an operation for correction. Br J Plast Surg 1949;2:78.
6. Baek SM, Kim S, Bindinger A. The prominent mandibular angle: preoperative management, operative technique and results. Plast Reconstr Surg 1989;83:272.
7. Moore AP, Wood GD. The medical management of masseteric hypertrophy with Botulinum toxin type A. Br J Oral Maxillofac Surg 1994;32:26–8.
8. Smyth AG. Botulinum toxin type A treatment of bilateral masseteric hypertrophy. Br J Oral Maxillofac Surg 1994;32:29–33.
9. Moss ML. The primacy of functional matrices in orofacial growth. Dent Pract Dent Rec 1968;19(2):65–73.
10. Moss ML, Rankow RM. The role of the functional matrix in mandibular growth. Angle Orthod 1968; 38(2):95–103.
11. Moss ML. The functional matrix hypothesis revisited. 2. The role of an osseous connected cellular network. Am J Orthod Dentofacial Orthop 1997;112(2):221–6.
12. Enlow DH. Facial growth. 3rd edition. Philadelphia: Saunders; 1990.
13. Kim ST, Choi JH, Park MY, et al. The change of the maximal bite-force after Botulinum toxin A injection for lower face contouring. J Korean Soc Aesthetic Plast Surg 2005;11(1):45–50.
14. Yu C, Chen PKT, Chen YR. Botulinum toxin A for lower facial contouring: a prospective study. Aesthetic Plast Surg 2007;5:445–51.

Traumatic Rhinoplasty in the Non-Caucasian Nose

David W. Kim, MD*, Harry S. Hwang, MD

KEYWORDS

- Traumatic injury • Rhinoplasty • Non-Caucasian
- Nasal deformity

Traumatic injury resulting in nasal deformity poses unique challenges to the surgeon. The goals of rhinoplasty are to correct both cosmetic and functional problems that may not have otherwise been an issue prior to the injury. As for all rhinoplasty patients, preoperative evaluation of posttraumatic nasal deformity requires attention to the observed deformities of the nose as well as the baseline anatomy. This baseline anatomy varies significantly from individual to individual, often owing to characteristic ethnic features. Although it is overly simplistic to group all individuals from one ethnicity as having one type of nose, the rhinoplasty surgeon must understand the common variations of nasal anatomy seen in various races of individuals. In addition, certain anatomic features may affect the pattern of injury or deformity following nasal trauma. The ethnic anatomic differences in the non-Caucasian nose in the context of posttraumatic nasal deformity are discussed in this article. The various rhinoplasty techniques and strategies to address these issues are reviewed.

NASAL ANATOMY

A comprehensive review of nasal anatomy is beyond the scope of this subject. In this section, the pertinent anatomy relevant to patterns of nasal trauma is discussed. In particular, the structural anatomy of the nasal bones and nasal septum has bearing on the patterns of injury following trauma. This section reviews this general anatomy.

The following section outlines variations of anatomy based on variable ethnic features.

The skeletal framework of the nose is often divided into 3 sections: the upper third consists of the osseous vault; the middle third consists of the upper cartilaginous vault; and the lower third consists of the lower cartilaginous vault. The nasal septum provides support in all 3 sections and divides the nasal cavity in half. The septum has 2 distinct portions, a cartilaginous portion anteriorly and a bony portion posteriorly.

The nasal septum is a sagittal midline structure that divides the nose into 2 cavities, and provides structural support to the osseous and cartilaginous vaults.[1] The septum is divided into 2 components. The cephalic-posterior osseous septum consists of the perpendicular plate of the ethmoid and the vomer. The caudal-anterior cartilaginous septum consists of the quadrangular cartilage. The dorsal aspect of the osseous septum is formed by the perpendicular plate of the ethmoid. The thickness of the perpendicular plate of the ethmoid varies considerably. This plate attaches superiorly to the frontal bone, anteriorly the nasal spine, and posteriorly the cribriform plate. The septum articulates with the inward projection of the nasal bones in the midline anterosuperiorly, and it borders the quadrangular cartilage anteroinferiorly. Posteroinferiorly it borders the vomer. The vomer is shaped like the keel of a boat. The vomer articulates with the perpendicular plate of the ethmoid superiorly. Along its inferior aspect, the vomer attaches to the midline nasal crest of

Department of Otolaryngology – Head and Neck Surgery, University of California, 400 Parnassus Avenue, A-730, San Francisco, CA 94143, USA
* Corresponding author.
E-mail address: drkim@dwkimmd.com (D.W. Kim).

Facial Plast Surg Clin N Am 18 (2010) 141–151
doi:10.1016/j.fsc.2009.11.011
1064-7406/10/$ – see front matter © 2010 Elsevier Inc. All rights reserved

the palatine bone posteriorly and the maxilla anteriorly. Anterior to its articulation with the vomer, the maxillary crest forms a groove into which the quadrangular cartilage sits.

The cartilaginous septum comprises the quadrangular cartilage. The inferior aspect of the septum rests within a groove in the nasal spine and maxillary crest. The ventral surface of the quadrangular cartilage is typically thickened in comparison to the remainder of the structure. The dorsal aspect of the quadrangular cartilage forms the external contour of the nasal bridge. The dorsum of the central third of the nose is formed by the upper lateral cartilages' articulation with the cephalic aspect of the quadrangular cartilage. The least rigid portion of the cartilage is the most caudal, which extends anterior to the nasal spine. The membranous septum is the soft tissue continuation of the cartilaginous septum. The membranous septum consists of a central layer of subcutaneous areolar tissue between the vestibular skin on each side, thereby bridging the caudal edge of the cartilaginous septum to the medial crura of the lower lateral cartilages and columella. Within the membranous septum are the ligamentous attachments of the medial crura to the caudal septum. The membranous septum is mobile, and displaces easily with manipulation of the columella due to the lack of cartilage.

The inner layer of the septum consists of either perichondrium or periostium, covered by an outer layer of mucosa. The vascular and nervous supply to the septum is contained within the 2 septal lining layers. In a traumatic septal hematoma, separation of the mucoperichondrium from the underlying cartilage may occur, which in turn may lead to ischemic necrosis of the affected septum and result in a perforation or a saddle nose deformity. This situation arises due to the fact that the perichondrial and periostial layers bear the majority of the biomechanical strength of the septal lining and bone.[2]

Septal deviations off the mid-sagittal plane often have both functional and cosmetic implications, especially in the setting of nasal trauma. Deviations along the floor of the nasal airway may cause considerable airway obstruction. Combinations of cartilaginous and osseous deformities often contribute to the obstruction. Portions of the septum may be jagged and angulated in the setting of nasal trauma. Surgical treatment may require removing or repositioning these deviated skeletal elements. If deviations of the perpendicular plate of the ethmoid and vomer are not adequately corrected, persistent posterior airway obstruction after septal surgery may result.

Deviations of the caudal and dorsal edge of the septum also have cosmetic and functional implications. Along the rhinion to the anterior nasal spine, septal deviations may manifest as visible external deformities. A crooked nose deformity at the upper cartilaginous vault, the nasal tip, the columella, or the columellar base may be due to a deviation of the mid-dorsal septum, anterior septal angle, mid-caudal septum, or posterior septal angle, respectively. These irregularities may originate from a traumatic event, and thus correction of a severely crooked nose may require surgical intervention.

Together with the bony septum, the osseous vault is a pyramidal structure that provides the principal structural support for the nose. The distance from nasion to rhinion defines the cephalic-caudal length of the osseous vault. This vault consists of the frontal process of the maxilla and the paired nasal bones. The osseous vault articulates cephalically with the frontal bone at the nasofrontal suture line. The nasal bones superiorly derive midline support from the perpendicular plate of the ethmoid. At the keystone area, the caudal edge of the nasal septum is joined by a connective tissue to the upper cartilaginous vault. Each nasal bone can be described as an elongated quadrangle, with its lateral long edge articulating with the frontal process of the maxilla and its medial long edge articulating in the midline with the contralateral nasal bone. The bones cephalically are narrow and thin at the nasofrontal suture line, and wider and thinner along its free caudal edge. Most traumatic nasal fractures occur in the caudal, more projecting portion of the nasal bones where they are the thinnest.

In brief, the upper cartilaginous vault consists of the paired, shieldlike upper lateral cartilages that are fused in the midline to the dorsal edge of the cartilaginous septum. The nasal bones provide the majority of reinforcement to the upper lateral cartilages at their cephalic margin, the keystone area. The key elements in the lower cartilaginous vault are the paired lower lateral (or alar) cartilages. With the septum, the lower lateral cartilages provide support to the nasal tip.

ETHNIC ANATOMIC DIFFERENCES

Ethnic variations that have been described to influence nasal morphology are categorized into 3 general forms: leptorrhine, platyrrhine, and mesorrhine.[3–5]

- The *leptorrhine* ("tall and thin") nose is associated with Caucasian or Indo-European descent. This type of nose has served as the basis of aesthetic ideal in Western culture. The leptorrhine nose has become the reference point for comparison when studying noses of different ethnicities, because it is the most extensively studied type of nose in modern nasal analysis.

- The *platyrrhine* ("broad and flat") nose is associated with African descent. Its characteristics include very thick skin, a low radix, a bulbous and lower projected tip, a short dorsum, and flared nostrils.

- The *mesorrhine* ("intermediate") nose has features of both the leptorrhine nose and the platyrrhine nose. The "typical" Asian or Latino nose is commonly regarded as mesorrhine, which is characterized by a low radix, rounded and less projected tip, variable anterior dorsal projection, and rounded nostrils. There is, however, considerable variation in this group.

Many of the functional and aesthetic ethnic differences in the nose is due to variations in the size and development of the nasal septum. Septal projection may be highly variable. Because the septum is attached to the cartilages that determine nasal shape (lower lateral and upper lateral cartilages), its overgrowth may lead to excessive projection of these structures. For example, the tension nose deformity is the situation whereby the septum pulls the cartilaginous elements of the nose under tension. These types of noses are characterized by a high cartilaginous dorsum, a low hanging columella that is created by a prominent caudal septal border, and a tip-defining point that is determined by a projecting anterior septal angle.

In a recent study, Asian noses were compared with Caucasian noses.[6] Overall, Asian noses were found to have less projection, in general, at all levels compared with Caucasian noses. The average Caucasian male nasal tip projection was 3.2 cm, whereas the average Asian male projection was significantly less than 2.5 cm ($P<.001$). The average Caucasian female nasal tip projection was 2.8 cm, whereas the average Asian female projection was 2.4 cm ($P = .010$). Similar significant findings were found of nasion projection between the Caucasian and Asian noses. Decreased nasal projection may protect Asian individuals from a greater degree of nasal trauma relative to Caucasian individuals. When comparing the width of the bony vault, Caucasian female noses on average were significantly narrower compared with their Asian counterparts.[6] In regard of variations in nasal bone length, differences in length may also be partially influenced by ethnicity. With the notion that the Asian nose, in general, is broader in appearance compared with the Caucasian nose, the Asian nose also tends to have a shorter nasal length relative to the Caucasian nose, as evident by a larger width-length ratio.[6] Furthermore, variations in the width and medial-lateral position of the nasal bones may be hereditary or acquired. Hereditary variations are more likely to manifest as a symmetric but unusually narrow or wide osseous vault; acquired traumatic injuries typically manifest in gross asymmetries. These observations reflect the generally accepted notions that the Asian nose is broader and shorter along the dorsum, the nasal tip is less projected, and the radix is low lying (ie, mesorrhine nose).[7]

Another aspect of the nasal anatomy that varies between ethnic groups is the thickness of the nasal skin-soft tissue envelope (SSTE). Individuals of African decent tend to have very thick, inelastic SSTE overlying the nasal skeleton, whereas individuals of Asian decent tend to have SSTE of intermediate thickness. In general, the SSTE of Caucasian individuals tends to be thinner. Thus, it is reasonable to consider that in the context of nasal trauma, skin thickness may influence the external appearance of the nose by camouflaging the apparent defects of the nasal skeleton. Furthermore, the thickness of the SSTE may influence the type of maneuvers that are feasible during operative repair of posttraumatic nasal deformities.

With regard to nasal trauma, it is the authors' opinion that the leptorrhine nose, with its greater projection along the osseous vault and dorsum, renders it more susceptible to significant distortion following nasal trauma. The flatter profile of the mesorrhine and platyrrhine nose provides relative protection against impact to the nose. In addition, when fractures to the bones of the nose do occur, it may be more apparent in the leptorrhine nose due to the greater prominence of the osseous vault and septum. The lower pyramidal geometry and thicker skin envelope of the non-Caucasian nose tends to mask whatever skeletal distortion may occur (**Fig. 1**).

Even with these 3 descriptions of ethnically based nasal morphology, caution is warranted if one were to overly generalize rhinoplasty for the non-Caucasian nose. To classify a non-Caucasian nose as an "ethnic" nose to which "ethnic rhinoplasty" principles apply may be overly simplistic. Significant variations may exist between 2 noses from the same ethnic background as well as 2 noses from 2 different ethnic backgrounds. For example, Latinos with Caribbean ancestry are more likely to have platyrrhine noses, whereas those of Central and South American descent have more leptorrhine noses.[8] It would be inappropriate to uniformly apply ethnic group characteristics to an individual patient based one's ethnic or racial background. However, possessing an awareness of the global differences

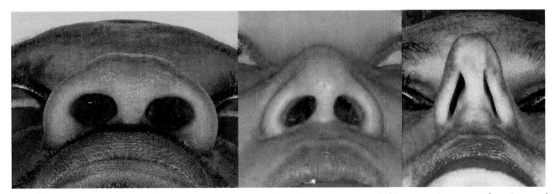

Fig. 1. Base view images showing the broad range of nasal geometries and skin types in noses of patients of different ethnicities.

between ethnic nasal morphologies will allow a rhinoplasty surgeon to be more sensitive to the needs of all patients. Ethnic anatomic nasal variations are important to understand to properly assess the nasal defects and plan the appropriate surgical management strategy for posttraumatic nasal deformities.

TREATMENT OF OSSEOUS NASAL VAULT DEFORMITIES

In the evaluation of posttraumatic nasal deformities, the preoperative interview and assessment should elicit the mechanism of injury. Posttraumatic nasal obstruction may help to determine if injury occurred to the nasal septum or the osseous or cartilaginous nasal skeleton. Cosmetic deformities that resulted from the injury should be distinguished from those that predate the injury. The goals of surgical repair should be clearly discussed and agreed on by the patient and the surgeon. Functional improvement to correct nasal airway obstruction is typically the main priority; however, aesthetic considerations must also be discussed and clarified.

Closed reduction is an option to treat the deviated bony vault in the early traumatic crooked nose. The procedure must be performed before rigid osseous union has occurred because reduction relies on the mobility of the fractured bony segments. This time point varies from patient to patient. This technique has the advantage of being minimally invasive and rapid, and may be performed under local anesthetic. Unless reduction can be performed within the first hours following injury before the onset of edema, the procedure should be delayed several days until swelling has resolved. The edema will impede mobilization of the bony fragments as well as create difficulty in

accurate assessment of final position of the osseous nasal vault. Because closed reduction is less precise than formal open reduction, it poses an increased risk of residual deviation and need for a second operation. As such, deformities with bony comminution, extensive cartilaginous injury, or severe septal deviations should be treated with other techniques.

After appropriate topical and local anesthesia, with or without intravenous sedation, reduction is performed with a strong, flat instrument such as a Boise elevator or the back of a scalpel handle. A lifting and levering motion will allow the bony segments to separate and mobilize into reduction. An occasional audible or palpable pop signals that reduction has been achieved. The bony nasal vault should be completely mobilized to ensure adequate reduction. If the opposite problem is encountered in which the bones do not easily mobilize, early osseous union may have occurred. Vigorous digital pressure will refracture the bones and allow movement of the bony nasal vault in most cases. If necessary, the surgeon may choose to perform osteotomies to create controlled fracture lines. An assortment of reduction forceps and instruments are available for closed septal mobilization and reduction; these techniques, however, are less likely to achieve precise and stable reduction.

Open reduction refers to fracture reduction through incisions and osteotomies, which can be performed either through an endonasal or external rhinoplasty approach.[9] The advantage of open reduction of nasal bone fractures is that it allows for more precise placement of osteotomies to achieve the most symmetric reduction. Any dorsal hump reduction should be performed before osteotomies. Medial osteotomies disconnect the 2 halves of the osseous vault so each may be moved independently, and lateral osteotomies free the anterior sidewall of the osseous vault from its attachment to the rest of the frontal process of the maxilla. The lateral osteotomy is made on the frontal process of the maxilla and preserves the naso-maxillary suture line. The lateral osteotomy should lie lateral to the bony deformity so that it may be incorporated into the segment of mobilized bone. In cases in which the nasal bone has a very convex, concave, or irregular topography, the bone may need to be mobilized in more than one segment to correct the contour irregularities. In such situations, an intermediate osteotomy may be necessary between the medial and lateral osteotomies. When several osteotomies are needed, they are performed medial to lateral so that the cuts are always made on stable bone (**Fig. 2**). The distance of osteotomies needed to mobilize the nasal bones are dictated by their length, which is also highly variable. There is a wide range of height, length, and width of the osseous vault, and these should be taken into account in the planning of osteotomies. Using an osteotome of inappropriate size can lead to excessive intranasal

soft tissue trauma, resulting in postsurgical aesthetic nasal deformity and asymmetry.[10] Osteotome selection is often dictated by the experience of the surgeon. For the Asian nose, a recent study discussed osteotome selection based on radiographic analysis of nasal and facial bone thickness.[11] The thickness of the facial bony lateral wall at 3 points along the track of a lateral osteotomy, and 2 points along the track of a medial osteotomy and intermediate osteotomy were measured. The average bony thickness along the track of a lateral osteotomy was 2.61 ± 0.66 mm at the low level, 2.75 ± 0.76 mm at the middle level, and 2.72 ± 0.53 mm at the high level in subjects. The average bony thickness along the track of an intermediate osteotomy was 1.26 ± 0.34 mm at the low level and 1.31 ± 0.32 mm at the high level in the subjects. The average bony thickness along the track of the medial osteotomy was 2.54 ± 0.31 mm at the low level and 2.77 ± 0.30 mm at the high level in subjects. Based on these results, the investigators recommended using 2.5-mm or 3.0-mm osteotomes to minimize trauma during osteotomies in the Asian nose. The caveat regarding the use of small osteotomes is that the instrument may slip in less experienced hands and may require repeated passes, thereby exacerbating soft tissue injury.[12] If necessary, larger osteotomes can be used for individuals who have larger, thicker nasal bones.

In treating nasal fractures of the non-Caucasian nose through either closed or open reduction, a few unique considerations come into play. First, due to the flatter geometry of the nasal pyramid, there will be generally less displacement from the midline than in leptorrhine noses of greater projection. In addition, the flatter geometry creates less contrast between the dorsum, which generally reflects light, and the nasal sidewall, which is in shadow; this renders deviations of the non-Caucasian nose less noticeable than an equivalent deviation in the Caucasian nose. Finally, a darker and thicker skin envelope also masks deviations of the nasal pyramid. Although the surgeon should strive for as precise a reduction as possible, these factors provide a margin of camouflage to hide slight imperfections following treatment (**Fig. 3**).

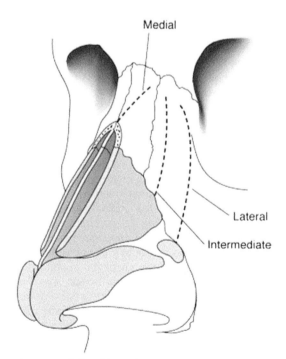

Medial

Lateral

Intermediate

Fig. 2. Medial and lateral osteotomies allow for repositioning of the nasal bone. If the bony segment is also misshapen (convex or concave), additional intermediate osteotomies can be placed to improve the contour as well as the position. (*From* Kim DW, Toriumi DM. Management of posttraumatic nasal deformities: the crooked nose and the saddle nose. Facial Plast Surg Clin North Am 2004;12(1):111–32; with permission.)

TREATMENT OF NASOSEPTAL L-STRUT DEFORMITIES

In certain traumatic nasal septal deformities, the cartilaginous middle vault and nasal tip move into a favorable position after osseous vault repositioning. This scenario is seen frequently when the nasal septum is tilted due to bony deviation, with a normal relationship between the upper lateral

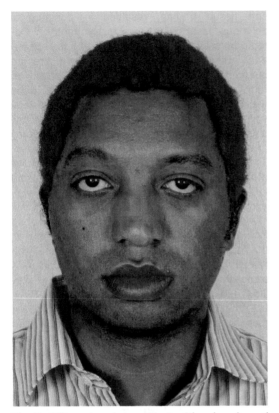

Fig. 3. African American patient with splayed nasal bones and deviation to left following trauma. These deformities are somewhat masked by overall lower projection and thicker, darker skin envelope.

cartilages and dorsal septum. With osteotomies, the tilted septum is returned to midline bringing along the dorsal margin of the septum and nasal tip. However, if the lower two-thirds of the nose do not straighten with bony vault correction, the deviations are likely related to more complex septal deformities with distortion of dorsal margin of the septum and the upper lateral cartilages. In general, the dorsal middle vault will parallel the dorsal deviations of the cartilaginous septum, the cartilaginous domes and nasal tip will follow deflections of the anterior septal angle, the medial crura and columella will parallel the caudal septal margin, and the columellar base (medial crural footplates) will mirror the posterior septal angle. Thus for the traumatic crooked nose, the adage, "where the septum goes, so goes the nose" is especially applicable. As such, correction of the deviated lower two-thirds of the nose may require modulation of the nasal septal L-strut.

The external rhinoplasty approach is preferable in cases of significant dorsal or caudal septal deviation. This approach provides direct visualization and wide exposure, to reposition, disassemble, and reconstruct the L-strut as deemed necessary to correct the deformity. This method involves elevating the SSTE and subsequently the bilateral mucoperichondrial flaps from the floor to the connection of the nasal septum with the upper lateral cartilages. Septal deformities from trauma as well as inherent bending of the cartilage can then be assessed. The areas of deviation should then be localized by region: dorsum, anterior septal angle, caudal margin, or posterior septal angle. The method of correction will depend on the site(s) involved and the severity of the deformity.

Harvesting of the posterior-cephalic cartilage may be performed through the external approach. At minimum, a 1.2-cm dorsal and caudal strut should be left to maintain support for the nose. Fractures, crush injury, or thinning of portions of the strut should be noted and may require suture reinforcement or graft support.

For isolated dorsal (anterior) cartilaginous septal deviations, placement of sutured in-place spreader grafts between the dorsal margin of the cartilaginous septum and upper lateral cartilages can be considered. Spreader grafts are useful to correct functional and cosmetic problems related to a narrow or asymmetric middle vault. The dimensions of spreader grafts will vary depending on specific needs and anatomy. In general, the grafts range from 6 to 12 mm in length, 3 to 5 mm in height, and 2 to 4 mm in thickness. More than one graft on each side may be needed depending on availability and thickness of grafting material and the degree of asymmetry. The grafts are usually placed from a dorsal approach after the upper lateral cartilages are freed from the septum. The dorsal profile of the spreader grafts, upper lateral cartilages, and septum should be coplanar and smooth. The grafts may need to be trimmed in situ to ensure an even dorsal surface. For relatively weak septal cartilage with mild to moderate deviation, spreader grafts serve to overcome the inherent curvature of the septum and result in straightening of the dorsal line. For stronger septal cartilage with more severe deviation, asymmetric or curved spreader grafts may be placed to compensate for the asymmetry of the middle vault (Fig. 4).

In cases of caudal septum deviation, multiple strategies can be used to correct and or camouflage these deformities. These methods include caudal septal repositioning, caudal extension grafting, caudal septal reconstruction, and subtotal septal reconstruction.

For cases in which the caudal septal margin is relatively straight, but the posterior septal angle is dislocated from the nasal spine, the columellar

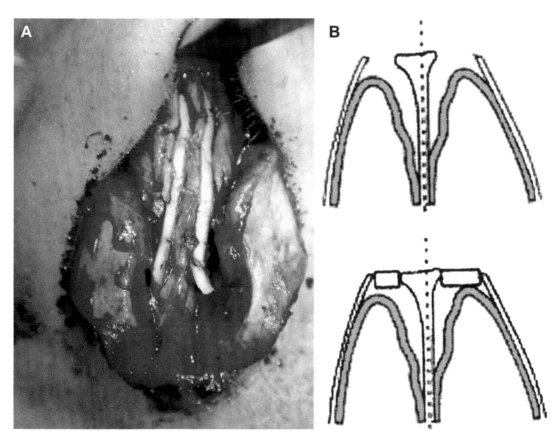

Fig. 4. (A) Spreader grafts placed between the upper lateral cartilage and dorsal septum to set middle vault width and symmetry. (B) Spreader grafts can be placed asymmetrically to overcome a pre-existing middle vault asymmetry. (From Kim DW, Toriumi DM. Management of posttraumatic nasal deformities: the crooked nose and the saddle nose. Facial Plast Surg Clin North Am 2004;12(1):111–32; with permission.)

base or medial crural footplates may appear shifted to one side. One method to correct this deformity is to trim the caudal septum inferiorly to shift over the nasal spine back to midline. The septum is then sutured into position through the posterior septal angle to the periosteum of the nasal spine. If excessive height at the caudal septal margin impedes reimplantation or causes buckling, a conservative trim of the posterior septal angle may be performed to create room for repositioning. Overreduction should be avoided as this will lead to loss of tip projection.[13]

Other strategies can be used to correct mild to moderate septal caudal deflections. The caudal septum can be cross-hatched on the concave side to minimize the cartilage memory then the septum can be splinted with thin septal cartilage splinting grafts to keep the caudal septum in a straight orientation. A caudal extension graft can be used to lengthen the nose and set the tip in the midline in patients with a foreshortened nose. Patients with a relative caudal septal

deficiency may present with columellar retraction and an underprojected, overrotated nasal tip. The graft should overlap the existing caudal septum and be stabilized with sutures to the medial crura. By adjusting the shape and position of the caudal extension graft and the relative medial crural position, the surgeon can impart changes in projection, rotation, nasolabial angle, and columellar show.

For patients with severe caudal septal deflections, simple camouflaging or repositioning techniques are likely to result in incomplete correction in these cases. The best technique for such deformities is to reconstruct the caudal strut by removing the deviated segment of caudal septum by replacing it with a straight autologous cartilaginous graft. This procedure assumes the availability of a segment of intact, straight cartilage from the remainder of the septum. In cases where there is deficiency of septal cartilage that may be used for reconstruction, alternative graft options include autologous auricular cartilage, autologous carved costal cartilage, and cadaveric costal cartilage. To reconstruct the caudal strut, the deviated caudal portion of the strut is incised and removed to where enough cartilage of the remaining dorsal remnant of the septum is in a relatively midline position. A minimum of 1.5 cm of dorsal-caudal strut should remain intact. A flat rectangular piece of cartilage is then placed in the desired position for the new caudal septum. The shape and orientation of this graft should be placed to set the new anterior septal angle, caudal free margin, and posterior septal angle in a favorable midline position. It is critical that the surgeon anticipate the 3-dimensional relationship of this graft to the dorsal septal remnant, lower lateral cartilages, nasal spine, and nasolabial angle. Careful assessment of this aspect of the reconstruction is critical to a good outcome. Proper execution allows the surgeon to correct severe caudal septal deviations as well as provide excellent functional outcomes (**Fig. 5**).

In more severe septal deviation in which both the dorsal and caudal components of the L-strut are deviated, a subtotal septal reconstruction may be necessary. In these cases, both the middle vault and nasal tip are asymmetric. In subtotal L-strut reconstruction, the deviated portion of the dorsal septum is removed en bloc with the caudal septum. Enough dorsal septal remnant should remain to allow for suture fixation to the replacement graft. In addition, to ensure stability for the entire reconstruction, it is critical that the

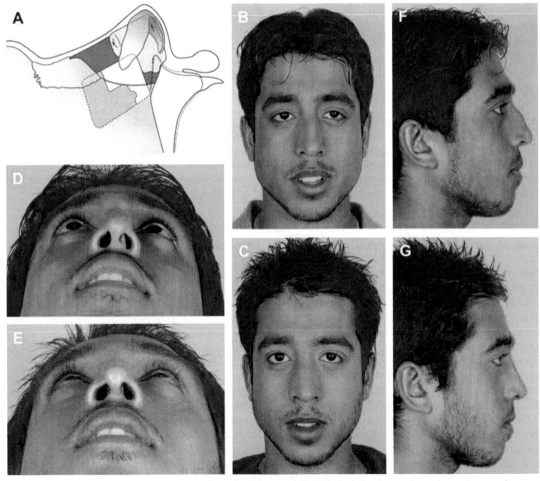

Fig. 5. (*A*) Caudal septal replacement graft with suture stabilization of the lower lateral crura onto the new caudal septum. (*B*) Preoperative frontal view of patient with severe caudal septal deviation and crooked nose from traumatic injury. (*C*) Postoperative frontal view. (*D*) Preoperative base view. (*E*) Postoperative base view. (*F*) Preoperative lateral view. (*G*) Postoperative lateral view. (*From* Kim DW, Toriumi DM. Management of posttraumatic nasal deformities: the crooked nose and the saddle nose. Facial Plast Surg Clin North Am 2004;12(1):111–32; with permission.)

attachments of the dorsal remnant to the septal bone are stable. Positioning of the reconstructed L-strut from harvested cartilage is determined by the relationship to the dorsal cartilaginous remnant, the bony dorsum, the desired anterior septal angle and tip position, the nasal spine, and the upper lateral and lower lateral cartilages. Other techniques such as shield grafts or crushed cartilage onlay grafts may then also be performed to provide additional camouflage or refinements to the reconstruction (**Fig. 6**). As previously mentioned, in cases in which septal or auricular cartilage is insufficient to correct a relatively larger dorsal deficiency, costal cartilage may be harvested and carved into an appropriate graft. In the most severe of nasal trauma cases in which all septal and tip support is lost and global collapse of the nose has ensued, a costal cartilage dorsal onlay graft may be integrated in a tongue-in-groove manner to an extended columellar strut (**Fig. 7**).

In the non-Caucasian nose, several considerations must be kept in mind in approaching treatment of deformities of the L-strut. First, because there tends to be less cartilage available in the nasal septum in non-Caucasian patients, there may be a need to harvest grafting material from outside of the nose. Rib cartilage is a favorable material for L-strut reconstruction, as it is strong and can be carved into straight segments. Ear cartilage tends to be too soft and curved to bear the structural load of a reconstructed L-strut. Second, because many non-Caucasian noses are less projected and wider, deviations of the nose may be visually less apparent than when they occur in more projected, narrow noses. This may prompt the surgeon to forgo a complete L-strut deconstruction and reconstruction, and opt instead for camouflaging techniques such as asymmetric spreader grafts or onlay grafts. Finally, non-Caucasian patients may wish to create other changes to the appearance of the nose, which

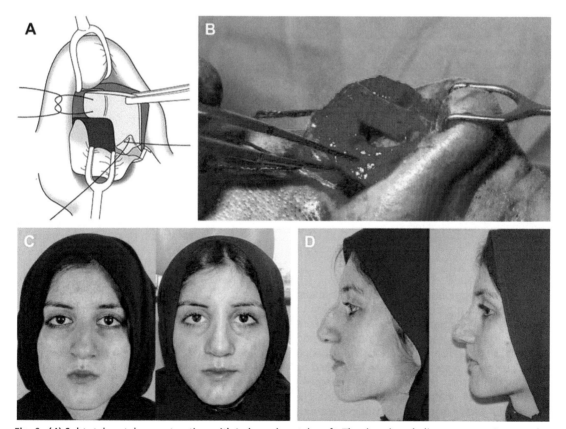

Fig. 6. (A) Subtotal septal reconstruction with L-shaped septal graft. The dorsal-cephalic component is sutured to the septal cartilage remnant at the keystone area. The ventral-caudal aspect is sutured to periosteum around the nasal spine. (B) Intraoperative photo of L-shaped strut (*courtesy of* Dr Dean Toriumi). (C) Preoperative and post-operative frontal views of patient with severe dorsal-caudal septal deviation. (D) Preoperative and postoperative lateral views.

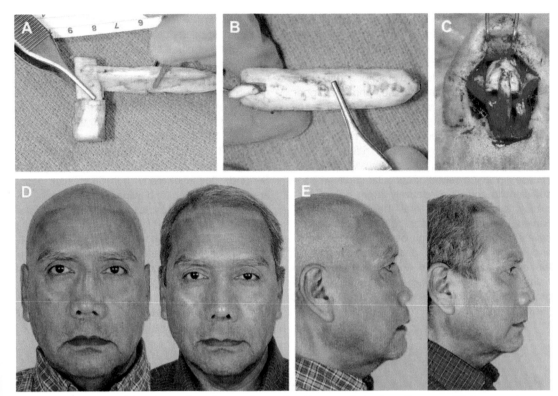

Fig. 7. (A–C) Integrated dorsal costal cartilage onlay graft with extended columellar strut. (D) Preoperative and postoperative frontal views of patient with total nasal collapse. (E) Preoperative and postoperative lateral views.

can be affected by the manner in which the L-strut is reconstructed. For example, a flat, low dorsum can be elevated if the dorsal component of the L-strut is constructed to extend dorsally above the level of the native dorsum. Alternatively, an underprojected or flat nasal tip may be able to be augmented by advancing the nasal tip tripod relative to the caudal component of the L-strut reconstruction.

SUMMARY

Traumatic nasal deformities that lead to cosmetic and functional complications pose a challenge to the rhinoplasty surgeon. Optimal management requires careful preoperative analysis and thoughtful surgical planning. Thorough knowledge of the nasal anatomy, which is in part influenced by the patient's ethnicity, is critical. By understanding the complicated anatomy of dorsal-caudal L-shaped strut and its relationship to the other structural components of the nose, the surgeon can best determine which techniques to use to achieve functional stability and integrity, and at the same time correct difficult cosmetic nasal deformities.

REFERENCES

1. Beeson W. The nasal septum. Otolaryngol Clin North Am 1987;20:743–67.
2. Kim DW, Toriumi DM. The Biomechanical strength of human nasal septal lining: a comparison of the constituent layers Presented at the American Academy of Otolaryngology—Head and Neck Surgery Fall Meeting in New York, September 21, 2004.
3. Papel ID, Capone RB. Facial proportions and esthetic ideals. In: Behrbohm H, Tardy ME, editors. Essentials of septorhinoplasty. Stuttgart: Thieme; 2004. p. 65–74.
4. Rohrich RJ, Muzaffar AR. Rhinoplasty in the African-American patient. Plast Reconstr Surg 2003;111: 1322–39.
5. Ofodile FA. Nasal bones and pyriform apertures in blacks. Ann Plast Surg 1994;32:21–6.
6. Leong SCL, White PS. A comparison of aesthetic proportions between the Oriental and Caucasian nose. Clin Otolaryngol Allied Sci 2004;29:672–6.
7. Zingaro EA, Falces E. Aesthetic anatomy of the non-Caucasian nose. Clin Plast Surg 1987;14:749–65.
8. Milgrim LM, Lawson W, Cohen AF. Anthropometric analysis of the female Latino nose. Revised aesthetic

concepts and their surgical implications. Arch Otolaryngol Head Neck Surg 1996;122:1079–86.

9. Toriumi DM, Hecht DA. Skeletal modifications of rhinoplasty. Facial Plast Surg Clin North Am 2000;8:413–32.

10. Murakami CS, Younger RAL. Managing the postrhinoplasty or post-traumatic crooked nose. Facial Plast Surg Clin North Am 1995;3:421.

11. Lee HM, Kang HJ, Choi JH, et al. Rationale for osteotome selection in rhinoplasty. J Laryngol Otol 2002;116(12):1005–8.

12. Tardy ME, Denneny J. Micro-osteotomies in rhinoplasty. Facial Plast Surg 1984;1:137.

13. Toriumi DM, Becker DG. Rhinoplasty dissection manual. Philadelphia: Lippincott; 1999.

Asian Rhinoplasty

Paul S. Nassif, MD[a,b,*], Kimberly J. Lee, MD[c,d]

KEYWORDS

- Asian rhinoplasty • Asian nose • Ethnic rhinoplasty
- Westernization rhinoplasty • Structural grafting
- Rhinoplasty • Primary rhinoplasty • Alar base reduction

Asian rhinoplasty is one of the most challenging ethnic rhinoplasties that plastic surgeons face primarily secondary to the lack of nasal dorsum and weak cartilaginous framework in combination with thick skin and soft-tissue envelope. Three goals that should be achieved are as follows:

1. Pleasing the patient
2. Achieving an aesthetically pleasing and functional result
3. Maintaining a natural look.

Of these goals, pleasing the patient can prove to be the most difficult to achieve, because many patients possess unrealistic expectations and a desire to achieve an aquiline Caucasian nose. The patients may envision noses similar to those of models or celebrities, even though it may not be suitable for their faces, because of their lack of awareness of the underlying nasal structures. The surgeon's most important task is to attempt to convince the patient that this result is unrealistic, nonfunctional, aesthetically unpleasing, and difficult to achieve with his or her thick skin. Only when this task is accomplished, with good communication and understanding of realistic outcomes between the surgeon and patient, may the surgery proceed with caution.

One of the most common problems in Asian rhinoplasty is the desire to achieve a less bulbous, Westernized nasal tip. To attain a defined nasal tip, aggressive over-resection of lower lateral cartilages is usually performed. When aggressive lower lateral cartilage reduction occurs, this usually causes the following problems: loss of projection, counterrotation (ptosis), loss of support, nasal obstruction, more bulbous nasal tip, and possible long-term nasal tip contour irregularities.

Modern rhinoplasty practices suggest that less is more and that aggressive cartilage removal is antiquated. Less cartilage removal, additional nasal support through structural grafting, and tip-suturing techniques are being advocated at national and international facial plastic meetings, suggesting that these techniques may lead to decreased revision rhinoplasties.

This article describes the Asian nasal anatomy, rhinoplasty goals, preoperative nasal evaluation and surgical planning, surgical sequence and techniques, postoperative care, risks and complications, and pearls.

ANATOMY

A brief description of the Asian nose is discussed and the descriptions described are present in most, but not all, typical Asian noses (**Fig. 1**A, B). These include the following:

- Thick skin with abundant fibrofatty tissue
- Deep, low, and inferiorly set radix

[a] Department of Otolaryngology, University of Southern California School of Medicine, Los Angeles, California, USA
[b] Spalding Drive Cosmetic Surgery and Dermatology, 120 South Spalding Drive, Suite 315, Beverly Hills, CA 90212, USA
[c] Department of Surgery, Division of Head & Neck Surgery, David Geffen School of Medicine at University of California, Los Angeles, California, USA
[d] Division of Otolaryngology, Cedars-Sinai Medical Center, Beverly Hills, California, USA
* Corresponding author. Spalding Drive Cosmetic Surgery and Dermatology, 120 South Spalding Drive, Suite 315, Beverly Hills, CA 90212.
E-mail address: drnassif@spaldingplasticsurgery.com (P.S. Nassif).

Facial Plast Surg Clin N Am 18 (2010) 153–171
doi:10.1016/j.fsc.2009.11.018
1064-7406/10/$ – see front matter © 2010 Published by Elsevier Inc.

154

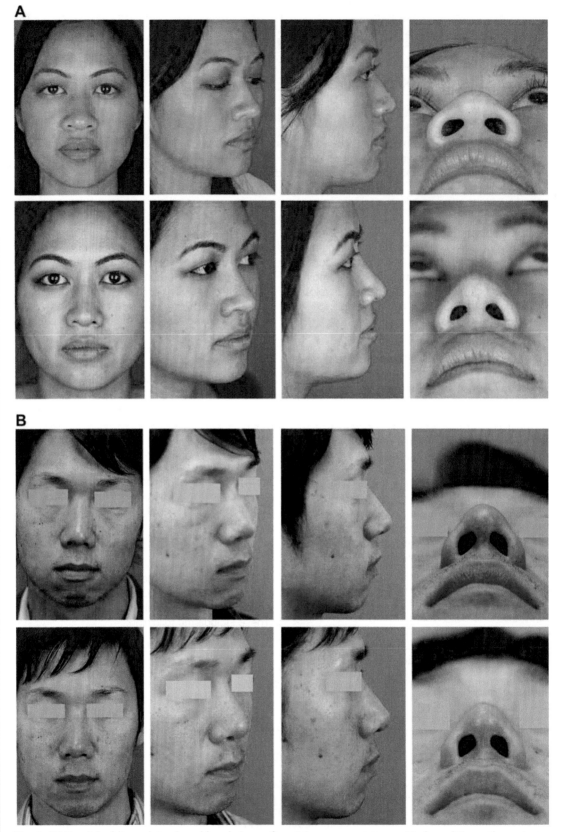

Fig. 1. (A) Frontal, oblique, lateral, and basal views of an Asian woman preoperatively and 7 months postoperatively. (B) Frontal, oblique, lateral, and basal views of an Asian man preoperatively and 6 months postoperatively.

- Short, broad, and flat nasal bones with low nasal bridge and dorsum
- Wide, bulbous, thick-skinned, deficient, ptotic, nasal tip with abundant, fibrous, nasal superficial muscular aponeurotic system (SMAS), broad domes, minimal tip definition, flimsy and weak lower lateral cartilages
- Short and retracted columella
- Wide, thick, horizontal ala with flaring nostrils
- Retracted, acute nasolabial angle (less than 90 degrees) nasolabial junction with under-developed nasal spine.

GOALS

The primary goals in Asian rhinoplasty are as follows:

1. Thinner nasal bridge
2. Augmented dorsum
3. Refined tip with increased projection and rotation
4. Vertically oblique nostrils and triangular nasal base
5. Increased columellar length
6. Obtuse nasolabial angle (greater than 90 degrees)
7. Moderate skin and soft-tissue envelope thickness for aesthetically pleasing tip definition.

PREOPERATIVE NASAL EVALUATION AND SURGICAL PLANNING

Excellent physician-patient communication is critical. During the consultation process, it is paramount to concentrate carefully on the patient's desires and goals. It is important to assess whether or not the patient has realistic expectations and to determine the cause of the patient's unhappiness with his or her nose. During this process, the plastic surgeon needs to assess whether the patient is a good candidate for ethnic surgery. Can your conservative rhinoplasty achieve the patient's goals and make them satisfied with the overall result? Poor patient selection can lead to an unhappy patient and a significant amount of stress to the surgeon regardless of how successful the surgery is.

Furthermore, during the history and physical examination, special attention must be directed to determine if there is a component of nasal airway obstruction. If so, is the nasal airway obstruction static or dynamic and what are its characteristics? What factors alleviate or worsen this? For the physical examination, the authors use a nasal analysis

worksheet (**Fig. 2**) while performing a detailed visual and tactile evaluation of the nose.

During the physical examination, it is important to look, listen, and feel. First, the bilateral paramedian vertical light reflexes along the dorsum should be carefully inspected visually for symmetry.

Next, it is important to listen and observe the patient during normal and deep inspiration on frontal and basal views. Often, the diagnosis is easily identifiable, such as supra-alar, alar, or rim collapse (slitlike nostrils) during static or dynamic states. External valve collapse (lower lateral cartilage pathology) can be ascertained using a cotton-tipped applicator, while manually obstructing the contralateral nostril, to elevate the area of nasal obstruction, such as the alar rim, midalar cartilage, or supra-alar region. Often, nasal obstruction in the supra-alar region may identify an extremely narrow pyriform aperture secondary to low lateral osteotomies. By elevating the ptotic nasal tip, one can easily identify improvement of nasal airway obstruction. As the internal valve is the narrowest region of airflow, the Cottle maneuver can easily detect internal valve collapse. External visualization of the medial crura feet in the basal view can also reveal any contribution to nasal airway obstruction.

The nose should be palpated while examining the bony and cartilaginous skeleton, the tip, and skin and soft-tissue envelope to assess for any underlying asymmetries or lack of structure.

Following a thorough external nasal evaluation, the endonasal examination ensues with anterior rhinoscopy. The nasal septum is inspected for perforations, septal deviation, and for quantity of septal cartilage, because Asians often have short septums with insufficient cartilage. Other important causes of nasal obstruction are hypertrophic turbinates, obstructive synechiae between the lateral nasal wall and septum, nasal masses or polyps, and congenital abnormalities (concha bullosa).

During the physical examination, a problem list with solutions should be clearly documented on the nasal analysis sheet. For example, common problems include

1. Bulbous, poorly projected tip with a plan of open rhinoplasty with structural grafting
2. Low dorsum with a plan of augmentation with diced costal plan of augmentation with diced costal cartilage wrapped in costal perichondrium.
3. Wide ala with a plan of bilateral alar base reduction.

If structural grafting is indicated, plan for the constituent material. A thorough knowledge of

NASAL ANALYSIS

Patient Name:_____Date: _____

- **Skin Quality:**   Thin   Medium   Thick   Sebaceous
- **Primary Description:**   Big   Twisted   Large Hump   Boxy   Pinched   Bulbous

FRONTAL VIEW

- **Dorsum:** Twisted   Deviated   Straight   Convex: **R L**   Bony   Bony-Cartilaginous   Cartilaginous
- **Width:**   Narrow   Wide   Normal   Wide-Narrow-Wide   Depressed L R
- **Tip:**   Deviated   Bulbous   Asymmetric   Amorphous   Pinched   Parenthesis Deformity
- **Support:**   Normal   Weak
- **Medial Canthal-Alar Relationship:**   Wide   Normal   Narrow   Sill   Weir
- **Tip Defining Points:**   Uni   Double   Narrow
- **Nasal Bones:**   Short   Normal   Long
- **Middle Vault/Upper Lateral Cartilages:** Narrow   Normal   Subluxed   Asymmetric

BASE VIEW

- Trapezoidal   Triangular
- **Tip:**   Deviated   Bulbous   Wide   Bifid   Asymmetrical
- **Base:**   Wide   Narrow   Normal   Dislocated Caudal Septum: No   Yes   R   L
- **Rim Aperture:**   Narrow   R   L   Normal
- **Columella:**   Columellar/ Lobule Ratio (2:1)   Normal   Abnormal
- **Medial Crural Footplates:**   Wide   Normal

LATERAL

- **Nasofrontal Angle:**   Shallow   Deep   Normal
- **Nasal Starting Point:**   High   Low   Normal
- **Nasal Length:**   Normal   Short   Long
- **Dorsal Hump:**   Y   N   Bony   Cartilaginous   Over-Resected   Bone   Cartilage
- **Tip Projection:** Normal   Decreased   Increased   Ratio (.55-.60)_____   (TDP-AFJ/Nasion-TDP)
- **Alar-Columellar Relationship:**   Normal   Abnormal   A-C Show _____mm
- **Naso-Labial Angle:**   Obtuse   Acute   Normal   _____ degrees
- **Infratip Lobule:**   Over-rotated   Counter-rotated
- **Supratip Break:**   Y   N
- **Nasal Ptosis:**   Y   N   With Smiling: Y   N
- **Infratip Break:**   Y   N

Fig. 2. Nasal analysis worksheet.

- **Chin:**   Normal   Microgenia   Macrogenia

- **Columella:**   Normal   Hanging   (Septum   Medial Crura   Soft Tissue)   Retracted   (Base)

- **Ala:**   Normal   Hanging   Retracted   R   L

-
- **Pollybeak:**   Y   N   Cartilaginous   Soft Tissue

Intranasal

- **Septum:**   **Deviated**   **Y   N   Spur   R   L**

          Caudal Deviation   Y   N   R   L

          _____% **Obstruction   R**

          _____% **Obstruction   L**

          Edematous Mucosa   Y   N   Erythematous Mucosa   Y   N

          Perforation   Y   N   If yes, where _____

- **Turbinates: Hypertrophic   Y   N   R   L   Normal**

- **Internal Nasal Valve: Narrow   Normal**

- **External Nasal Valve: Collapsed   Intact**

- **More Prominent Ear: R   L**

PROBLEM LIST/PLAN:

          Alar Batten Grafts   L   R   Alar Rim Grafts   L   R   Lateral Crura Strut Grafts   L   R

          Columellar Strut   Infratip Lobule Graft   Dome Graft   Shield Graft   Plumping Grafts

          Composite Grafts   L   R   Medial Crural Overlay   Lateral Crural Overlay   Dome Sutures

          Tongue-In-Groove   Spreader Grafts   L   R

          Conchal Cartilage   L   R   Costal   Temporalis Fascia   L   R

          Onlays: Lateral Nasal Wall   L   R   Radix   Bony Vault   Middle Vault

          Alar Base Reduction: Sills   Weir   I   II

          Osteotomies   Double   R   L   Hump Reduction   Bone   Cartilage

          Septoplasty   Turbinoplasty

          Functional: Cosmetic:

Paul S. Nassif, MD, FACS   Date _____

Fig. 2. (*continued*)

the types of autologous (septal, conchal, costal cartilage, and deep temporalis fascia) or alloplastic grafting and of harvesting techniques is needed.

In addition to standardized rhinoplasty preoperative photographs, computer imaging is useful to improve communication between surgeon and patient and visually solidify the end result. This strategy is useful only if patients are notified that the final image is not a *guarantee* of results. However, despite proper notification and consent, there have been reports of lawsuits filed by patients for results that are inconsistent with what was generated during the consultation. Computer imaging can help identify the patient's expectations and unrealistic expectations can be identified through these images. Therefore, computer imaging is a powerful tool that further enhances patient evaluation for surgery. There have been numerous instances when computer morphing has identified patients with unrealistic expectations. Furthermore, the computer image can be used as a guide during surgery.

Often in Asian rhinoplasty, the patient has microgenia, and a chin implant would benefit the overall a esthetic appearance. Computer imaging will help the patient make a decision to undergo a chin implant.

SURGICAL SEQUENCE AND TECHNIQUES

Initially, attention is directed toward septoplasty and septal cartilage harvesting, with possible inferior turbinate reduction. This stage is followed by external rhinoplasty incisions and skeletonization for the external approach, or an endonasal approach if minimal tip work is to be performed, then nasal tip surgery with harvest/placement of autologous grafts, osteotomies if indicated, and next dorsal augmentation with autologous or alloplastic grafts, and lastly alar base reduction.

SEPTOPLASTY AND INFERIOR TURBINATE REDUCTION

Asian noses rarely exhibit a deviated septum. If a deviated septum is identified, a standard septoplasty is performed. If the septum is not deviated, septal cartilage is harvested, leaving approximately 10 mm for the caudal and dorsal strut. Often, only a small amount of cartilage is harvested, which is insufficient for grafting, and auricular cartilage or costal cartilage for structural and dorsal grafting is often necessary. The patients are always informed preoperatively that this is a possibility. The literature notes multiple techniques and approaches to correct a deviated

septum, so this is not discussed in detail here. If indicated, conservative turbinate reduction by your method of choice can be performed.

OPEN RHINOPLASTY
Injection

Most Asian rhinoplasties require an external approach to maximize exposure to the underlying framework and access to the nasal tip. After infiltrating the nose with ample lidocaine with epinephrine to help hydrodissect the skin from the skin and soft-tissue envelope and for control of hemostasis, a subdermal dissection over the nasal tip is performed, leaving the superficial muscular aponeurotic system (SMAS) dorsal to the cartilage mucoperichondrium. Once the nose has been opened, additional local anesthetic is injected to hydrodissect the mucoperichondrium from the lower lateral cartilages (**Fig. 3**). Hydrodissection aids in dissecting SMAS/mucoperichondrium en bloc (**Fig. 4**A–E) from the nasal tip to use as an onlay or camouflage a tip graft. A subperiosteal dissection over the nasal dorsum is performed if dorsal augmentation is required or if a bony hump is present.

NASAL TIP SURGERY

Tip surgery is the most difficult part of rhinoplasty, especially because the goals are improved definition, narrowed tip, increased projection, and rotation. If adequate projection is present with an over-rotated infratip lobule, a bruised cartilage infratip lobule graft **Fig. 5** may be placed. **Fig. 6** are often employed in most Asian rhinoplasty because poor tip projection is often identified.

A conservative cephalic trim is performed leaving approximately 6 to 7 mm as the caudal

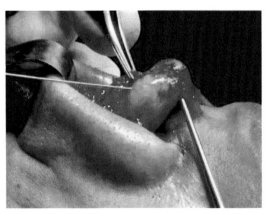

Fig. 3. Local injection used to hydrodissect the mucoperichondrium from the right lower lateral cartilage.

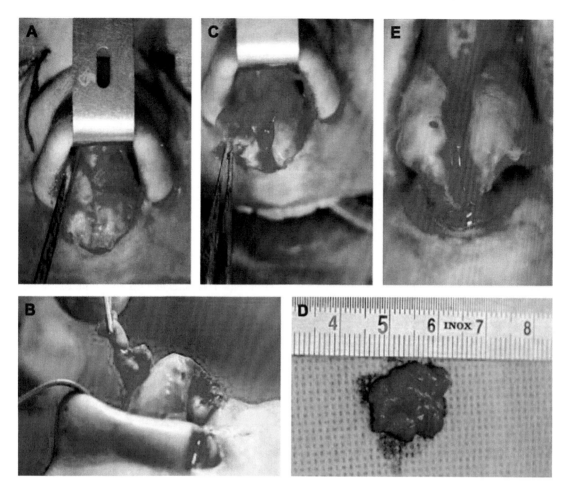

Fig. 4. Nasal SMAS/mucoperichondrium excised from the nasal tip.

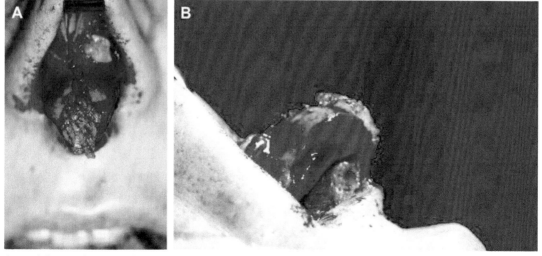

Fig. 5. (*A*) Lateral and (*B*) frontal view of a bruised infratip lobular graft.

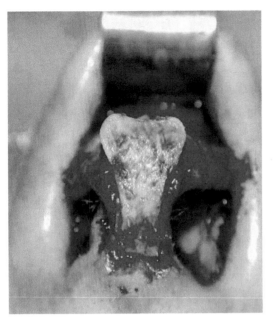

Fig. 6. Shield graft carved from septal cartilage.

increases nasal tip projection and tip rotation. The lateral crura are advanced onto the medial crura to project the nasal tip and to rotate the tip. The lateral crura are advanced adjacent to the dome medially (**Fig. 9**). A bilateral interdomal suture and a transdomal suture are placed using 5-0 polydioxanone suture. The tongue-in-groove technique may also be used to elevate a hanging columella and to increase tip projection and rotation as desired (**Fig. 10A–F**). In this technique, the medial crura are advanced on the anterior caudal septum using 5-0 polydioxanone suture.

Releasing the lower and medial lateral cartilages from the adherent vestibular tissue with placement of an extended or basic columellar strut may be all that is required instead of structural grafting to increase tip projection. Numerous grafts may modify tip projection such as a basic columellar strut (**Fig. 11A,B**), shield tip graft (**Fig. 6**), bruised onlay dome or infratip lobular grafts (**Fig. 5**), or a combination of any of these grafts. The authors place a columellar strut in nearly 100% of ethnic rhinoplasties to provide the foundation for projection as the nasal tip is reconstructed. Columellar struts may be carved from septal cartilage (authors preference), auricular cartilage (least preferred), or rib cartilage **Fig. 12**. In many instances, cartilage is

remnant (**Fig. 7**). Next, the vestibular tissue is undermined from the posterior surface of the alar cartilage (lateral and medial crura) (**Fig. 8**). This technique will release any constraints from the cartilage and may increase the natural projection and allow a lateral crural steal.[1,2] This technique

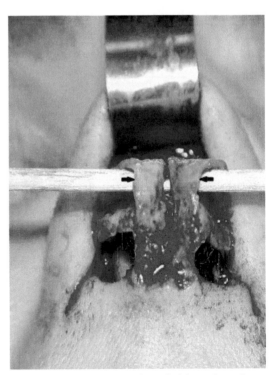

Fig. 8. Released lower and medial lateral cartilages (*arrows*) from the adherent vestibular tissue to aid in increasing tip projection.

Fig. 7. Cephalic trim marked leaving a 7 mm caudal remnant of left lower lateral cartilage (*arrow*).

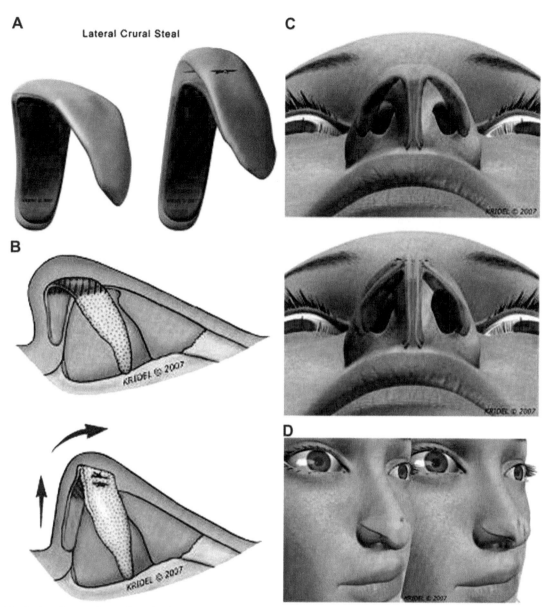

Lateral Crural Steal

Fig. 9. (*A–D*) Lateral crural steal aids in increased nasal tip projection and rotation. The lateral crura are advanced onto the medial crura to project the nasal tip and to rotate the tip. The lateral crura are advanced adjacent to the dome medially. A bilateral interdomal and a transdomal suture are placed with a 5-0 suture of your choice (*Courtesy of* Russell W.H. Kridel, MD, Houston, TX).

present along the dorsal septum for revision rhinoplasty. In addition to the endonasal septoplasty approach, the dorsal septal cartilage may be obtained via open approach by elevating the middle vault mucoperichondrium from the septum, after release of the caudal end of the upper lateral cartilage. Dorsal septum may be harvested without lack of dorsal support provided that at least a 1

cm dorsal caudal septal strut of cartilage is protected. If the harvested septal cartilage is short 2 segments can be sutured to one another (**Fig. 12**). To augment the nasolabial or subnasal regions, plumping grafts or a posterior septal extension graft may be considered. The authors also use diced cartilage injected through a tuberculin syringe for plumping grafts (**Fig. 13**).

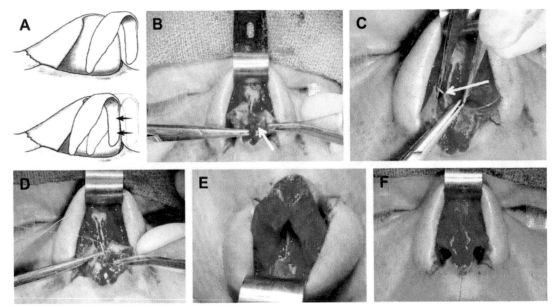

Fig. 10. (*A*) Tongue-in-groove technique (*From* Kridel RW, Scott BA, Foda HM, et al. The tongue-in-Groove technique in septorhinoplasty: Arch Facial Plast Surg 1989;1:246–56). (*B*) A 5-0 polydioxanone suture is passed through the posterior caudal medial crural ligament (*arrow*) from the outside to the inside (toward the septum). The suture can also be passed through the posterior medial crural cartilage (*arrow*). (*C*) The suture is passed through the anterior septal angle (*arrow*). (*D*) The suture is finally passed in the opposite direction exiting the medial crural ligament or the medial crural cartilage. (*E*) Overhead and (*F*) frontal view of the tip with increased tip projection.

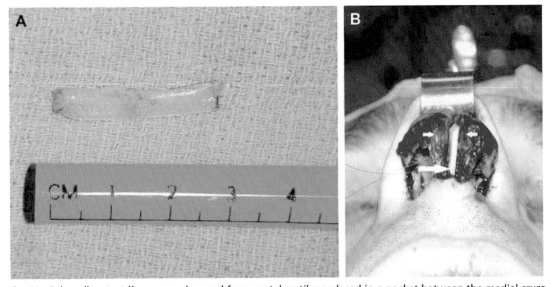

Fig. 11. Columellar strut (*large arrow*) carved from septal cartilage placed in a pocket between the medial crura (*small arrows*).

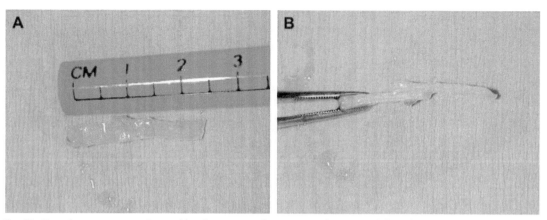

Fig. 12. Two short segments of septal cartilage sutured to one another toward their distal ends creating a longer columellar strut.

In addition to using septal cartilage, a columellar strut may be created from auricular cartilage by suturing a double-layered segment with the concave sides facing each another (**Fig. 14**). A shield graft or infratip lobular graft can extend the infratip lobule and create proper domal highlights. Shield grafts made from auricular cartilage are usually less rigid than septal grafts but either is sufficient. If the graft extends a moderate amount above the native tip, a buttress graft (**Fig. 15A, B**) is placed posterior to the shield graft to prevent warping of the graft. In addition, lateral alar contour grafts can be placed to camouflage the lateral edges of the shield graft. With shrink wrappage, you can see the contour of an unsightly graft; these grafts give a smooth transition to create a balanced alar-dome contour. With placement of a shield graft, the infratip lobule is usually over-rotated. One or 2 infratip lobule grafts with bruised cartilage can be placed to correct this over-rotation.

Once all grafts are sutured into place, nasal SMAS/mucoperichondrium (**Fig. 16**), rib perichondrium, see **Fig. 17** or deep temporalis fascia

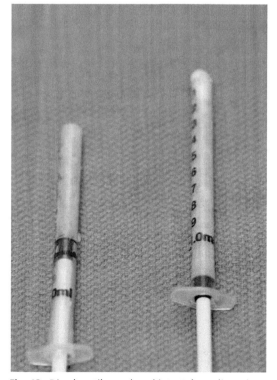

Fig. 13. Diced cartilage placed into tuberculin syringe for plumping grafts.

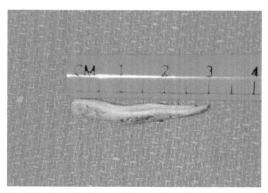

Fig. 14. An auricular cartilage columellar strut created by suturing a double-layered segment with the concave sides facing one another.

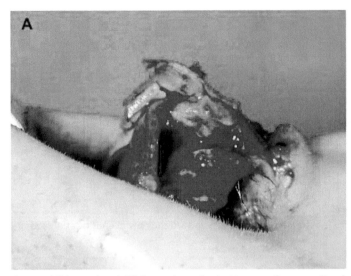
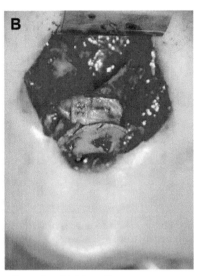

Fig. 15. (*A*) Lateral and (*B*) front view of a buttress graft preventing bending of a shield graft.

(**Fig. 18**) is placed over the tip complex (**Fig. 19**) to prevent long-term visibility of the grafts through the skin.

If additional cartilage is needed, autologous cartilage is preferred. Auricular cartilage (**Fig. 20**)

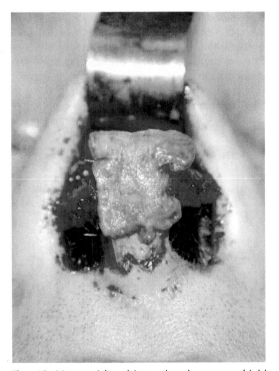

Fig. 16. Mucoperichondrium placed over a shield graft to prevent visibility of the graft through the skin.

harvesting from the concha cavum and cymba may be approached from the anterior (**Fig. 21A–C**) or posterior (**Fig. 22**) surface. Costal cartilage (**Fig. 23**), which has been well described in the literature, is the preferred autologous cartilage for Asian rhinoplasty. If using costal cartilage, the perichondrium from the rib is used.

OSTEOTOMIES

Conservative management of the nasal bones is essential, because many Asian patients have low nasal bones, and because of the high risk of asymmetric nasal fractures. If osteotomies are indicated, the nasal mucosa inside the lateral nasal wall is infiltrated with local anesthetic to help achieve vasoconstriction and hemostasis.

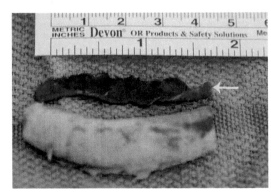

Fig. 17. Coastal cartilage is shown below rib perichondrium (*white arrow*).

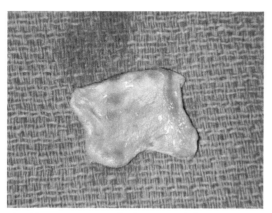

Fig. 18. Deep temporalis fascia used for augmentation or to cover cartilage grafts.

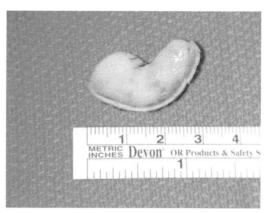

Fig. 20. Convex auricular cartilage used for tip reconstruction.

The author prefers low to low osteotomies followed by fading medial osteotomies or infracturing.

RADIX AND DORSAL AUGMENTATION

For radix and dorsal augmentation, the surgeon needs to create an adequately sized pocket for

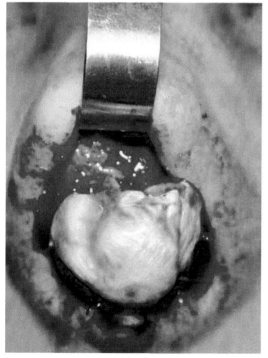

Fig. 19. Deep temporalis fascia draped over the nasal tip and grafts.

the grafts, while ensuring that the pockets are just barely larger than the graft. Anything larger will encourage graft displacement with unpleasing results. Autologous grafts (septal, conchal, or costal cartilage) are preferred to alloplastic grafts such as layered 1- to 2-mm polytetrafluoroethylene sheeting (**Fig. 24**). Because of the high risk of infection and subsequent extrusion, silicone implants (**Fig. 25**) are not used. For minimal radix or dorsal augmentation, nasal SMAS/mucoperichondrium, rib perichondrium, or deep temporalis fascia (see **Fig. 16**) is preferred. For moderate radix or dorsal augmentation, bruised cartilage (septal, conchal, or costal) is placed posterior to the harvested nasal scar tissue/mucoperichondrium, rib perichondrium, or wrapped in temporalis fascia (**Fig. 26**A–D). Diced cartilage wrapped in fascia (DCF) (**Fig. 27**), popularized by Calvert [3] and Daniel, has become the authors' preference for considerable dorsal augmentation. The diced cartilage is placed in a 1-mL tuberculin syringe with the distal end removed, which allows the diced cartilage to easily pass through the syringe into the temporal fascia (**Fig. 27**). The temporalis fascia is wrapped around the syringe and secured with a running 5-0 chromic suture. An alternative method is to place the perichondrium posterior to the nasal soft-tissue/skin envelope in the region of augmentation and to inject the diced cartilage along the dorsum posterior to the perichondrium. The perichondrium may also be placed via percutaneous sutures posterior to the nasal soft-tissue/skin envelope. To create a smooth dorsal augmentation, the DCF graft should extend to the cephalad supratip region. En bloc cartilage grafts placed over the dorsum may warp and look unnatural; therefore, the authors do not favor them.

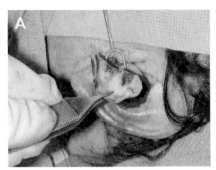
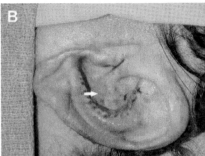
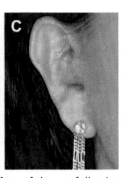

Fig. 21. (*A*) Auricular cartilage harvested from the anterior approach. (*B*) Anterior surface of the ear following incision closure and coapting sutures placed through the concha cavum and cymba (*arrow*). (*C*) Healing anterior auricular incision.

ALAR BASE REDUCTION

Alar base reduction can be simply divided into narrowing the ala with or without the vestibular component, nasal sill/floor, or a combination of both. Nasal sill excision alone is rarely used in the authors' practice for Asian rhinoplasty, because this narrows the nostril and nasal floor with subsequent narrowing of the airway without reducing the alar lobule (**Fig. 28**A, B). With this technique, the only way to achieve alar reduction is to create a standard sill incision at the junction of the ala and nostril as shown in **Fig. 29**. If the Asian patient refuses this, this technique may be used with limited results. In most patients, the alar lobule needs to be reduced to achieve harmony and balance with the Asian rhinoplasty.

Sheen and Sheen[4] have described numerous ways to reduce the alar lobule and nostril, which if performed properly, will create an aesthetically pleasing result with a minimally visible scar (**Fig. 32**A–D). To simplify this, vestibular reduction decreases nostril size, and cutaneous reduction of the alar lobule modifies the size and contour of the alar lobule. Two types of alar bases (**Fig. 30**A, B) are described:

- Type I: excessive alar lobule with normal-sized nostrils
- Type II: large nostrils and excessive alar lobules.

Type I excises the alar lobule (cutaneous) only without any vestibular skin. This process entails an external alar excision along the entire border of the alar lobule. Photos of a patient with type I weir with a nasal sill component are shown.

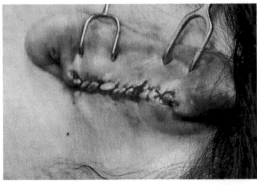

Fig. 22. Postauricular closure following conchal cartilage harvesting.

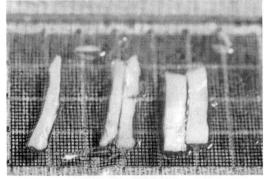

Fig. 23. Costal (rib) cartilage carved into a columellar strut (*left*), rim grafts (*middle*) and alar batten grafts (*right*).

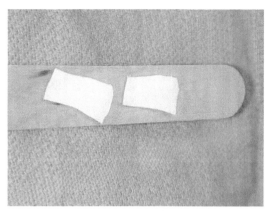

Fig. 24. Layered 1- to 2-mm polytetrafluoroethylene sheeting.

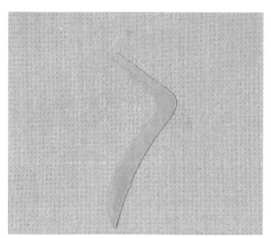

Fig. 25. Typical silicone L-strut used for dorsal augmentation.

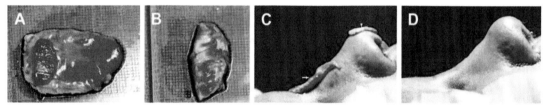

Fig. 26. (*A*) Crushed cartilage placed in temporalis fascia. (*B*) Crushed cartilage wrapped in temporalis fascia. (*C*) Before: crushed cartilage wrapped in deep temporalis fascia used as a radix/cephalad dorsal graft (*arrow*) and fascia placed over the dome (*arrowhead*). (*D*) After.

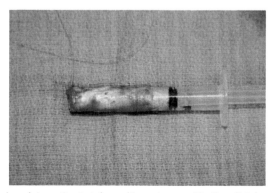

Fig. 27. Diced cartilage is placed in a 1-mL tuberculin syringe with the distal end of the syringe removed. Enlarging the distal end of the syringe will allow the diced cartilage to flow easily through the syringe. Deep temporalis fascia is wrapped around the syringe and secured with a running 5-0 chromic suture.

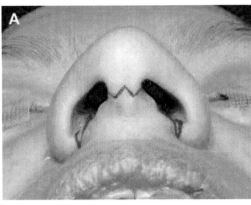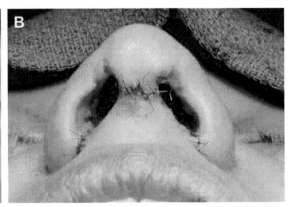

Fig. 28. (*A*) Preoperative base view of the standard nasal sill incision. (*B*) Postoperative view of the nasal sill procedure revealing a narrowed nostril and nasal floor with subsequent narrowing of the airway without reducing the alar lobule.

(**Fig. 31**A–D). In general, a 3- to 4-mm reduction will lead to a significant reduction. However, in certain patients, the authors have removed as much as 5 to 6 mm of alar lobule, which is not common practice. Additionally, patients with I type I alae with nasal sill components can also undergo excision of the alar lobule extending into the nasal sill to reduce the alar base (**Fig. 33**A–C).

Type II primarily excises the alar lobule (cutaneous) with some vestibular tissue (less than cutaneous). The same type of incision and resection are performed as in type I. The exception is that the incision enters the internal vestibular lining of the nose with an excision of a small to moderate amount of vestibular tissue. The techniques described do not include routine nostril sill/floor

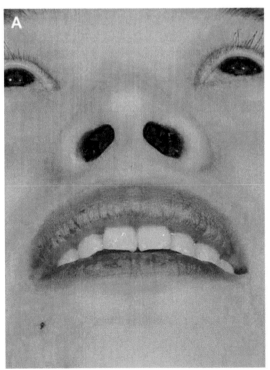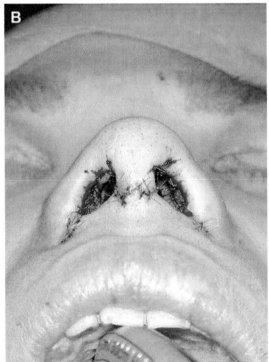

Fig. 29. (*A*) Preoperative base view of the lateral nasal sill/alar incision. (*B*) Postoperative view of the lateral nasal sill/alar incision with a mild to moderate amount of alar lobule reduction. The nostril is also narrowed with subsequent narrowing of the airway.

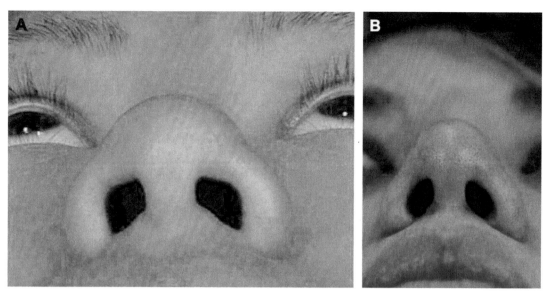

Fig. 30. (*A*) Base view of type I: excessive alar lobule with normal-sized nostrils. (*B*) Base view of type II: large nostrils and excessive alar lobules.

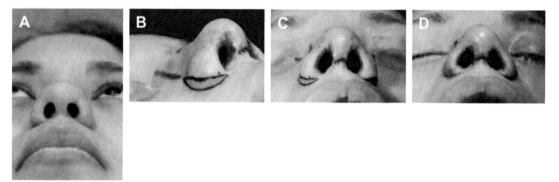

Fig. 31. (*A*) Base view of type I: excessive alar lobule with normal-sized nostrils. (*B*) Lateral view of surgical markings showing the alar lobule (cutaneous) excision without vestibular skin. It involves an external alar excision along the entire border of the alar lobule. (*C–D*) Base view of the surgical markings.

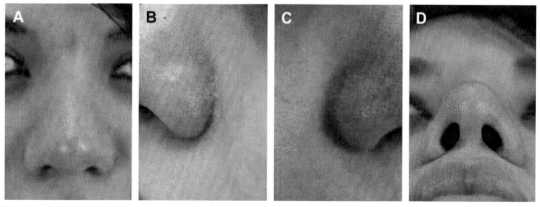

Fig. 32. (*A–D*) Postoperative photos of alar base reduction scar.

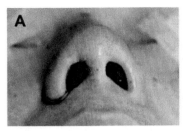
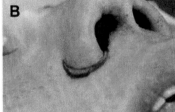
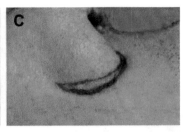

Fig. 33. (*A*) Preoperative front, (*B*) base, and (*C*) lateral views of type I with surgical marking showing the alar lobule excision including extension into the nasal sill.

excisions that may be incorporated into either of the described alar base reduction techniques.

To obtain the most aesthetically pleasing scar, the following pearls should be heeded. Traditional teaching instructs the incision to be approximately 1 mm on the nasal side of the alar-facial junction. After noticing a few visible scars at the cephalad alar lobule due to the placement of the incision despite meticulous closure techniques, the authors now make the incision in the alar-facial junction, which is less noticeable postoperatively. The incision is beveled and a medial flap technique is used when vestibular tissue is resected. The medial flap technique (**Fig. 34A–D**) involves making the alar-facial incision initially while extending medially along the alar base and stopping short of the last 2 to 3 mm. A back cut that preserves a small triangular (medial) flap is made before the superior cut. The wedge of tissue is excised and the natural continuity of the lateral nasal sill is preserved.

Gentle bipolar cautery is used for hemostasis followed by subcutaneous closure with 5-0 Vicryl and a running 6-0 Prolene for the skin closure. If vestibular resection is performed, 5-0 chromic is used in a running or interrupted pattern, with suture removal in 7 days.

POSTOPERATIVE NASAL CARE

- Meticulous cleansing of incisions
- Basic saline nasal sprays
- Suction bulb to suction nose pro re nata (PRN)
- Head elevation
- Ice compresses
- Postoperative nighttime taping for 6 to 10 weeks
- Kenalog 10 mg/mL after 4 weeks PRN

RISKS AND COMPLICATIONS

- Over-aggressive cartilage removal; causing loss of tip projection and tip ptosis
- Prolonged bruising or hyperpigmentation
- Infection
- Prominent alar scarring
- Excessive alar reduction
- Abnormal-appearing ala
    - Flat ala with loss of natural base curves
- Nasal asymmetry, graft irregularity, displacement and extrusion
- Graft absorption
- Prolonged swelling.

PEARLS

- Carefully evaluate the nasal anatomy and physiology and patient's mental state
- Establish realistic aesthetic and functional goals for the patient and for yourself
- Prepare a detailed preoperative evaluation and surgical plan
- Maintain nasal airway function

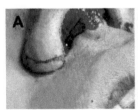
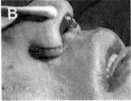
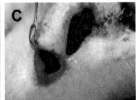
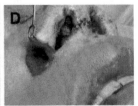

Fig. 34. (*A, B*) The medial flap technique involves making the alar-facial incision initially while extending medially along the alar base and stopping short of the last 2 to 3 mm. (*C*). A back cut that preserves a small triangular (medial) flap is made before the superior cut. (*D*) The wedge of tissue is excised and the natural continuity of the lateral nasal sill is preserved.

- Perform revision procedures only when truly warranted.

REFERENCES

1. Kridel RWH, Konior RJ, Shumrick KA, et al. Advances in nasal tip surgery: the lateral crural steal. Arch Otolaryngol Head Neck Surg 1989;117:1206–12.

2. Kridel RWH, Scott BA, Foda HMT. The tongue-in-groove technique in septorhinoplasty. Arch Facial Plast Surg 1989;1:246–56.

3. Calvert JW, Brenner K, DaCosta-Iyer M, et al. Histological analysis of human diced cartilage grafts. Plast Reconstr Surg 2006;118(1):230–6.

4. Sheen JH, Sheen AP. Aesthetic rhinoplasty. St Louis (MO): The Mosby Company; 1987.

Hispanic/Mestizo Rhinoplasty

Roxana Cobo, MD[a,b],*

KEYWORDS

- Hispanic rhinoplasty • Mestizo facial characteristics
- Thick skin • Bulbous tip • Acute nasolabial angle

There are many different ethnic groups in the world. Wars and the search for better working opportunities have changed migration patterns around the world. Rich developed countries are constantly receiving immigrants from poor countries who seek opportunities for a better quality of life for themselves and their families.[1] This has changed the racial composition of many countries and pure races are being replaced by more mixed multiracial groups.

The United States, Spain, and, in a lesser proportion, Canada and the European countries have had big migrations from Latin American countries. The largest minority ethnic group in the United States is the mestizos or Hispanics.[2]

Cosmetic rhinoplasty has grown in demand over the years and today, with the exception of minimally invasive cosmetic procedures, it is the most frequently performed facial plastic surgery around the world. Through the ages, the ideal facial characteristics have been defined following the characteristics of whites whereby the ideal nose is defined as moderately thin, with a strong bony dorsum, and a tip that is angular and slightly projecting. Each ethnic group has its own defined beauty patterns that are influenced by cultural backgrounds and religious upbringing, but globalization and communication media have popularized the white or western look worldwide.

Today, facial plastic surgeons are faced with patients who come from many different ethnic groups, and they find that what had been established as a standard of beauty when performing rhinoplasty does not necessarily give these patients what they want. Mestizo patients are not the exception and, for surgeons, it has become a priority to define exactly what the patient wants and whether the surgical result is attainable.[3]

MESTIZO RACE

The term *Hispanic* is defined as coming from a Spanish-speaking country (Larousse American Pocket English Dictionary). Most Latin American countries are Spanish-speaking countries, and patients who come from these countries are commonly referred to as Hispanic, Latino or mestizo.[4]

Mestizo is a definition that takes into account racial characteristics. It literally means a mixture of races. The history of Latin American mestizos started more than 30,000 years ago when people with Asian and Mongolian features crossed the Bering Strait and formed the different Indian tribes that inhabited the region when the Spanish discovered America in the fifteenth and sixteenth centuries. Africans were brought over as slaves during the eighteenth century. For this reason mestizo is defined as a mixture of 3 predominant races: Indian, white, and negroid.[5–7]

In Latin America, mestizos do not have a specific racial pattern, and the predominant features vary depending on the geographic zone from which the patient originates. People from Mexico, Peru, Bolivia, and many of the Central American countries exhibit stronger Indian facial characteristics, whereas in Argentina and Chile there is a strong influence from the different European countries.

a Private Practice, Facial Plastic Surgery, Centro Médico Imbanaco, Carrera 38A #5A-100, Consultorio 231A, Cali, Colombia, South America
b Service of Otolaryngology, Centro Médico Imbanaco, Carrera 38A #5A-100, Consultorio 231A, Cali, Colombia, South America
* Service of Otolaryngology, Centro Médico Imbanaco, Carrera 38A #5A-100, Consultorio 231A, Cali, Colombia.
E-mail address: rcobo@imbanaco.com.co

Facial Plast Surg Clin N Am 18 (2010) 173–188
doi:10.1016/j.fsc.2009.11.003
1064-7406/10/$ – see front matter © 2010 Elsevier Inc. All rights reserved.

Furthermore, in countries such as Brazil, the Caribbean islands, and the coasts of Colombia and Venezuela, there is a stronger African influence. Today, the mestizo race is characterized by diversity and mixtures; and one cannot find a single element, culture, or racial feature predominating over the rest in a persistent pattern.[5]

In the United States the Hispanic or Latin population comes mainly from Mexico, Central American countries, Colombia, Venezuela, Ecuador, and Peru. This population is concentrated in the southwestern border area (California, Texas, Arizona, New Mexico), Florida, and New York City, some of which are the main ports of entry into the country. Once established, the mestizo population has blended with the surrounding environment, and they can be found in all states of the nation.[2]

MESTIZO NASAL CHARACTERISTICS

Mestizo nasal characteristics differ from the accepted ideal white or western nose. The faces of these patients tend to be broad with a nose that looks small, undefined, and slightly flattened. The skin in these patients is thicker, resulting in a heavier skin–soft tissue envelope (S-STE).

The underlying structural support of these noses tends to be poor and unsupportive: bones are small and wide, cartilaginous structures tend to be flimsy and weak. Nasal bones tend to be small, although it is common to find patients with a deep radix and a small hump. Cartilaginous vaults can be weak. Tip support mechanisms are usually poor because of a weak caudal septum, small nasal spine, and flimsy unsupportive alar cartilages.

Externally, these noses can have a wide nasal bridge, low radix, wide nasal base, short columella, acute nasolabial angle, and nostrils that tend to have a more flaring and horizontal shape. The external appearance of these noses is the reflection of a poor underlying architectural framework and a thick and heavy S-STE (Table 1) (Fig. 1).[4]

PREOPERATIVE EVALUATION

During the preoperative consultation, additional to the standard consultation and physical examination, several questions must be answered with the help of the patient.[8]

1. Is it possible to establish a predominant racial feature?
   a. What nasal characteristics are present in the patient?
2. What is the patient's ethnic and racial background?
   a. Does he or she want to preserve these features
3. Is there a clear understanding between surgeon and patient of desires and expectations?
4. Has a realistic surgical plan been outlined and shown to the patient?
5. Have possible limitations, complications, and undesirable results been discussed with the patient?

Table 1
Mestizo nasal characteristics

Characteristics	Mestizo	Caucasian
Skin type	Normal to thick/sebaceous	Normal to thin
S-STE	Thick	Thin
Nasal dorsum	Normal to low radix Wide nasal bridge	Normal radix Normal nasal bridge
Nasal bones	Short	Long
Middle third of nose/ cartilaginous nasal vault	Weak, wide	Strong, normal trapezoid shape to narrow
Lower third of nose/nasal tip	Flimsy/unsupportive	Strong
Alar cartilages	Wide, flimsy, undefined	Normal width, strong, defined
Columella	Normal to short	Normal to long
Nasolabial angle	Normal to acute	Normal to obtuse
Nasal spine	Normal to short	Normal to long
Tip recoil	Poor	Strong
Nostril shape	Horizontal shape	Oval shape
Alar base	Normal to wide	Normal to narrow

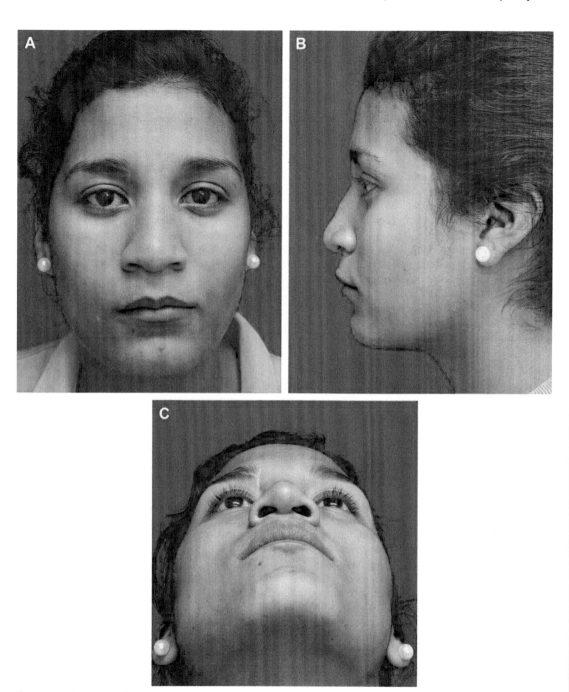

Fig. 1. Mestizo nasal characteristics: (*A*) Front view. Patients have broad faces with skin that can be thick and oily. Noses tend to have short nasal bones that are flattened with a wide bridge. Tips look bulbous and undefined. (*B*) Lateral view. A low radix associated with a small bony hump is often found. Nasolabial angles tend to be more acute. (*C*) Base view. Columellas can be short. Nostrils have a more horizontal shape with a tendency to flare.

STEP-WISE APPROACH TO THE MESTIZO NOSE

It is common to find anatomic variations within the mestizo population that depend on the different racial features that are found: white, Indian, and African. The mestizo ethnic group comprises an enormous geographic territory and the different migration patterns and political circumstances that have occurred through time make it difficult to categorize these patients into a specific racial group. Once an accurate anatomic diagnosis is made, problems can be defined and categorized and surgical approaches and techniques can be elaborated (**Box 1**).

This step-wise approach can be organized if the surgeon has a clear understanding of what the patient wants. Mestizo patients usually want a nose that looks smaller and more defined. Surgically, this translates into techniques that provide structural support but without making the nose look much bigger.

Anatomically, what is frequently encountered in these patients is as follows:

- Thick S-STE
- Weak bony and cartilaginous support structures of the nose.

SURGICAL TECHNIQUES IN THE MESTIZO PATIENT

Mestizo rhinoplasty is a real challenge because there are no standard surgical techniques that can be applied in all cases. The problems encountered in each patient must be individually and carefully defined and the surgical solutions applied. All cases are performed under general anesthesia and the external approach is used in most patients.[4] Surgical techniques are defined using a structural approach in these patients: conservative tissue excision, preservation of support structures of the nose, and structural

---

Box 1
Step-wise approach to the mestizo nose. Great anatomic variations can be encountered in the mestizo population. A step-wise approach will help the Surgeon identify problems and propose surgical solutions

Anatomic diagnosis

↓

Definition of existing problem

↓

Definition of surgical approaches and techniques

---

grafting to increase strength and define anatomic structures.[9,10]

One of the big problems encountered when this philosophic approach is used is that large amounts of cartilage are usually needed for structural grafting. In mestizo patients, the amount of quadrangular septal cartilage is not plentiful and is usually not thick. Techniques must be chosen wisely, and it is important to define the use of this limited cartilage: to augment, to strengthen, to fill in, and to smooth out regions of the nose (**Table 2**).

UPPER THIRD OF THE NOSE

The bony dorsum in mestizo patients tends to be low and wide and can frequently have a small dorsal convexity.

The following problems are encountered in the upper third of the nose:

1. Wide dorsum without hump
2. Low radix with small dorsal convexity
3. Low nasal dorsum.

Surgical Solutions

1. Medial and lateral osteotomies: will help narrow a wide bony dorsum
2. Radix graft: in those cases in which there is a low shallow radix with a small dorsal convexity, a morcelized radix graft can be used to fill in this space and avoid lowering the convexity of the dorsum. This technique helps build up the dorsum without making the nose look much bigger, and is an excellent alternative to the use of implants on the nasal dorsum (**Fig. 2**).[9,11]
3. Dorsal augmentation: if there is enough cartilage to cover all the patient's needs, dorsal onlay grafts can be used. In the author's experience, for the dorsum these are ideally carved from septal cartilage, taking care to bevel the edges so they will not become visible over time. If the augmentation that is needed is significant, alloplastic material such as expanded polytetrafluoroethylene (Gore-Tex) or porous high-density polyethylene (Medpor) can be used with a low complication rate and good cosmetic, long-term results (**Fig. 3**).[1,12]

MIDDLE THIRD OF THE NOSE

Mestizo patients frequently have short nasal bones with weak upper lateral cartilages (ULCs). If any dorsal work is going to be performed in which the ULCs will be dissected from the dorsal edge of the nasal septum, the structure of the

Table 2
Surgical techniques in mestizo patients

Anatomic Region	Procedure Performed
Upper third of nose	• Medial osteotomies • Lateral osteotomies • Radix grafts • Implants (Gore-Tex, Medpore)
Middle third of nose	• Spreader grafts • Morcelized cartilage over upper lateral cartilage

Lower third of nose	• Grafts
	  ○ Columellar strut
	  ○ Caudal extension graft
	  ○ Shield graft
	  ○ Alar rim grafts
	  ○ Lateral crural strut grafts
	  ○ Morcelized cartilage over nasal tip
	  ○ Alar batten grafts
	• Sutures
	  ○ Lateral crural steal
	  ○ Transdomal suture narrowing techniques
	  ○ Double dome unit
	  ○ Lateral crural overlay
	  ○ Medial crural overlay
	  ○ Fixation of medial crura to caudal septal border (tongue in groove technique)
	  ○ Septocolumellar suture
	• Resection
	  ○ Cephalic trim of lateral crura

middle third of the nose will be weakened. Preventive structural grafting must be performed to avoid postsurgical complications such as inverted-V deformities of the ULCs, collapse of any of the cartilaginous walls, or compromise of the internal nasal valve.[13]

The following problems are encountered in the middle third of the nose:

1. Short nasal bones with weak ULCs that have been dissected from the dorsal edge of the septum
2. Flattened middle third of nose caused by inherent weakness of the ULCs.

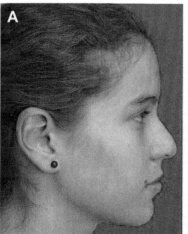
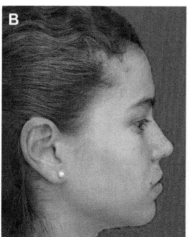
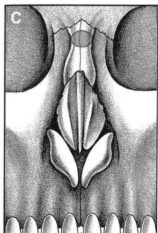

Fig. 2. Radix graft. (*A*) Lateral presurgical view showing a patient with small nasal bones, a low radix, and a small osteocartilaginous hump. (*B*) Lateral postsurgical view after placement of a morcerized cartilage radix graft harvested from septum and conservative rasping of the dorsum. (*C*) Placement of radix graft.

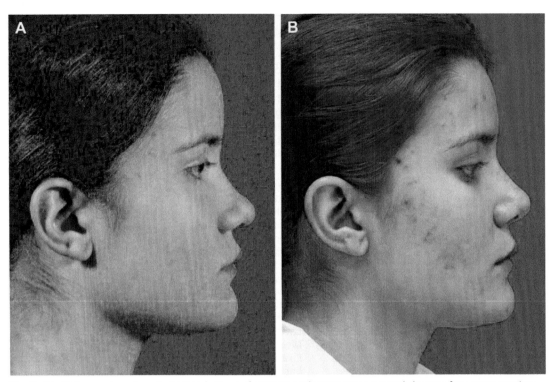

Fig. 3. (*A, B*) Pre- and postsurgical lateral views of patient with Gore-Tex on nasal dorsum for augmentation.

Surgical Solutions

Spreader grafts are rectangular pieces of cartilage that can measure 2 to 3 mm in thickness, 3 to 5 mm in height and 15 to 20 mm in length. These spreader grafts help give structural support to the middle third of the nose, maintaining its anatomic trapezoidal contour, and help prevent the appearance of an inverted-V deformity in this area (**Fig. 4**). Bilateral or unilateral spreader grafts can help correct any dorsal septal deviations. They can extend from the nasal bones to the nasal tip or can be fixated only in the middle third of the nose. In the cases in which there is a persistent depression on one side, bilateral spreader grafts can be placed, or dorsal onlay grafts of morcelized cartilage can be used to camouflage these defects.

LOWER NASAL THIRD OF THE NOSE

A practical way of planning surgery on the lower nasal third of the nose is first to understand the tripod, or pedestal, concept. The tripod is formed by the conjoined medial crura and both lateral crura. These flexible structures sit on a pedestal that is basically the caudal septum. Covering this tripod-pedestal skeleton is the -S-STE. Together these 3 structures give the final shape of the nasal tip.[14]

In mestizo patients, the lower third of the nose often has poor structural support and a thick S-STE. If this pedestal is not structured properly the nasolabial angle will become more acute and the tip will lose its support, resulting in a loss of projection and rotation. If work is going to be performed on the lower third of the nose, the nasal base should be stabilized before any tip work is done. The techniques used more frequently are the columellar strut or the caudal septal extension graft.[4,9]

The following problems are encountered in the nasal base:

1. A caudal septum that tends to be short and weak
2. Medial crura that tend to be short and weak, resulting in a short columella
3. Horizontally shaped nostrils that are the result of a weak tripod and pedestal structure
4. Disproportion in the alar-columellar relationship.

Surgical Solutions

Columellar strut

This strut is normally used in all open rhinoplasties because the approach itself produces disruption of the minor support structures of the nose that should be reconstructed to avoid postsurgical

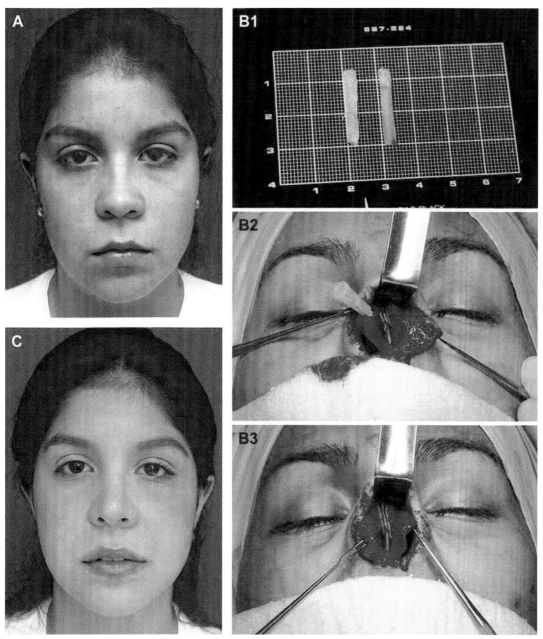

Fig. 4. Bilateral spreader grafts. (*A*) Frontal view of mestizo patient with short nasal bones, narrow middle third of nose with weak ULCs. (*B*) Surgical views of placement of bilateral spreader grafts. (*C*) Postsurgical view after placement of bilateral spreader grafts, medial and lateral osteotomies.

loss of tip projection. The strut ideally should be carved from a straight piece of cartilage and shaped depending on the needs of the patient. It is fixed in place in a pocket that is dissected between the medial crura. If the natural double break of the columella is to be preserved, the sutures should not be placed too high in the medial crura or near the domes. Ideally, the strut should sit a few millimeters above the nasal spine and

its superior portion should be cut 1 to 2 mm below the existing domes. Care should be taken not to leave the inferior portion of the strut touching or overlapping the anterior portion of the caudal septum or the nasal spine because, if it is not fixed properly, a clicking sensation on the base of the nose will result. The strut is designed to give additional support to the tripod and pedestal, helps maintain or increase tip projection and rotation, and corrects buckling or asymmetries that may be found in the medial crura.[4,9]

Caudal extension graft

The caudal extension graft has a special indication in mestizo rhinoplasty patients. In many patients, a columellar strut will not provide the necessary support to the pedestal. This graft is indicated in patients with acute nasolabial angles, under-projected tips, caudal septums that can be normal or short but with poor tip support, or inadequate alar-columellar relationships.[15,16] This graft ideally should be harvested from septal cartilage and should be a straight piece of cartilage. When septal cartilage is not available, conchal cartilage can be used, taking care to straighten the piece that is used. The graft is placed overlapping the caudal edge of the patient's nasal septum and is fixed securely with 3-0 vicryl sutures superiorly and inferiorly at the level of the nasal spine. The feet of the medial crura are then fixed to the caudal edge of this graft and its height set depending on how much tip rotation and projection the patient requires (**Fig. 5**).

Once the pedestal has been strengthened properly, the nasal tip lobule can be addressed in a proper fashion. Tip grafts should only be used with a stable nasal base. The STE of mestizo patients tends to be heavier and, if a stable base is not created, underlying structures will tend to collapse with time.

CONTOURING THE NASAL TIP

Tip-defining techniques in mestizo patients are a challenge. There are no standard tip procedures for mestizo patients, and those used are focused in increasing rotation, projection, and definition of the tip lobule without compromising support. Techniques should be conservative and predictable, reserving the more aggressive techniques for more prominent deformities.

The following problems are encountered in the nasal tip:

1. Alar cartilages that tend to be wide, flimsy, and collapse easily
2. Domes that lack definition
3. Weak medial crura.

Surgical Solutions

Surgical techniques can be divided into different categories.

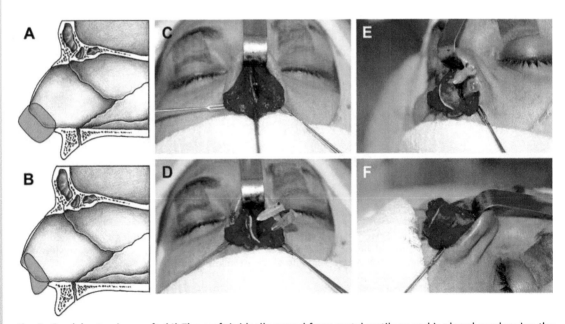

Fig. 5. Caudal extension graft. (*A*) The graft is ideally carved from septal cartilage and is placed overlapping the caudal edge of the septal cartilage and fixed in place with 5-0 vicryl sutures. The rectangular shape helps give support to a weak caudal septum. (*B*) A graft that is wider in its inferior portion helps correct an acute nasolabial angle and increases tip rotation and projection. (*C–F*) Surgical views of placement of caudal extension graft harvested from patients cartilaginous septem. Graft is fixed with needles and sutured in place with absorbable sutures. Graft must have stability superiorly and inferiorly. The nasolabial angle is pushed out resulting in a less acute angle. The feet of the medial crura are then fixed to this stable graft. Rotation and projection will depend on where the feet of the medial crura are placed.

Suturing techniques

Sutures are the first step in managing the bulbous undefined tip. These techniques help refine, project, and rotate. The ones that are used most routinely are lateral crural steal, dome-defining sutures, transdomal suture narrowing technique, and double dome unit. These are usually done with 5-0 nonabsorbable suture material.

Lateral crural steal This is one of the most useful techniques for mestizo noses.[4] Lengthening the medial crura at the expense of the lateral crura results in an increase of projection and rotation. The vestibular skin is dissected at and around the dome area; the new lateral position of the domes is marked and a nonabsorbable 5-0 continuous transdomal mattress suture is placed, fixing the domes in their new position. This technique rotates the tip superiorly, increases projection, and creates a more triangular base (**Fig. 6**).

Dome-defining sutures Dome-defining sutures are placed around the existing dome area. Mattress sutures define the dome area and narrow the domal angle. Special care must be taken to prevent pinching of the domal area with a resulting convexity of the lateral crus and buckling. If this occurs, placement of a lateral crural strut graft will help correct the buckling and pinching of the cartilage.

Transdomal suture narrowing technique This technique is used in broad boxy tips, improving support and enhancing tip projection. A 5-0 prolene suture is passed through the domes and knotted in the midline. This suture makes the tip shape more triangular (**Fig. 7**). Care must be taken not to tie the suture too tightly or to place the domes too close together. An adequate interdomal distance must be maintained to preserve the double light at the dome.[17]

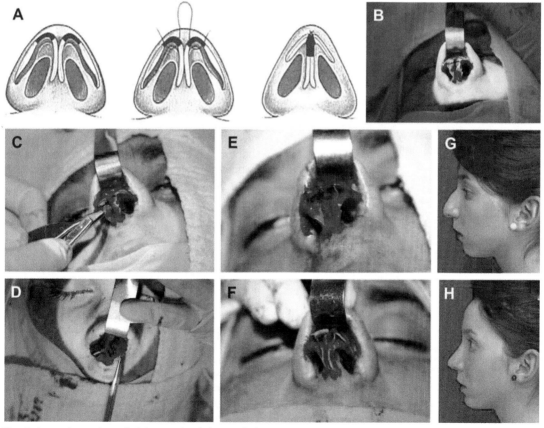

Fig. 6. Lateral crural steal. (*A*) Length of the medial crura is increased by shortening the length of the lateral crura. This technique results in an increase in rotation and projection of the nasal tip. (*B–F*) Surgical case in which a columellar strut has been sutured in place and lateral crural steal has been performed. There is an increase in tip rotation and projection at the expense of the lateral crura. (*G, H*) Pre- and postsurgical views of a patient after conservative hump removal with placement of a radix graft and rotation of the nasal tip using the lateral crural steal technique.

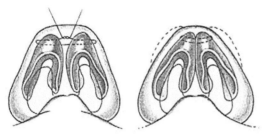

Fig. 7. Transdomal suture narrowing technique. A continuous polypropylene (proline) mattress suture is passed slightly lateral to the existing domes and knotted in the midline. This maneuver brings the domes together in the midline creating an adequate interdomal distance. This technique creates a more triangular-looking tip and base. Tip projection is usually increased slightly or maintained.

Double dome unit This technique combines suturing techniques. It increases tip projection and support and is more aggressive in lobular refinement. A 5-0 mattress dome-defining suture is used to define each dome independently, resulting in a more acute interdomal angle. A third continuous mattress suture is passed through these domes, securing them in the midline (**Fig. 8**). The same recommendations are followed when the transdomal suture narrowing technique must be used.[18]

Resection of alar cartilages
In patients with excessively wide alar cartilages, a conservative cephalic trim, leaving 9 to 10 mm

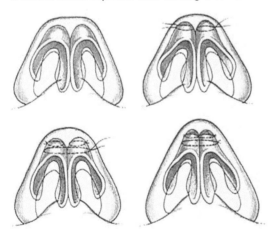

Fig. 8. Double dome unit technique. This technique is used with tips that are bulbous, undefined, and with a thick STE. Each dome is defined and sutured independently. A third continuous horizontal mattress suture is passed slightly lateral to the newly defined domes and sutured in the midline. This technique creates a triangular-looking tip and base and increases projection and rotation slightly.

at the lateral crus and 5 to 7 mm at the dome, can be performed. Care must be taken not to extend the excision into the lateral portion of the lateral crus. Avoidance of this excision prevents supra-alar pinching or collapse of the lateral nasal wall that tends to get worse with time. Cephalic trim is not performed routinely, and tip bulbosity is dealt with using suturing techniques that define the dome area without losing structural support.

Division of alar cartilages
Mestizo patients often have long plunging tips. These patients have acute nasolabial angles, and long alar cartilages with the lateral crus much longer than the medial crus. Suturing techniques alone are often not enough to increase rotation and, even if this is achieved, the nose looks large. The technique used more frequently is the lateral crural overlay technique. It is an excellent option to increase rotation and to shorten an over long nose without losing support.[19] The lateral crus of the alar cartilages is divided, and the cut segments are superimposed and fixed in place with 5-0 nonabsorbable mattress sutures. This technique reconstructs the alar cartilage, creating a new intact strip with increased support at the lateral crus, which is where the cartilaginous incision was made. Domes should be defined and fixed in place with any of the different suturing techniques mentioned earlier (**Fig. 9**).

Grafts in the nasal tip
Tip grafts are used to improve definition, increase support, and increase projection in many of the bulbous, undefined, thick-skinned mestizo tips.[9] Using grafts indiscriminately can create postsurgical problems because any graft used in the nose can shift, reabsorb, or become noticeable over time. In general, mestizo patients want a nose that look narrower and more defined. Because of inherent anatomic characteristics, often the only way to achieve this result is by using grafts to help build up the support structures that lie under a thick S-STE. Because the availability of cartilage grafting material is limited, surgery must be planned carefully and a judicious selection of where grafting material is going to be used becomes imperative. Grafts should be placed carefully and, when possible, sutured in place to avoid any postsurgical shifting that could create an unesthetic result (see **Table 2**).

Shield graft This graft is useful in patients with thick bulbous tips that need additional projection and definition. Grafts are carved according to a patient's needs. Septal cartilage is the ideal grafting source, although ear cartilage can also be used with good results. All edges of the graft

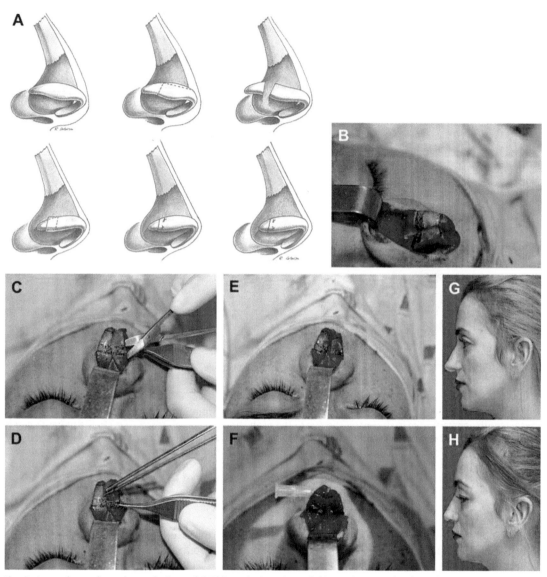

Fig. 9. Lateral crural overlay technique. (*A*) This technique is useful in patients with a long horizontal component of their alar cartilages, which creates long ptotic noses with an acute nasolabial angle (long plunging tips). The alar cartilage is dissected from the vestibular skin. If necessary, a conservative cephalic trim of the lateral crura is performed leaving at least 9 to 10 mm of cartilage in its vertical component. The cartilage is transected 10 mm lateral to the dome-defining point. The transected fragments are superimposed with the long medial segment placed on top of the short lateral segment. The segments are fixed with 5-0 prolene sutures. The edges are beveled and irregularities trimmed away. (*B–F*) The final result is a new intact strengthened strip that rotates the tip upward and shortens the long nose, as seen in the pre and post surgical result (*G, H*).

should be carefully beveled and then fixed in place to the caudal margins of the medial/intermediate crural strut complex with 6-0 nonabsorbable sutures. No matter how thick the overlying S-STE is, the leading edge of the graft is usually left at the level of the existing domes or only slightly above. In the cases in which the superior leading edge of the shield graft is 2 to 3 mm above the existing domes, a small buttress graft should be placed behind to avoid postsurgical cephalic rotation of the graft. The leading edge of the graft is then covered with morcerized cartilage or perichondrium to prevent visibility in the future (**Fig. 10**). Today, although many of our mestizo patients have a thick S-STE, shield grafts are reserved for those cases in which the other

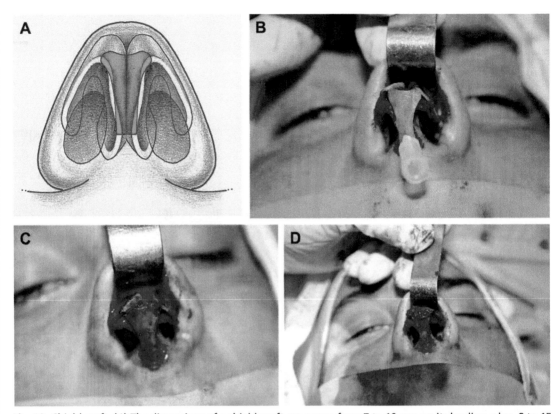

Fig. 10. Shield graft. (*A*) The dimensions of a shield graft can range from 7 to 10 mm on its leading edge, 8 to 15 mm in length and 2 to 4 mm in thickness. The size of the graft should be tailored according to the patient's needs. If possible it should be carved from nasal septal cartilage but auricular conchal cartilage can also be used with good results. (*B–D*) The graft is sutured to the caudal margins of the medial/intermediate crural strut complex with 6-0 prolene, taking care to bevel edges. The superior edge of the shield graft is usually covered with morcelized cartilage or temporalis fascia to avoid postsurgical visualization of any edges.

tip-defining techniques are not enough to produce a long-term esthetic result.

Alar rim grafts These grafts are long thin pieces of cartilage (10–15 mm in length and 2–3 mm in width) that are placed in a pocket made at the marginal incision along the alar cartilage.[15] The graft is fixed in place with a 5-0 absorbable suture, and the superior edge of the graft is gently crushed so that it will not become visible postsurgically. In mestizo patients, after dome binding sutures and other tip work are performed, a small concavity in the lateral crus of the alar cartilage that can later result in pinching of the tip and notching of the alar margin due to the natural weakness of the cartilage in these patients can easily be seen. These alar rim grafts help to fill in the concavity that can be produced in the alar margin after using suturing techniques, and help to give the lobule and the nostrils a more symmetric appearance (**Fig. 11**). In cases in which flaring is produced as a result

of using these grafts, small alar base reduction can be performed.

Morcelized cartilage Pieces of cartilage for this purpose are ideally harvested from septum. They are crushed using a bone/cartilage crusher. This cartilage can be placed in any area of the nose and is used to fill in concavities, smooth out irregularities, or cover edges of grafts or implants. The final result should be a piece of cartilage that has the texture of a mat, is completely pliable, but will not disintegrate into small pieces when manipulated. The cartilage should be placed into precise pockets so that it will not move and, when used over the nasal tip lobule, it is usually fixed into place with sutures (**Fig. 12**).

ALAR BASE REDUCTION

Alar base reduction is not a routine procedure in mestizo patients and should only be performed if

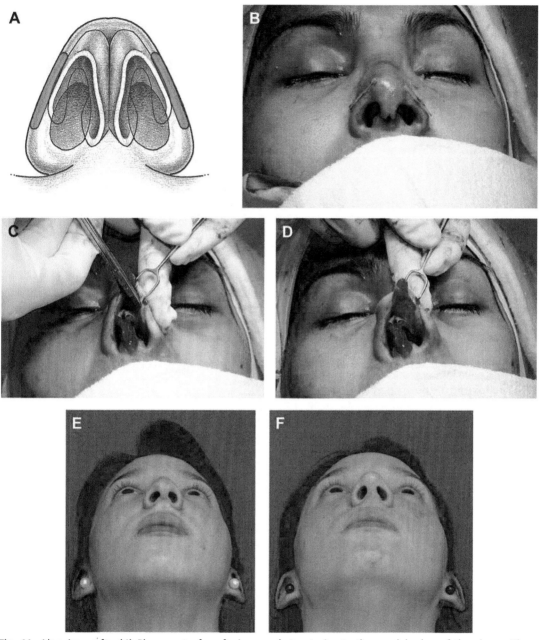

Fig. 11. Alar rim grafts. (*A*) Placement of grafts in a pocket anterior to the caudal edge of the alar cartilage following the marginal incision. (*B–D*) Surgical images showing the carved pieces of cartilage that will be used. A pocket is made following the marginal incision of the caudal edge of the alar cartilage. Once the graft has been introduced, it should be fixed in place with a 5-0 absorbable suture. (*E, F*) Pre- and postsurgical basal view of patient with placement of shield graft and alar rim grafts.

necessary at the end of the operation. Often, after the desired projection, rotation, definition, and structural support in the nasal lobule are achieved, the horizontal orientation of the nostrils changes to a shape that is more oval looking and the base reduction becomes unnecessary. Alar base reduction should be performed to decrease alar flare, alar base width, or both. The medial incision is placed at the natural crease that is formed at the junction of the nasal sill and the ala. The lateral incision should not extend into the alar facial groove, as this could leave an unsightly scar,

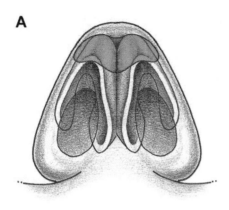
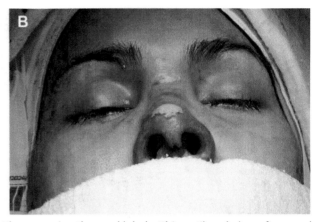

Fig. 12. Morcelized cartilage. (*A*) Morcelized cartilage covering the nasal lobule. This cartilage helps soften nasal tip contours and hides any irregularities that could become visible with time. (*B*) Patient with morcelized cartilage that is going to be placed in the radix area and over the nasal lobule.

especially in patients with thick oily skin. Incisions are closed with 6-0 prolene or nylon sutures, and sutures are removed after 8 days (**Fig. 13**).

S-STE

The S-STE in mestizo patients tends to be thicker, oilier, and have less elasticity than other patients. When performing the open approach, care is taken to keep dissection in the appropriate plane. The soft areolar tissue that is found covering the alar cartilages is usually resected but no defatting of the subcutaneous tissue is done, as this can seriously compromise the skin flap.

POSTSURGICAL FOLLOW-UP

The ethnic characteristics of our mestizo patients make follow-up a necessity. Skin types vary but, in general, they tend to have skin that is thicker and oilier. Because of this tendency, skin care is a priority in these patients. Sutures are removed 1 week postsurgery along with the cast that is used on the dorsum. Additional taping is left on

for another week; excessive taping worsens the oily skin. Patients should understand that it is normal for edema of the nasal tip to be present for several months after surgery. The nasal tip will feel stiff and, because of the skin coloring, dark circles under the eyes can be accentuated and can remain prominent for several months after the surgery. Sun exposure can worsen the edema and the dark circles under the eyes.

Patients with a thick S-STE or with persistent edema in the supratip region can be effectively treated with 1 to 2 mg of triamcinolone acetonide injections (Kenalog) subdermally. If necessary, these injections can be started as early as 2 weeks postsurgery and can be repeated every 6 weeks, taking care to tape the nose immediately after injection. Care should be taken not to inject too frequently, as this can produce permanent cutaneous atrophy. Dermatologic skin treatment with products that can help control the presence or worsening of acne, oily skin, and blackheads will diminish inflammation and will aid in the healing process.

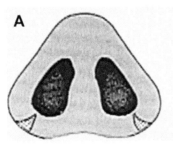
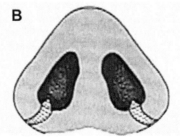
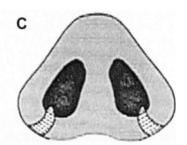

Fig. 13. Alar base reduction. (*A*) Reduction of alar flare: reduction of the lateral portion of the alar base without resecting nasal sill. (*B*) Resection of the more medial segment of the alar base will decrease the width of the nasal sill or base but with less reduction in flare. (*C*) Combined resection will decrease alar flare and the width of the base, giving the nostrils a more elongated look.

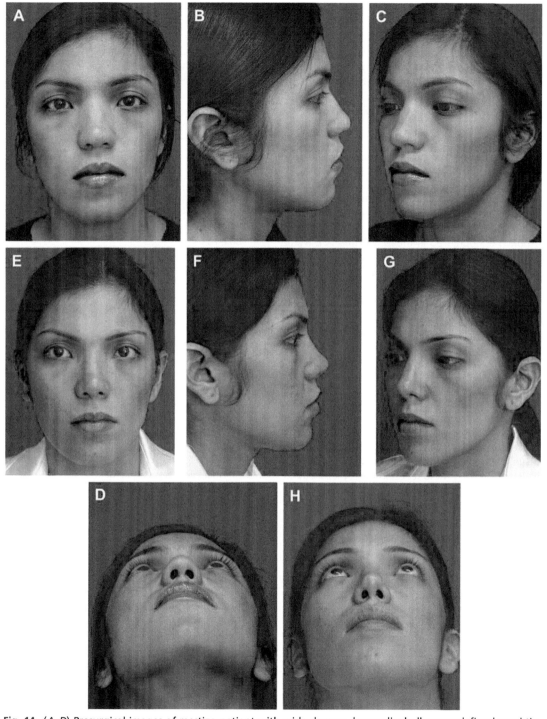

Fig. 14. (*A–D*) Presurgical images of mestizo patient with wide dorsum, low radix, bulbous undefined nasal tip, acute nasolabial angle and thick skin-soft tissue envelope. (*E–H*) Postsurgical images after placement of radix graft of morcelized cartilage, medial and lateral osteotomies, septal extension graft, shield graft, lateral crural steal suturing technique, and morcelized cartilage over nasal tip and supratip area.

Patients should be followed in a proper manner. Facial plastic surgery patients often desire immediate results. It is important to explain to them several times that edema will not resolve quickly, and that real postsurgical results will not be appreciated before 6 to 12 months. Establishing good communication channels will help strengthen the relationship with the patient and will help optimize the final results (**Fig. 14**).

SUMMARY

Mestizo patients are a growing ethnic group in the United States and, like all other groups, are constantly seeking rhinoplasties. The major problem encountered in these patients is a weak bony and cartilage framework associated with an S-STE that tends to be thick. The resulting anatomic structure is a nose that lacks support and definition. Surgical techniques should be focused on increasing and strengthening the existing bony and cartilaginous framework and creating definition, rotation, and projection of structures, but without increasing size and volume dramatically. Little tissue is resected in these patients, and sutures and grafts are used in a precise manner. The final desired result is a balanced-looking nose that blends in with the patient's face and can withstand the natural healing process. As surgeons we need to give our patients a surgical result that will bring them closer to their aesthetic ideal without changing their ethnic features in a dramatic fashion.

REFERENCES

1. Romo T III, Abraham MT. The ethnic nose. Facial Plast Surg 2003;19(3):269–77.
2. Leach J. Aesthetics and the Hispanic rhinoplasty. Laryngoscope 2002;112(11):1903–16.
3. Leong S, White P. A comparison of aesthetic proportions between the healthy Caucasian nose and the aesthetic ideal. J Plast Reconstr Aesthet Surg 2006;59:248–52.
4. Cobo R. Mestizo rhinoplasty. Facial Plast Surg 2003; 19(3):257–68.
5. Ospina W. América Mestiza-El país del Futuro. Bogotá, Colombia: Villegas Editores; 2000. p. 23–38.
6. Milgrim L, Lawson W, Cohen AF. Anthropometric analysis of the female Latino nose. Arch Otolaryngol Head Neck Surg 1996;122:1079–86.
7. Ortiz Monasterio F, Olmedo A. Rhinoplasty on the mestizo nose. Clin Plast Surg 1977;4:89–102.
8. Cobo R, Nolst Trenité G. Ethnic rhinoplasty. In: Nolst Trenité GJ, editor. Rhinoplasty, a practical guide to functional and aesthetic surgery of the nose. 3rd Edition. The Hague, Netherlands: Kugler Publications; 2005. p. 309–20.
9. Cobo R. Facial aesthetic surgery with emphasis on rhinoplasty in the Hispanic patient. Curr Opin Otolaryngol Head Neck Surg 2008;16(4): 369–75.
10. Toriumi D, Johnson C. Open rhinoplasty — featured technical points and long-term follow-up. Facial Plast Surg Clin North Am 1993;1:1–22.
11. Becker D, Pastorek NJ. The radix graft in cosmetic rhinoplasty. Arch Facial Plast Surg 2001;3(2): 115–9.
12. Godin MS, Waldman SR, Johnson CM. Nasal augmentation using Gore-Tex: a 10 year experience. Arch Facial Plast Surg 1999;1(2):118–21.
13. Toriumi D. Management of the middle nasal vault in rhinoplasty. Operat Tech Plast Reconstr Surg 1995; 2(1):16–30.
14. Johnson CM, To WC. The tripod-pedestal concept. In: Johnson CM Jr, Wyatt C, editors. A case approach to open structure rhinoplasty. 1st edition. Philadelphia: Elsevier Saunders; 2005. p. 9–20.
15. Toriumi DM. New concepts in nasal tip contouring. Arch Facial Plast Surg 2006;8(3):156–85.
16. Swartout B, Toriumi DM. Rhinoplasty. Curr Opin Otolaryngol Head Neck Surg 2007;15(4):219–27.
17. Tardy ME, Cheng E. Transdomal suture refinement of the nasal tip. Facial Plast Surg 1987; 1(4):317–26.
18. McCollough EG, English JL. A new twist in nasal tip surgery: an alternative to the Goldman tip for the wide or bulbous lobule. Arch Otolaryngol Head Neck Surg 1985;111:524–9.
19. Konior RJ, Kridel R. Controlled nasal tip positioning via the open rhinoplasty approach. Facial Plast Surg Clin North Am 1993;1:53–62.

Rhinoplasty in the Patient of African Descent

Monte O. Harris, MD[a,b,c],*

KEYWORDS

- African American rhinoplasty • Ethnic rhinoplasty
- African American • Black American • Culture • Ancestry

We are in the midst of truly changing times, as patients of African descent actively embrace facial cosmetic surgery. The Eurocentric aesthetic platform is slowly evolving to embrace a more global standard of beauty. This enlightened perspective has provided much-needed breathing room for populations with skin of color to seek facial enhancement without the accompanying claims of "trying to look Caucasian." As a result, stigma surrounding cosmetic nose reshaping has noticeably decreased in the African American community. Rhinoplasty is now more commonly perceived as a means to achieve greater harmony and balance in the face and not as a denial of ethnic heritage. In the 2006 American Academy of Facial Plastic and Reconstructive Surgery Member Survey, African Americans were more likely to seek rhinoplasty than any other facial plastic surgery procedure.[1] Modern rhinoplasty surgeons have the unique opportunity to redefine surgical logic and classification schemes to be more anatomically sophisticated and culturally sensitive.

Gaining surgical consistency in patients of African descent has proven to be elusive, unpredictable, and challenging for many rhinoplasty surgeons. In general, rhinoplasty necessitates a thorough appreciation for key surgical anatomy as well as a high degree of technical skill. These prerequisites are increasingly important even for the skillful surgeon who is not accustomed to operating on patients of African descent, as anatomic variables may often be misleading.[2] The author would further assert that identifying pertinent surgical anatomy and operative skill are not the only hurdles to overcome in achieving consistent favorable rhinoplasty outcomes in this population of patients. Anatomy and operative techniques can indeed be taught. Cultivating an aesthetic consciousness for Afrocentric nasal harmony, however, is a more nuanced endeavor. Here, surgical success relies on the surgeon's ability precisely to identify anatomic variables and reconcile these anatomic realities with the patient's expectations for aesthetic improvement and ethnic identity. To do this successfully, surgeons need not only a clear understanding of their patient's expressed aesthetic goals but, as importantly, the knowledge and understanding of the often unexpressed cultural influences that undergird these expectations. This knowledge is amongst the most challenging aspects of rhinoplasty surgery in patients of various cultures and ethnic groups. Yet, a surgeon's ability to "culturally connect" with the patient is essential to establishing a foundation for the creation of a shared aesthetic vision.

Much of the interruption in the progression to favorable rhinoplasty aesthetic outcomes occurs preoperatively during the consultation and nasal examination. There are 3 major areas of

[a] Center for Aesthetic Modernism, 5530 Wisconsin Avenue, Suite 612, Chevy Chase, MD 20815, USA
[b] Department of Otolaryngology–Head and Neck Surgery, Georgetown University Medical Center, 3800 Reservoir Road, Washington, DC 20007, USA
[c] Department of Dermatology, Howard University Hospital, 2041 Georgia Avenue, NW, Washington, DC 20060, USA
* Corresponding author. Center for Aesthetic Modernism, 5530 Wisconsin Avenue, Suite 612, Chevy Chase, MD 20815.
E-mail address: drharris@aestheticmodernism.com

Facial Plast Surg Clin N Am 18 (2010) 189–199
doi:10.1016/j.fsc.2009.11.012
1064-7406/10/$ – see front matter © 2010 Published by Elsevier Inc

breakdown that occur before the surgeon sets foot in the operating room.

1. Patient not confident that the surgeon understands his or her aesthetic goals.
2. Flawed nasal analysis and surgical plan based on Eurocentric nasal beauty standards.
3. Unrealistic expectations held by surgeon or patient without consideration of pertinent anatomic variables and nasal skin envelope limitations.

This article aims to provide insight for and raise the comfort level of rhinoplasty surgeons operating on patients of African descent. The article highlights the significance of exploring ancestry in the rhinoplasty consultation; identifies key anatomic variables in the nasal tip, dorsum, and alar base; and reviews surgical logic that has facilitated achieving consistent balanced aesthetic outcomes in the author's practice.

THE CULTURE CONNECTION: WHY EXPLORE ANCESTRY?

An appreciation for underlying heritage provides a link to culturally connect with prospective patients and serves as a tool for establishing realistic aesthetic goals. This cultural journey can be initiated by simply inquiring about a patient's family background. The author asks patients "where did your family originate?" This question opens a nonthreatening pathway to establish authentic dialog regarding ancestry and ethnicity. This cultural conversation can be the ultimate tool in surgical decision making as it may shed light on how much or how little change a patient desires, or in understanding what anatomic variables a patient associates with ethnic identity, or simply positioning the clinician in the patient's mind as someone who cares about his or her individuality.

WHO IS AN AFRICAN AMERICAN ... OR BLACK AMERICAN

Previous rhinoplasty literature has often discussed rhinoplasty in patients of African descent under the generic headings of "non-Caucasian"[2–4] and "ethnic."[5,6] Whereas some reports have taken a more focused and individualized approach using the terms "African American"[7,8] or "Black American,"[9,10] active debate exists regarding the definition and inclusiveness of the term African American that is beyond the scope of this article.[11] Much of the debate focuses on who actually falls under the umbrella of African American terminology. Arguments have included diverse opinions

regarding the inclusion of "white-skinned Caucasian" Africans and distinctions between Black Americans and African Americans. Being aware of the nuances of this particular debate, however, serves to heighten a surgeon's cultural sensitivity. From a pragmatic point of view, the most common categories of so-called African Americans who may present to the office for rhinoplasty are

1. Multiethnic descendants of the transatlantic slave trade born and raised in the United States
2. Immigrants of African countries now residing with citizenship in the United States
3. Children of an African immigrant parent or parents born in the United States (**Fig. 1**).

African American terminology has relevance from an anatomic, geographic, and cultural perspective. Racial admixture in the African American population has resulted in a diverse array of anatomic and morphologic nasal presentations. Psychosocial impressions of ethnic identity may be quite different for a Nigerian patient who immigrated by choice to the United States compared with the patient born and raised in America with remote African ancestry originating from the transatlantic slave trade. Ironically, many American-born descendants of slavery can more aptly identify European (such as Irish, Scottish) and Native American (such as Cherokee, Powhatan) lineage, over the nonspecific African heritage that defines their ethnic identity in American culture. A large segment of the African American cultural story has been motivated by an underlying desire to reconnect the links severed by slavery to a distinct African ancestral past. The past 30 years have seen a renaissance of sorts with respect to African American economic empowerment and the influence of uniquely African American culture on global society. African American influenced music (jazz, blues, hip hop), dance (Alvin Ailey American Dance Theater), and fashion have been embraced worldwide. The author's prospective rhinoplasty patients of African descent (most commonly between 20 and 40 years old) have nurtured their sense of self-identity in this accepting, globally inclusive environment. As a result, many of these patients hold preservation of ethnic identity in high regard as they seek to enhance facial attractiveness. These are cultural nuances of which ideally an aesthetic surgeon should be aware. Such awareness will not change the technical approach, but it may facilitate an enlightened conversation with the patient regarding ideal aesthetic outcomes, and allow surgeons to fine tune surgical logic regarding the amount of change the patient will find acceptable and pleasing. The "cultural

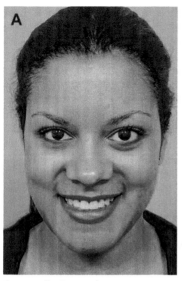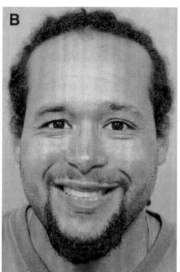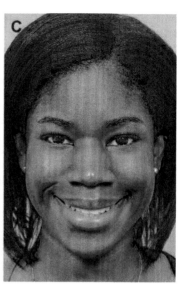

Fig. 1. Who is an African American? These photographs illustrate common categories of African Americans. (*A*) American-born citizen (African ancestry as a descendant of slavery). (*B*) Multiethnic (Sierra Leone/Russia) African immigrant now residing in the United States. (*C*) American-born citizen with African (Nigerian) parents.

connection" is yet another universal means to formulate a shared vision between surgeon and patient with regard to defining aesthetic ideals. Once the aesthetic vision is defined, it is up to the surgeon to formulate a surgical plan whereby the vision can be made a reality.

THE RHINOPLASTY CONSULTATION: AN EDUCATIONAL OPPORTUNITY (A TEACHING MOMENT)

The rhinoplasty consultation is an opportunity for both surgeon and patient to share and learn from each other. A major complaint that the author receives from patients of African descent who have visited other surgeons for consultation is a lack of confidence with the surgeon's ability to internalize their desired cosmetic goals with cultural sensitivity. As discussed previously, exploring ancestry is a means to set the stage whereby surgeons can learn from their patients. In the same regard, the nasal examination is an opportunity for the surgeon to take the lead and teach, creating an educational atmosphere for patients to learn from the surgeon. This educational platform between patient and surgeon creates an environment for the "sharing of knowledge," which will ultimately facilitate the creation of a shared aesthetic vision for rhinoplasty.

In the consultation, the author asks each patient what concerns he or she has with the appearance of their nose. To be more specific, each patient is given a cotton-tip applicator, is told it is a magic

wand, and is asked what he or she would change if it were that simple. The rhinoplasty consultation for patients of African descent sometimes comes with a bit of psycho-social baggage. African Americans have often rejected facial cosmetic surgery seeing it as a way of conforming to European ideals of beauty. In many instances the patients are on their own, without the benefit of family support or close associates who have already undergone the procedure with whom they can relay concerns. The magic wand exercise works to alleviate anxiety. The exercise also encourages patients to be more specific in identifying desired changes with a focus on key anatomic variables. The author then reviews the anatomy of the nose with the patient. In this teaching moment, the nose is separated into 3 major areas: upper, comprising the nasal bones; middle, comprising the upper lateral cartilages; and lower, comprising the paired tip lower lateral cartilages and the fibro-fatty framework of the nostrils. In a simplistic manner, the prospective rhinoplasty patients are informed that aesthetic complaints typically fall into 3 boxes. For some individuals a check can be placed in all 3 boxes, for some, 2 boxes, and others, only one. The first box includes complaints related to the overall contour of the bridge (shape, projection). The second box contains complaints associated with the width of the nose. The third box relates to concerns regarding the shape of the nasal tip and nostrils. The consultation then proceeds with surgeon and patient symbolically placing checks in the appropriate box or boxes, and together outlining a shared aesthetic plan incorporating specific techniques to modify their particular anatomy.

KEY TECHNIQUES RELATED TO SURGICAL ANATOMY

Given the vast morphologic diversity of patients of African descent, surgical approaches and techniques must be directed toward modifying specific anatomic variables. Previous reports have offered generalized descriptions regarding surgical anatomy in the African American patient without regard for geographic differences and ethnic makeup of the study population. For instance, Stucker notes that the lower lateral cartilages are thinner and more flaccid than those found in the Caucasian race.[12] Rohrich comments that "The African American nose typically has a short columella, broad flat dorsum, slightly flaring alae, and a rounded tip with ovoid nares."[7] Ofodile and Bokhari reviewed harmonious anthropometric indices and normal baseline measurements for the African American patient.[13] This article now comments on a few surgical concepts and technical pearls that have facilitated achieving consistent and natural results in patients of African descent.

MODIFYING THE NASAL TIP

Patients of African descent frequently present with concerns regarding the appearance of the nasal tip. Common complaints include bulbous shape, lack of tip projection, and poor tip definition. The lack of tip definition and broad, bulbous lobule appearance are often multifactorial, resulting from a combination of a thickened skin envelope, increased subcutaneous fibro-fatty tissue overlying the lower lateral cartilages, and a rounded/convex contour of the lower lateral cartilages.

Improving the appearance of the nasal tip should be approached from the perspective of contour modification and not simply narrowing. To do this reliably, it is important to comprehend the relationship between the external nasal contour and shape of the underlying tip structures.[14] This exercise can be exceedingly difficult in the subset of patients of African descent who possess a thick skin envelope, excessive fibro-fatty subcutaneous tissue, and fragile lower lateral cartilages. By understanding the correlation between the external tip morphology and the underlying structure, the surgeon can simplify nasal tip surgery to preserve the favorable contours of the lower lateral cartilages and modify those that are unfavorable.[14] With this goal in

mind, developing a cultural sensitivity for a broad range of aesthetically pleasing anatomic contour relationships becomes important. The author wholeheartedly concurs with Toriumi's position that "even broad tips that possess favorable shadowing can look very good."[14] Rhinoplasty surgeons are strongly urged to peruse the pages of ESSENCE magazine, a monthly women's health and beauty publication, on a regular basis to familiarize themselves with the range of aesthetically pleasing nasal tip contours in women of African descent.

Ofodile and James have reported that the alar cartilages in African American patients are similar in size to those of Caucasian patients.[15] Given the inherent morphologic diversity in African American patients, it should be further added that the full spectrum of cartilage shape, size, and thickness can be present, depending on the underlying multiethnic racial ancestry. A critical point of distinction is that in patients of African descent, it can be quite difficult to predict the shape of the cartilage framework without actual visualization. Digital palpation to assess cartilage strength is not as helpful as in individuals of European descent, due to the masking effect of the thickened skin and subcutaneous fibro-fatty tissue. In Ofodile's study of the Black American nose, the presence of a heavy layer of fibro-fatty tissue was a consistent finding in all the subjects.[13] The author has been surprised to find extremely weak and fragile lower lateral cartilages in patients despite a firm tip with digital palpation. Improved visualization with an external rhinoplasty approach has consequently proven to be a more reliable means to assess the anatomic contributions to external tip morphology in patients of African descent.

For external rhinoplasty, the skin envelope elevation is often performed just under the subcutaneous tissue, allowing for controlled tip debulking. A particular effort is made to preserve the fibro-fatty subcutaneous material overlying the lower lateral cartilages so that it can be used later for soft-tissue graft material, usually to soften the appearance of cartilaginous shield grafts (**Fig. 2**). Although patients and surgeons may harbor reservations with the transcolumellar incision of the external approach, it has been found to heal in an imperceptible manner when executed proficiently and closed with meticulous surgical technique. The author use a 6-0 polypropylene suture in a vertical mattress fashion to reapproximate the columellar skin at the peaks of the inverted-V columella incision. The marginal incisions are closed with 5-0 fast-absorbing gut.

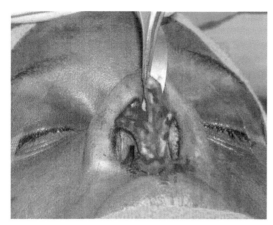

Fig. 2. Subcutaneous fibro-fatty soft tissue overlying lower lateral cartilages.

The prolene sutures are removed at postoperative day 6. Two-layer closure with a single deep 5-0 monocryl is recommended if significant tension is present as a result of increased tip projection from cartilaginous tip grafts.

The columellar strut is the primary workhorse for nasal tip modification in patients of African descent. As an essential support graft, the columellar strut is placed to offset intrinsic alar cartilage weakness. A particular effort is made to harvest a strong resilient cartilage graft from the maxillary crest to be used for the columellar strut (**Fig. 3**). The vestibular skin adjacent to the intermediate and medial crura is elevated in a limited fashion to create a space for burying the fixation stitches. Multiple 5-0 PDS stitches in a horizontal mattress fashion are used to secure and stabilize the columellar strut. Fixation of the columellar strut between the medial crura provides a stable foundation for a "ground up" approach to improving tip contour and projection.

Much attention has been placed on the presence of a supratip break point as a marker for a balanced elegant relationship between tip and

dorsum. It should be stressed that preservation of the infratip breakpoint has equal relevance in achieving a natural unoperated-appearing outcome. Care should be taken to place shield grafts in a manner that does not obliterate the infratip break point. The author recommends preserving the fibro-fatty tissue of the interdomal space when present and leaving it attached inferiorly (**Fig. 4**A). This tissue can be repositioned as a pedicled overlay soft tissue graft to improve the contour of the infratip region (**Fig. 4**B).

MODIFYING THE NASAL DORSUM

The majority of complaints in patients of African descent with regard to the nasal dorsum center on the presence of wide nasal bones, dorsal underprojection, and lack of aesthetic continuity

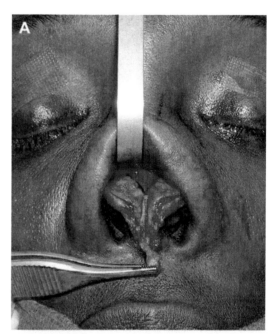

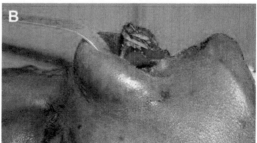

Fig. 4. (*A*) Inferiorly based medial crura soft tissue graft. This graft material can be helpful to soften the infratip breakpoint. (*B*) Infratip graft complex with pedicled soft tissue graft in place over surface of shield graft.

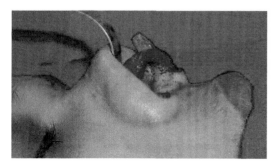

Fig. 3. Strong columellar strut positioned between medial crura.

between the brow and tip. In occasional cases, there is a dorsal convexity that may benefit from reduction (**Fig. 5**A, B). Patients of African descent commonly present with unfavorable nasal bone architecture for osteotomy induced narrowing.[9] Although there is significant diversity in the thickness and shape of the nasal bones, very few approach a classic leptorrhine configuration even in cases where there is recognized European ancestry. The pyriform aperture is often oval in shape with short, thickened nasal bones. As a result, lateral osteotomy tends to have little visual impact on narrowing the bony vault.[15]

The author spends a fair amount of time with the patient, reviewing the shape of the dorsum and its relationship with a continuous brow-tip aesthetic line. Female patients of African descent are usually aware of the impact of contour shadowing and highlighting, as a result of their familiarity with makeup techniques, to give the illusion of a more refined bridge. A high dorsum is not essential for a continuous brow-tip aesthetic line. The author has several patients with a low, flat bridge who have a pleasing, elegant brow-tip aesthetic line. In this subset of patients, dorsal augmentation is indicated only as a measure to maintain a harmonious profile line in situations when tip projection has been surgically increased. Ideal dorsal height is ultimately dependent on tip projection. It is widely appreciated that nasal harmony features tip projection being slightly higher than the dorsum along with the presence of a slight supratip break. As Stucker states, "a nasal dorsum that is augmented beyond what the tip projection can accommodate loses its aesthetic harmony."[12]

Conservative dorsal augmentation has the dual benefit of creating the appearance of a more contoured bridge while establishing continuity of the brow-tip aesthetic line. Onlay grafts are fashioned with an aesthetic goal of maintaining a harmonious profile line. Excessive dorsal elevation in patients of African descent disrupts nasal harmony, as the high bridge typically falls outside of the normal range of ethnic variation in patients with otherwise broad facial features.

For primary rhinoplasty in patients of African descent, the dorsum is rarely elevated greater than 3 mm beyond the preoperative baseline. Although autologous material is considered safer, the amount that can be normally harvested without using autologous rib cartilage is often inadequate for the extent of dorsal augmentation required. Expanded polytetrafluoroethylene (ePTFE) is the alloplastic material of choice for dorsal augmentation.

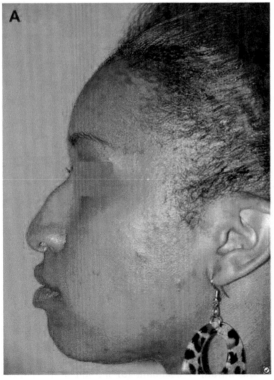 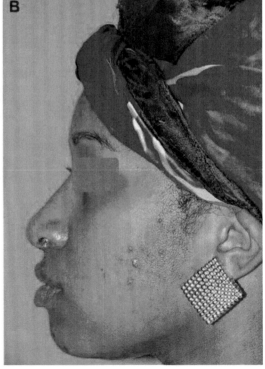

Fig. 5. (*A*) Preoperative profile view of patient of African descent with dorsal convexity. (*B*) Postoperative profile view following reduction rhinoplasty.

The author has found it to be an aesthetically exceptional material, with ease of sculpting, excellent blending with the dorsal contour, and a low complication rate. Conrad and colleagues[16] recently reported a 1.9% incidence of biologic complications such as soft tissue reaction, infection, and extrusion in a 17-year retrospective review. The author most often uses ePTFE sheeting (ePTFE-SHEET-061 [Implantech Associates, Inc, Ventura, CA]) to elevate the bridge and autologous septal cartilage for tip cartilage grafting. The ePTFE sheeting is carved in a manner to create an onlay implant encompassing the full length of the dorsum from the nasion to the region cephalad of the supratip breakpoint. Osteotomy is reserved for those situations where the nasal bones are long and more vertically oriented or in situations, as Rohrich defines, where the width of the bony vault is greater than 80% of the intercanthal width.[17]

MODIFYING THE NOSTRILS (ALAR FLARE) AND NASAL BASE

The majority of patients of African descent presenting for rhinoplasty will complain that their nostrils are too wide or that "my nose spreads when I smile." There needs to be renewed thinking for both the patient and the surgeon with regard to surgical modification of the nostrils and nasal base. Professional and popular culture has programmed patients and many surgeons to believe that an aesthetically pleasing rhinoplasty outcome should include reduction of alar flare. Traditional Eurocentric nasal aesthetics has promoted that the lateral attachment of the ala to the cheek should lie within the vertical line drawn through the medial canthus. As a surgical goal, Rohrich states that by bringing the elements of the nose to lie closer to this boundary, nasal features can be enhanced without altering ethnic appearance.[7] The author disagrees with this surgical logic, particularly for patients of African descent. Investigators have demonstrated that the normal index for African American patients is actually a nostril attachment to the face lateral to the medial canthus.[13] Surgeons must be sensitive to this Afrocentric anatomic variable and avoid attempting to surgically modify African American nasal morphology to fit into a Caucasian aesthetic standard. It is also important to be sensitive to the aesthetically harmonious relationship between the tip lobule and alar rims to avoid creation of unnatural shapes as a result of surgery. For instance, McCurdy stresses that extreme caution is indicated in noses exhibiting a wide lobule in association with a wide alar base.[18] In such cases, alar reduction often results in a rectangular or square configuration of the lobule that is aesthetically less desirable than the original lobular shape.[18]

Excessive nostril narrowing in patients of African descent is the most easily recognized tell-tale sign of nasal disharmony (**Fig. 6**). The efficacy of alar base modification is also debatable because significant tissue removal does not necessarily guarantee a long-term improvement in flare.[19] In

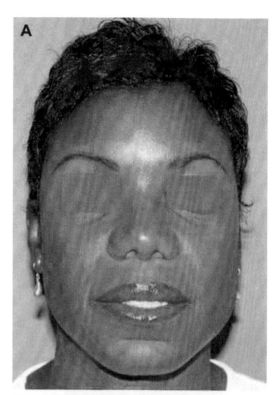

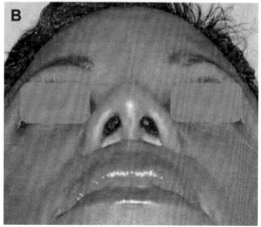

Fig. 6. (A) Excessive narrowing of the nasal ala. (B) Triangular "tent pole" configuration resulting from reduction of alar flare in association with increased tip projection.

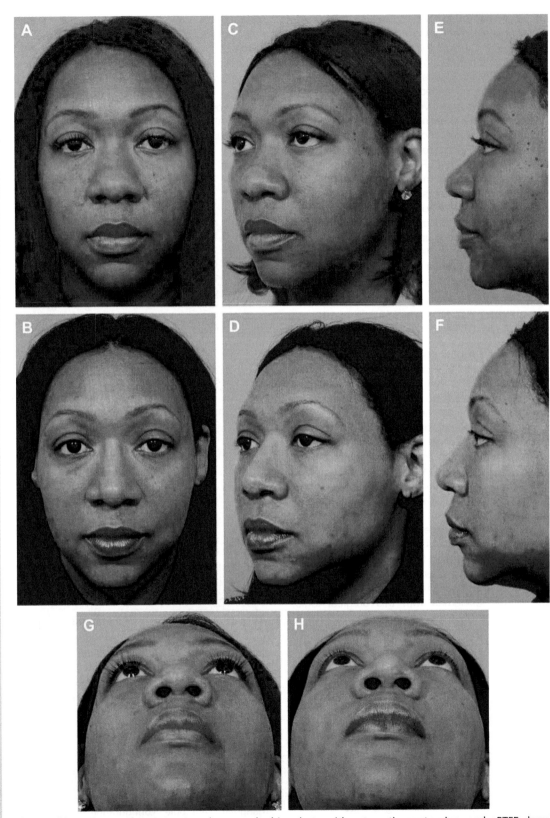

Fig. 7. This patient underwent external approach rhinoplasty with suture tip contouring, and ePTFE dorsal augmentation without direct modification of the nostrils. (*A, C, E, G*) Preoperative views; (*B, D, F, H*) 6-month postoperative views. Note preoperative horizontal nostril orientation.

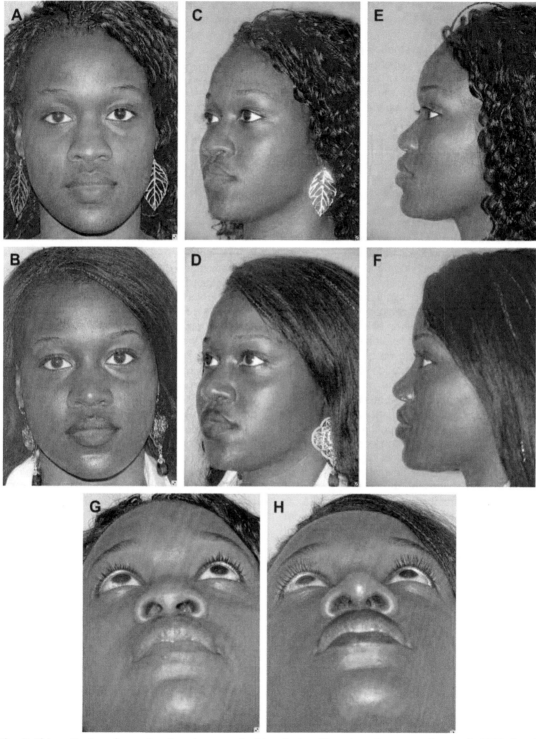

Fig. 8. This patient underwent external approach rhinoplasty with suture tip contouring, and ePTFE dorsal augmentation without direct modification of the nostrils. (*A, C, E, G*) Preoperative views; (*B, D, F, H*) 6-month postoperative views. Note improved appearance of the nasal base as a result of increased tip projection.

most cases with appropriate modification of the tip and dorsum, Weir excision type alar narrowing becomes unnecessary.

To broaden the aesthetic perspective of prospective rhinoplasty patients in reference to alar modification, a series of "before and after" results for cases in which the nostrils were not manipulated in a direct manner is reviewed,(- **Fig. 7**) thus allowing illustration of the pleasing effects of modifying tip projection and its secondary beneficial impact on nostril shape/width (**Fig. 8**). The author asserts that direct alar rim and base modification is overused in patients of African descent and contributes only in a limited capacity, if at all, to an improved long-term aesthetic outcome.

When indicated, successful reduction of the wide nasal base and alar flare is primarily dependent on sound clinical judgment and a culturally sensitive aesthetic sensibility. The author has found Porter's simplified nostril orientation classification system to be a clinically useful tool for determining which patients of African descent are more likely to have a favorable outcome with alar wedge resection narrowing.[20] In the study, 3 categories of nostril orientation were described: inverted, vertical, and horizontal (**Fig. 9**). In the author's experience, those patients with a horizontal nostril orientation benefit from alar wedge resection and nasal base reduction in a substantive way. The horizontal orientation lends itself to more predictable surgical reduction. Lateral alar wedge excisions in patients with an inverted nostril orientation tend to accentuate the inverted configuration in an unnatural way. In patients of African descent with a vertical nostril orientation, additional narrowing is not necessary. In patients with a horizontal nasal base without alar flare, resection of the nostril sill with medialization of the ala is an effective technique, as described by Stucker and colleagues.[12] In patients with horizontal base with alar flare, resection of the sill along with wedge excision of alar flare can be achieved as described by Foda.[21] Caution is necessary in noses lacking a well-defined nostril sill, because

scarring and notching are potentially more problematic.[18]

AN AVOIDABLE COMPLICATION: NASAL DISHARMONY

An abundance of scientific rigor has been placed on the integral aspect of nasal analysis as a key to successful rhinoplasty. In rhinoplasty surgical planning, nasal analysis has primarily focused on linear surface measurements, photographic review, and clinical nasal examination. As we move further into the 21st century, a modern approach to rhinoplasty should feature a more sophisticated appreciation for nasal contour aesthetics beyond anthropometric linear measurements.

In patients of African descent, the author sees iatrogenic nasal disharmony as the most common complication of rhinoplasty. A review of the previous rhinoplasty literature focusing on patients of African descent illustrates many examples of less than optimal aesthetic outcomes. In many instances, the preoperative photograph is more balanced aesthetically than the postoperative result. This nasal disharmony is most frequently seen as an overly narrowed dorsum packaged with a wide tip; overly narrowed nostrils associated with a wide tip lobule; or an excessively narrowed tip, dorsum, and nostrils in a patient with otherwise broad/full ethnic features. Most of these poor aesthetic outcomes could easily be avoided by adopting less of a surgical emphasis on narrowing. The author's gut feeling is that poor outcomes are more often a result of poor aesthetic judgment rather than failures in surgical technique. Surgeons must undergo a mental paradigm shift in rhinoplasty logic for patients of African descent. Low, flat, and broad can indeed be beautiful. Surgeons must keep in mind that a wide nose is not inherently unattractive. However, one can very effectively make it unattractive by artificially packaging wide features with overly narrow modifications, thus creating nasal disharmony and imbalance. Modern rhinoplasty should be

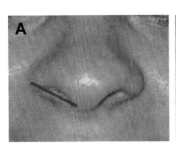 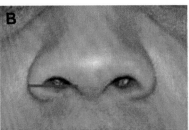 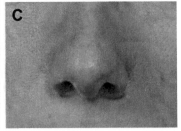

Fig. 9. Nostril Axis of Orientation classification. (*A*) inverted, (*B*) horizontal, (*C*) vertical.

undertaken from a mindset of maintaining or establishing pleasing surface contour relationships.

SUMMARY

Rhinoplasty surgeons have a unique opportunity to adopt a modern approach to rhinoplasty through redefining surgical logic to be more anatomically sophisticated and culturally sensitive. Technical expertise is not the most significant hurdle to overcome in achieving favorable rhinoplasty outcomes in patients of African descent. Cultivating a renewed aesthetic consciousness for Afrocentric beauty aligned with technical competence is paramount. Exploring ancestry provides a pathway to "culturally connect" with prospective patients, and serves as a tool for establishing a shared aesthetic vision between patient and surgeon.

REFERENCES

1. American Academy of Facial Plastic and Reconstructive Surgery. American women are not alone—men embracing self improvement through facial plastic surgery. March 8, 2006. Available at: http://www.aafprs.org/media/press_release/030806.htm. Accessed September 4, 2009.
2. Matory WE, Faces E. Non-Caucasian rhinoplasty: a 16-year experience. Plast Reconstr Surg 1986; 77(2):239–52.
3. Zingaro EA, Falces E. Aesthetic anatomy of the non-Caucasian nose. Clin Plast Surg 1987;14(4):749–65.
4. McCurdy JA. Aesthetic rhinoplasty in the non-Caucasian. J Dermatol Surg Oncol 1986;12(1):38–44.
5. Nolst Trenite GJ. Considerations in ethnic rhinoplasty. Facial Plast Surg 2003;19(3):239–45.
6. Romo T, Abraham MT. The ethnic nose. Facial Plast Surg 2003;19(3):269–77.
7. Rohrich RJ, Muzaffar AR. Rhinoplasty in the African American patient. Plast Reconstr Surg 2003;111(3): 1322–41.
8. Slupchynskyj O, Gieniusz M. Rhinoplasty for African American patients. Arch Facial Plast Surg 2008; 10(4):232–6.
9. Ofodile FA, Bokhari FJ, Ellis C. The Black American nose. Ann Plast Surg 1993;31:209–19.
10. Baker HL. Anatomical and profile analysis of the female Black American nose. J Natl Med Assoc 1989;81(11):1169–75.
11. "African American". Available at: http://en.wikipedia.org/wiki/African_American. Accessed Aug 19, 2009.
12. Stucker FJ, Lian T, Sanders K. African American rhinoplasty. Facial Plast Surg Clin North Am 2002; 10:369–76.
13. Ofodile FA, Bokhari F. The African-American nose: part II. Ann Plast Surg 1995;34:123–9.
14. Toriumi DM. New concepts in nasal tip contouring. Arch Facial Plast Surg 2006;8:156–85.
15. Hubbard TJ. Bridge narrowing in ethnic noses. Ann Plast Surg 1998;40:214–8.
16. Conrad K, Torgerson CS, Gillman GS. Applications of GORE-TEX implants in rhinoplasty reexamined after 17 years. Arch Facial Plast Surg 2008;10(4):224–31.
17. Rhorick RJ. Rhinoplasty in the black patient. In: Daniel RK, editor. Rhinoplasty. Boston: Little, Brown; 1993. p. 659–76.
18. McCurdy JA. Asian rhinoplasty. In: McCurdy JA, Lam SM, editors. Cosmetic surgery of the Asian face. 2nd edition. New York: Thieme Medical Publishers, Inc; 2005. p. 65.
19. Bennett GH, Lessow A, Song P, et al. The long-term effects of alar base reduction. Arch Facial Plast Surg 2005;7:94–7.
20. Porter JP, Olsen KL. Analysis of the African American female nose. Plast Reconstr Surg 2003;111: 620–6.
21. Foda HT. Nasal base narrowing: the combined alar base excision technique. Arch Facial Plast Surg 2007;9(1):30–4.

Middle Eastern Rhinoplasty

Babak Azizzadeh, MD[a,b,c],*, Grigoriy Mashkevich, MD[d]

KEYWORDS

• Middle Eastern • Ethnic • Rhinoplasty

DEMOGRAPHICS AND SCOPE

In the United States, the estimated size of the Middle Eastern diaspora ranges from 1.2 to 3.5 million people, depending on the census source.[1,2] Most of this ethnic group (94%) reside in large metropolitan areas, particularly in the cities of Los Angeles, Detroit, and New York.

Patients of Middle Eastern extraction can trace their roots to 1 of the many countries in a vast geographic area of the Middle East. As ethnic and cultural borders of this part of the world have been blurred over the centuries by migration and intermixing of various populations, it is not surprising that people living in the Middle East and neighboring countries (Afghanistan, Pakistan, and India) have many of the nasal characteristics found in the Middle Eastern nose.

Because Middle Eastern extraction implies a wide range of ethnicities and religions, aesthetic needs and desires for rhinoplasty vary subtly between various geographic regions of the Middle East (and, by extension, within the diaspora presently living in the United States). For instance, people living outside the Arabian Peninsula and Gulf regions (Saudi Arabia, Kuwait, Qatar, UAE, Oman, and Iran) desire a greater change with rhinoplasty, in terms of dorsal reduction and tip projection.[3]

THE MIDDLE EASTERN NOSE

Several distinct surface features define the Middle Eastern nose (**Table 1**). These features can be readily identified on photographs of people of Middle Eastern descent (**Fig. 1**).

The upper two-thirds of the Middle Eastern nose is dominated by a high radix and a strong dorsum, with an associated dorsal hump. The dorsal hump is almost always accentuated by an under projected, hanging nasal tip, which creates the illusion of increased dorsal height. As a result, tip elevation is an important surgical maneuver in reducing this illusion and visually lowering the dorsum.

The cartilaginous framework of the lower one-third of the nose consists of weak lower lateral cartilages, resulting in varying degrees of nasal tip ptosis. The medial crura are typically thin and add minimal structural integrity toward nasal tip support. The lateral crura tend to have a cephalic orientation and contribute variably to supratip and supra-alar fullness. Overactive depressor septi nasi muscle and alar flaring can also be seen.

A thick overlying skin–soft tissue envelope (SSTE) covers the osseo-cartilaginous framework of the Middle Eastern nose. This property of the SSTE significantly influences the appearance of the lower one-third of the nose by blunting tip definition and adding fullness to the supratip and supra-alar regions. Around the nasal tip, numerous pilosebaceous units give the skin an oily texture and further contribute to increased skin thickness. In the postoperative period, pilosebaceous content of the SSTE promotes tissue scarring and pollybeak formation, caused by increased vascularity in the region.

a The Center for Facial & Nasal Plastic Surgery, 8670 Wilshire Boulevard, Suite 200, Beverly Hills, CA 90211, USA
b Facial Plastic & Reconstructive Surgery, Cedars-Sinai Medical Center, USA
c Division of Head & Neck Surgery, David Geffen School of Medicine at UCLA, CA, USA
d Division of Facial Plastic Surgery, New York Eye & Ear Infirmary, 310 East 14th Street, New York, NY 10003, USA
* Corresponding author. The Center for Facial & Nasal Plastic Surgery, 8670 Wilshire Boulevard, Suite 200, Beverly Hills, CA 90211.
E-mail address: md@facialplastics.info (B. Azizzadeh).

Facial Plast Surg Clin N Am 18 (2010) 201–206
doi:10.1016/j.fsc.2009.11.013

Table 1
Common visual features associated with a Middle Eastern nose

Upper third	High radix, overprojecting bony dorsum, excessive dorsal width
Middle third	Widening of the osseous and cartilaginous vaults, straight of the brow-tip aesthetic line
Nasal tip	Amorphous hanging nasal tip, cephalically orientated lower lateral crura, weak medial crura, acute nasolabial configuration
Nostrils	Variable degree of alar flaring
SSTE	Thick oily skin, high density of pilosebaceous units, amorphous tip appearance, supratip fullness

complement ethnic facial features. Changes resulting in westernization of nasal appearance may lead to dissatisfaction by the patient and the family.

It is generally a good idea to include a family member in the consultation process. Their opinion may represent important feedback and help avert potential misunderstanding within the family. Digital photography and morphing can greatly assist in conveying the proposed changes and help communicate more effectively. Digital morphing should be used as a point of reference, without implicit guarantees as to the surgical result. The various points discussed in the previous and later sections of this article should be kept in mind when altering patient images. If requested, before and after photographs of previously operated patients can be presented. This review of photographs may also help clarify the differences in rhinoplasty goals between white and Middle Eastern noses.

CONSULTATION DYNAMIC

The initial consultation for rhinoplasty on Middle Eastern patients allows the surgeon to learn about the patient's concerns, goals, and motivations for surgery. During this visit, the concept of maintaining ethnic identity should be clearly communicated to the patient. Requests for an extreme change in appearance should warn the surgeon of unrealistic goals or a lack of understanding that significant changes in nasal appearance may not

SURGICAL CONSIDERATIONS IN RHINOPLASTY ON MIDDLE EASTERN PATIENTS

One of the guiding principles of rhinoplasty on Middle Eastern patients is preservation of ethnic appearance through avoidance of over resection.[4,5] Westernization of nasal proportions, by attempting to achieve the established standards for an aesthetically pleasing nasal configuration for white people, must be avoided in patients of

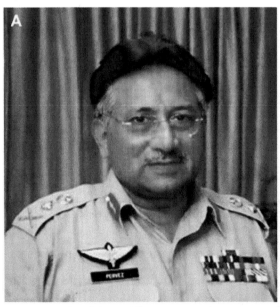
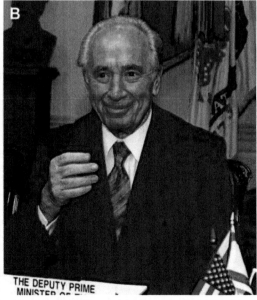

Fig. 1. Examples of the Middle Eastern nasal appearance, highlighting typical visual features outlined in Table 1. Well-known political figures in the Middle East: (*A*) Pervez Musharraf; (*B*) Shimon Perez.

Middle Eastern descent. Failure to do so can lead to an incongruous nasal-facial relationship and, potentially, to an unsatisfied patient. Basic surgical principles include a conservative reduction of the radix and dorsum, adequate tip projection, and sufficient tip rotation that maintains a hint of an acute nasolabial angle (less than 95°). These and other essential objectives for rhinoplasty on Middle Eastern patients are listed in **Table 2**.

The authors prefer an external rhinoplasty approach because of superior visualization of internal structures and access for the open grafting techniques described in this section. An endonasal approach is used in patients with satisfactory tip appearance and support, and who thus requiring only dorsal modification. In the authors' experience, the columellar scar from an external approach heals exceptionally well in this patient population. A similar conclusion has been also reached by Foda,[6] who analyzed the columellar scar in 600 patients of Arabic extraction. In this series, only a small fraction (1.5%) of patients found their final scar to be unacceptable in appearance; the reasons cited were widening, pigmentary changes, and columellar rim notching.

The philosophy of open structure rhinoplasty underlies the basic surgical tenets of rhinoplasty on Middle Eastern patients. Addition of structure to the native cartilaginous framework is critical in the context of weak native cartilages and a thick overlying SSTE. Due to its thickness and propensity to contract, the SSTE can easily overwhelm any unaltered native cartilage in the postoperative period. Hence, addition of strong support mechanisms to the cartilaginous framework are an important long-term preventive strategy.

Following open rhinoplasty exposure, conservative dorsal hump reduction should be carried out on the upper two-thirds of the nose. Maintenance of sufficient dorsal height is critical in preserving the ethnic appearance of a Middle Eastern nose. Compared with a white nose, the radix and the dorsum must be conserved to a greater extent. In addition, in most cases of dorsal hump reduction, the authors reinforce the middle vault by performing spreader grafting. This procedure prevents collapse of the upper lateral cartilages and avoids internal valve narrowing and an inverted V deformity.

As previously discussed, a dependent position of the nasal tip partially contributes to the appearance of excessive dorsal height. Tip projection, in turn, creates an illusion of a lowered dorsum. This maneuver, almost always necessary during rhinoplasty on Middle Eastern patients, allows for a more conservative reduction of the nasal dorsum. Similarly, low radix accentuates the dorsal height. Correction of a disproportional radix-dorsum relationship improves the overall dorsal balance and reduces its prominence. Crushed cartilage grafts are an effective means of filling the radix bed and can be guided into position with a 4-0 chromic suture on a Keith needle. A knot is then tied over the skin at the site of the transcutaneous suture placement, further securing the graft in the postoperative period. This suture can be removed in approximately 1 week without consequence.

After dorsal hump modification and middle nasal vault repair, the lower lateral cartilages are examined for inherent weakness. Nasal tip reconstruction begins by placing a columellar strut and securing it to the medial crura. A septal extension graft can be used instead.[7] When projecting the tip, it should be kept in mind that the supratip break should never be as prominent as in the ideal white nose. In male patients, it is especially desirable to have a minimally visible break in the supratip region. Cartilage suturing techniques (interdomal sutures, lateral crural steal dome sutures, and so

Table 2	
Essential surgical concepts and techniques in rhinoplasty on Middle Eastern patients	
Upper third	Conservative dorsal reduction (with concomitant tip elevation), maintenance of a high radix, medial and lateral osteotomies
Middle third	Medial and lateral osteotomies, spreader grafts to prevent valve collapse and mid-vault narrowing
Nasal tip	Cartilage sparing maneuvers with preferential use of suture techniques, placement of supporting grafts (columellar strut or septal extension grafts, shield or cap grafts), consideration for lateral crural strut grafts and alar rim grafts
Nostrils	Alar base modification on an as-needed basis
SSTE	Conservative subcutaneous tissue removal (especially in the supratip region), postoperative monitoring and conservative steroid (triamcinolone acetonide) injections to counter pollybeak formation

forth) and additional grafting as necessary (shield or cap grafts) are used to improve tip projection and definition.[8-10] Judicious nasal skin defatting may be undertaken at this point, in the subdermal plane.

Minimal resection of the cephalic margin of the lower lateral cartilages should be performed. Lower lateral cartilages are typically weak structures and contribute minimally to tip fullness. The authors prefer to reinforce lateral crura with lateral crural strut grafts and alar rim grafts.[11,12] These maneuvers provide an additional layer of protection against postoperative collapse of the vestibule, and against alar rim notching and retraction. The key factor is to create a straight, structurally sound, lateral crura avoiding excessive convexity or concavity.

Tip rotation should be conservative with the aim of creating a nasolabial angle of approximately 95° or smaller. This result can be achieved in most instances with a combination of strut placement, dome suturing, and a conservative triangular caudal septal excision with the base at the anterior septal angle. Vertically oriented lateral crura may prevent cephalic rotation of the nasal tip tripod, necessitating an additional lateral crural overlay[13] or caudal repositioning of the lateral crura. If either scenario is encountered, lateral crural strut grafts are used for reinforcement.

At the end of the procedure, medial and lateral osteotomies are performed. Medial osteotomies are performed in a lateral fading fashion at the osseo-cartilaginous junction. If the patient has an

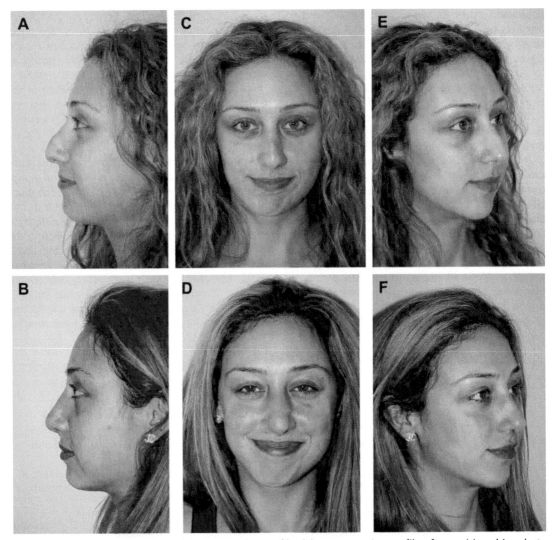

Fig. 2. Middle Eastern rhinoplasty. (A) Preoperative profile; (B) postoperative profile after revision rhinoplasty; (C) preoperative frontal view; (D) postoperative frontal view after revision rhinoplasty; (E) preoperative view; (F) postoperative view after revision rhinoplasty.

open roof deformity, medial osteotomy is avoided. Lateral osteotomies are performed in a high-low-high fashion.

If necessary, alar base modification can be completed following the osteotomies, keeping in mind that mild alar flaring is an important feature of the Middle Eastern nose. The type of alar base modification depends on 2 key factors: alar flaring and interalar-intercanthal distance. If the patient has a normal interalar-intercanthal relationship (1:1), then alar wedge resection is performed. If the patient's interalar distance is significantly wider than the intercanthal distance, then a nasal sill incision becomes necessary. Middle Eastern patients can tolerate alar bases slightly wider than the intercanthal distance.[14] In clinical practice, the authors often perform alar base modification as a secondary procedure under local anesthesia about 6 months after the rhinoplasty. Prepoperative and postoperative clinical photos of a rhinoplasty are shown in **Fig. 2**.

POTENTIAL COMPLICATIONS AND PITFALLS

Rhinoplasty on Middle Eastern patients can result in several potential complications arising from a combination of surgeon- and patient-related factors.

In the upper two-thirds of the nose, excessive lowering of the dorsum and radix can lead to unwanted westernization. The need to lower the dorsum can be greatly diminished by restoring adequate tip projection during surgery, as discussed in the previous section.

In the lower one-third, increased skin thickness and high density of pilosebaceous units in the SSTE can contribute to postoperative pollybeak formation. Fat excision in the supratip region and close monitoring in the immediate postoperative period can help avoid this complication. Injections with triamcinolone acetonide (Kenalog-10; Bristol-Myers Squibb Co, Princeton, NJ) have been shown to counteract formation of tissue bulk in the supratip region.[15] These injections can be started as soon as 1 week postoperatively and repeated every 2 weeks until adequate soft tissue resorption occurs. A judicious use of small volumes and low concentrations of triamcinolone acetonide should avoid pigmentary skin changes. The authors rarely use steroid injections but do reserve them for this purpose.

Insufficient structural grafting of the columella, combined with overly aggressive resection of the native cartilage, can lead to the development of postoperative nasal tip ptosis. Adding sufficient structure during rhinoplasty, by placement of a strong columellar strut (or a caudal septal

extension graft), with concomitant medial crural binding sutures, effectively preserves nasal tip position in the postoperative period.

Excessive nasal tip rotation, with a resultant obtuse nasolabial angle, can lead to an unnatural appearance for this patient population. Whereas the tenets of rhinoplasty on white patients suggest an ideal nasolabial angle range of 95° to 110° in women, a similar configuration in a Middle Eastern patient may lead to an out-of-place appearance. A practical goal of less than 95° of rotation should avoid potential tip over rotation.

SUMMARY

Rhinoplasty on Middle Eastern patients presents several challenges inherent in ethnic nasal surgery. Preservation of native nasal harmony and avoidance of westernization are essential goals in this operation. Attainment of natural results depends on the surgeon's understanding of anatomy and relationships of intranasal and nasal-facial components in a Middle Eastern nose. Aesthetic surgical refinement in this patient group relies primarily on conservative dorsal resection and strengthening of the native cartilaginous framework. The concepts presented here underlie the basic tenets of rhinoplasty on Middle Eastern patients.

REFERENCES

1. US Census Bureau. Census 2000. Available at: http://www.census.gov/prod/2003pubs/c2kbr-23.pdf. Accessed March 15, 2009.
2. The Arab American Institute. Available at: http://www.aaiusa.org/arab-americans/22/demographics. Accessed March 15, 2009.
3. Bizrah MB. Rhinoplasty for Middle Eastern patients. Facial Plast Surg Clin North Am 2002; 10(4):381–96.
4. Rohrich RJ, Ghavami A. The Middle Eastern nose. In: Gunter JP, Rohrich RJ, Adams WP, editors. Dallas rhinoplasty: nasal surgery by the masters. St Louis (MO): Quality Medical Publishing; 2007. p. 1139–65.
5. Romo T 3rd, Abraham MT. The ethnic nose. Facial Plast Surg 2003;19(3):269–78.
6. Foda HM. External rhinoplasty for the Arabian nose: a columellar scar analysis. Aesthetic Plast Surg 2004;28(5):312–6.
7. Byrd HS, Andochick S, Copit S, et al. Septal extension grafts: a method of controlling tip projection shape. Plast Reconstr Surg 1997;100(4):999–1010.
8. Baker SR. Suture contouring of the nasal tip. Arch Facial Plast Surg 2000;2:34–42.
9. Rohrich RJ, Adams WP. The boxy nasal tip: classification and management based on alar cartilage

suturing techniques. Plast Reconstr Surg 2001; 107(7):1849–63.

10. Toriumi DM. New concepts in nasal tip contouring. Arch Facial Plast Surg 2006;8(3):156–85.

11. Gunter JP, Friedman RM. Lateral crural strut graft: technique and clinical applications in rhinoplasty. Plast Reconstr Surg 1997;99(4):943–52.

12. Rohrich RJ, Raniere J, Ha RY. The alar contour graft: correction and prevention of alar rim deformities in rhinoplasty. Plast Reconstr Surg 2002;109(7): 2495–505.

13. Foda HMT, Kridel RWH. Lateral crural steal and lateral crural overlay. An objective evaluation. Arch Otolaryngol Head Neck Surg 1999;125:1365–70.

14. Kridel RW, Castellano RD. A simplified approach to alar base reduction: a review of 124 patients over 20 years. Arch Facial Plast Surg 2005;7(2): 81–93.

15. Hanasono MM, Kridel RW, Pastorek NJ, et al. Correction of the soft tissue pollybeak using triamcinolone injection. Arch Facial Plast Surg 2002; 4(1):26–30.

Index

Note: Page numbers of article titles are in **boldface** type

Facial Plast Surg Clin N Am 18 (2010) 207–221
doi:10.1016/S1064-7406(10)00016-7
1064-7406/10/$ – see front matter © 2010 Elsevier Inc. All rights reserved

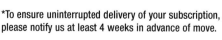